Playing by the Rules

An Update on Government Policies, Regulations and Acts for Practicing Obstetricians and Gynecologists

Second Edition

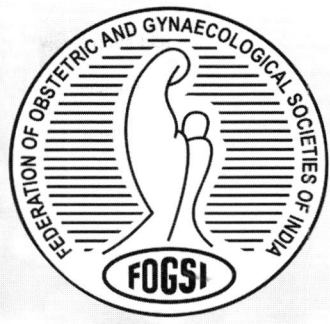
Federation of Obstetric and
Gynaecological Societies of India

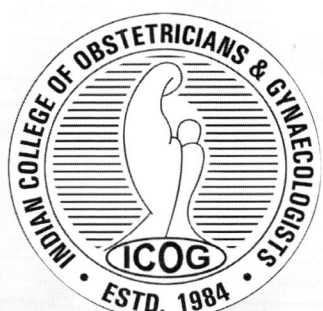
Indian College of Obstetricians
and Gynaecologists

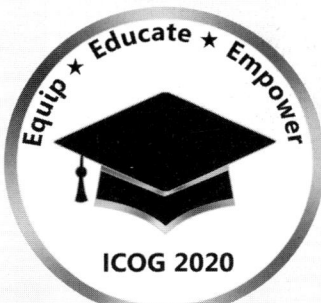
ICOG 2020

Playing by the Rules

An Update on Government Policies, Regulations and Acts for Practicing Obstetricians and Gynecologists

Second Edition

Chief Editor

Mandakini Megh MD DGO FICMCH FICMU FICOG
Chairperson ICOG-FOGSI
International Vice President, MWIA Central Asia
Consulting Obstetrician and Gynecologist
Director, Dr Megh's Gynaeo-care (a specialized clinic for women and adolescent girls)
Dean, Indian College of Medical Ultrasound (former); Vice President, FOGSI (2012-13)
Head, Cama and Albless Hospital (former); Deputy Director, Government of Maharashtra (former)
RCH, Family Welfare, World Bank, Maternal Health Consultant, UNICEF; Past President, IFUMB

Co-editor

Reena J Wani MD MRCOG FICOG DNBE FCPS DGO DFP
Professor (Addl) and Head, Department of Obstetrics and Gynecology
HBT Medical College and Dr RN Cooper Municipal General Hospital
Ex-Professor (Addl), I/C Family Welfare Program, Department of Obstetrics and Gynecology
TN Medical College and BYL Nair Ch Hospital, Mumbai
Chairperson, FOGSI Perinatology Committee, 2015–2017
Core Committee Member, FOGSI Violence Against Women Cell
Managing Committee Member, MOGS, UNESCO Bioethics
President, MBPC (Mumbai Breast Feeding Promotion Committee)
Section Editor, TIP; Peer Reviewer, JOGI

Associate Editors

Rajshree Dayanand Katke MD FICOG FMAS
Professor and Head, Department of Obstetrics and Gynecology, SRTR Medical College, Ambajogai
Ex-Professor, Grant Government Medical College, Mumbai, Ex-Superintendent, Cama and Albless Hospital, Mumbai

Rashmi Jalvee MS DGO DNB
Assistant Professor, Department of Obstetrics and Gynaecology
Dr RN Cooper Municipal General Hospital, Mumbai, Maharashtra

Preeti Deshpande MS (OBGY)
Consultant Obstetrician and Gynaecologist
Raheja-Fortis Hospital, Guru Nanak Hospital, Fellowship Infertility
Advanced Endoscopic Training, IRCAD (France), Mumbai

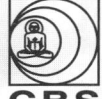

CBS Publishers & Distributors Pvt Ltd

New Delhi • Bengaluru • Chennai • Kochi • Kolkata • Mumbai
Bhopal • Bhubaneswar • Hyderabad • Jharkhand • Nagpur • Patna • Pune • Uttarakhand • Dhaka (Bangladesh) • Kathmandu (Nepal)

Disclaimer

Science and technology are constantly changing fields. New research and experience broaden the scope of information and knowledge. The editors and contributors have tried their best in giving information available to them while preparing the material for this book. Although, all efforts have been made to ensure optimum accuracy of the material, yet it is quite possible some errors might have been left uncorrected. The publisher, printer, editors or the contributors will not be held responsible for any inadvertent errors, omissions or inaccuracies.

Playing by the Rules
An Update on Government Policies, Regulations and Acts for Practicing Obstetricians and Gynecologists
Second Edition

ISBN: 978-93-89688-51-1

Copyright © Federation of Obstetrics and Gynaecological Societies of India and Publisher

Second Edition: 2020
First Edition: 2015
 Reprint: 2017

All rights are reserved. No part of this book may be reproduced or transmitted in any form or by any means, electronic or mechanical, including photocopying, recording, or any information storage and retrieval system without permission, in writing, from the editors, contributors and the publisher.

Published by Satish Kumar Jain and produced by Varun Jain for

CBS Publishers & Distributors Pvt Ltd
4819/XI Prahlad Street, 24 Ansari Road, Daryaganj, New Delhi 110 002
Ph: 011-23289259, 23266861, 23266867   Fax: 011-23243014   Website: www.cbspd.com
 e-mail: delhi@cbspd.com; cbspubs@airtelmail.in

Corporate Office: 204 FIE, Industrial Area, Patparganj, Delhi 110 092
Ph: 011-4934 4934   Fax: 011-4934 4935   e-mail: publishing@cbspd.com; publicity@cbspd.com

Branches

- **Bengaluru:** Seema House 2975, 17th Cross, KR Road, Banasankari 2nd Stage, Bengaluru 560 070, Karnataka
 Ph: +91-80-26771678/79   Fax: +91-80-26771680   e-mail: bangalore@cbspd.com
- **Chennai:** 7, Subbaraya Street, Shenoy Nagar, Chennai 600 030, Tamil Nadu
 Ph: +91-44-26260666, 26208620   Fax: +91-44-42032115   e-mail: chennai@cbspd.com
- **Kochi:** 42/1325, 1326, Power House Road, Opp KSEB Power House, Eranakulam 682 018, Kochi, Kerala
 Ph: +91-484-4059061-65   Fax: +91-484-4059065   e-mail: kochi@cbspd.com
- **Kolkata:** No. 6/B, Ground Floor, Rameswar Shaw Road, Kolkata-700014 (West Bengal), India
 Ph: +91-33-2289-1126, 2289-1127, 2289-1128   e-mail: kolkata@cbspd.com
- **Mumbai:** 83-C, Dr E Moses Road, Worli, Mumbai-400018, Maharashtra
 Ph: +91-22-24902340/41   Fax: +91-22-24902342   e-mail: mumbai@cbspd.com

Representatives

• Bhopal	0-8319310552	• Bhubaneswar	0-9911037372	• Hyderabad	0-9885175004
• Jharkhand	0-9811541605	• Nagpur	0-9421945513	• Patna	0-9334159340
• Pune	0-9623451994	• Uttarakhand	0-9716462459	• Dhaka (Bangladesh)	01912-003485
• Kathmandu (Nepal)	977-9818742655				

Printed at India Binding House, Noida, UP, India

to
the teachers who taught us, bureaucrats and policymakers
with whom I have worked extensively in Mantralaya
Public Health Department, Government of Maharashtra

and

Gorakh Megh, IAS, Ex-Principal Secretary, Government of Maharashtra
for his continuous support during my carreer

—Mandakini Megh

Message

Amongst the greatest freedoms we can have is the freedom from avoidable ill-health and escapable mortality....
—Amartya Sen, Nobel Laureate

As obstetricians we have a unique position in health care—we look after two patients (mother and fetus), we make the difference between life and death for both of them.... hence we have a double responsibility.

Looking at the Indian scenario, various Acts have been implemented like MTP, PCPNDT, domestic violence and other government rules and regulations like sterilization, laparoscopic ligation. Knowledge of all such government Acts and Policies is essential to every practising obstetrician and gynecologist.

FOGSI publication *Playing by The Rules* edited by Dr Mandakini Megh, Chief Editor and Vice President, FOGSI (2012–2013), Dr Reena J Wani (Co-editor), Dr Preeti Deshpande, Dr Rashmi Jalvee and Dr Rajshree Dayanand Katke (associate editors), along with the contributors from all over India, has discussed various acts, government policies and rules. I am sure this book will be a useful source of information for the practicing obstetricians and gynecologists.

I wish the team all the best for success of this FOGSI publication.

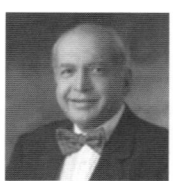

CN Purandare
President-Elect, FIGO

It gives me pleasure in writing a few words about the book *Playing by The Rules: An Update on Government Policies, Regulations and Acts for the Practicing Obstetricians and Gynecologists* by Dr Mandakini Megh.

This book was indescribable efforts by Dr Mandakini Megh who has been well assisted by co-editors to get experts in different fields of medicine to write the different sections of this book. All the sections are well-researched and give in-depth insights into the topics they cover.

I hope each reader will be able to find the guidance they need in *Playing by The Rules* to help them in their practice.

I wish the team all the best for success of this FOGSI publication.

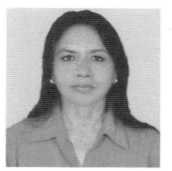

Shomita Biswas IFS
Member-Secretary
Maharashtra State Commission for Women, Mumbai

Foreword

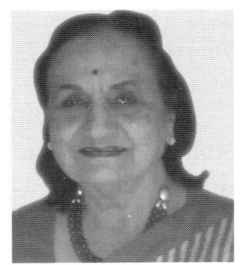

"Playing by the Rules" is what is inculcated in all young children. A dictum which stays with us all our lives. It forms the basis of a civilised society.

So this book with this apt title is the essence of a good practice. It is a necessity in today's world with its diversity and different value systems.

It is very comprehensive and duly updated from the previous edition which was also a resounding success.

The authors are all well-known and experts in their own fields. They have taken great pains to include all relevant documents so as to facilitate references.

The rules do change over time. It is due to changes in the society and the medical practices. One has to keep up with these changes in one's busy practice. The patients too have become more knowledgeable and question your statements. Hence it is very valuable to have your documentation ready at hand to discuss the complicated issues which govern our choice of treatment.

Today's medical fraternity is invariably "under stress" for various reasons. This book hopefully will reduce the stress levels by giving correct guidance and support.

It is with great pleasure that I send my greetings and best wishes to the editors and all authors for taking up this onerous task and presenting it to all FOGSI members at the inauguration of AICOG 2020 in Lucknow.

I would like to end with those few lines which are also a "truism" which cannot be challenged.

Never stop learning
Because LIFE
Never stops teaching

With warm personal regards

Usha Saraiya
MD DGO FIAC FICOG FRCOG (UK)
Consultant, Obstetrician-Gynaecologist
Breach Candy, Saifee, Elizabeth Hospitals
Conferred Hon. Fellowship by RCOG in 2012
Past President, MOGS and FOGSI
Chairman, Indian College of Obstetrician and Gynaecologist (2006–2009)
Award for "Outstanding Woman Obstetrician and Gynaecologist" at FIGO 2003
Chairman, Ethics Committee for Clinical Research of NIRRH and ICMR 2011–2018
Lifetime Achievement Award by AOGIN India in September 2017
Zur Hausen Oration delivered at Cuttack in March 2018
Delegate to WHO's 71st Assembly for discussions on Women's Health at Geneva in May 2018

Foreword

It is a great pleasure to write the Foreword to the unique book *Playing by the Rules: An Update on Government Policies, Regulations and Acts for Practicing Obstetricians and Gynecologists.*

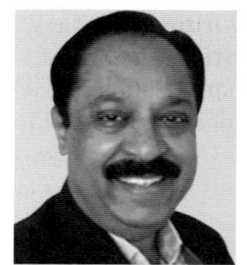

We are very busy in our routine practice and many times we forget to know the important aspects of the government's policies, regulations, and acts on women's health issues. It is the need of the hour for us to update ourselves for the same being the main health caregivers of Indian women. This book is an amalgamation of the government rules and regulations on various issues pertaining to women's health, women's safety, child protection, and medical ethics.

The various government policies and measures like the role of Women's Commission, Domestic Violence Act, Protection of Children against Sexual Offences Act, Janani Suraksha Yojna, Policies for Adolescent Reproductive Health and the National Rural Health Mission and Welfare Programmes have been put forward in a very precise and useful manner in this book. This will serve as a ready reckoner and guide for all of us, practising in the public and private sectors in India.

I congratulate the Chief Editor Dr Mandakini Megh and Co-editor Dr Reena J Wani and associate editors taking this important and very useful subject for publication.

I wish all the success to the book.

Alpesh Gandhi
President-Elect, FOGSI-2020

Preface to the Second Edition

During one of the FOGSI meetings, managing committee members were curious to know the update on Government guidelines for ligation and many issues of MTP, which was becoming a grave area of concern. I was asked to update the details about the same, the idea of updating my book *Playing by the Rules* just struck to me then.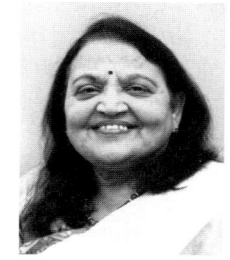

Having set upon this ambitious project, the journey was not easy. To get busy specialist to spend time and put down their thoughts was a challenge; to ensure that we got the facts and right and updated was our responsibility; and to serve this consolidated offering to you, dear readers, in time was herculean task. We hope this update serves its purpose and you find it helpful in day-to-day practice!

It was observed that there are many practical queries by practising obstetricians and gynecologists while implementing these programme, rules and regulations. Now the second edition contains 10 new chapters out of total 41 chapters, new additions are POCSO Act, medicolegal challenges as case discussion, IUI clinic set up protocols, Medical Councils for doctors, domestic violence, anti-ragging rules and something new on biomedical waste management and Clinical Establishment Act, etc.

Not only that all the 31 chapters from the previous edition have been completely rewritten according to the current rules and guidelines, some of the chapters even updated until December 2019 policies amended by the GOI and by the experts in the particular field.

My sincere thanks to Co-editor Dr Reena J Wani for her dedicated work to edit this book.

I wish to express my appreciation to all the contributors, without their support this book would not have been possible, and thanking them for timely submission of the manuscript as well in spite of a short notice. I particularly would like to appreciate the young associate editors, Dr Rashmi Jalvee and Dr Preeti Deshpande, for their continued and sincere efforts. I thank Dr Rajshree Katke as well for editing this book.

I thank CBS Publishers and Distributors, New Delhi, for their cooperation in bringing out this book in a stipulated time, especially Ramesh Krishnamachari, for his coordination.

Finally a word of thanks to our families and support staff who have been very patient with us as we have spent many long hours of personal time getting this handbook to you!

Mandakini Megh

Preface to the First Edition

"Goals are the fuel in the furnace of achievement"
—Brian Tracy

The genesis of this book was nearly three years ago when there was so much upheaval and discussion about medicolegal and malpractice issues related to our speciality, especially regarding family planning. We decided to put together this update to give each practising obstetrician and gynecologist a "ready reckoner" they could look at whenever they had any doubts regarding any particular aspect of their practice.

Having set upon this ambitious project, the journey was not easy. To get busy specialists to spend time and put down their thoughts was a challenge; to ensure that we got the facts right and updated was our responsibility; and to serve this consolidated offering to you, dear readers, in time was a herculean task. We hope this update serves its purpose and you find it helpful in day-to-day practice!

The idea about the books on guidelines strikes us when posted as Deputy Director, Family Welfare, RCH public health department, Government of Maharashtra, handled important subjects like medical termination of pregnancy, PCPNDT, tubal ligation and laparoscopic, recognition of clinical trainings. It was observed that there are many practical queries by practising obstetricians and gynecologists while implementing these programmes.

"Nothing is permanent but change" said Heraclitus. It is possible that there will be revision, additions and modifications which may come into effect after we have compiled this book— we welcome feedback from the readers and look forward to your inputs. Also a few more policies which are in consideration will also likely to appear in the next editions to come.

Finally a word of thanks to our families and support staff who have been very patient with us as we have spent many long hours of personal time getting this handbook to you!

Mandakini Megh

Contributors

Alka Kuthe MBBS DGO LLM
Consultant Obstetrics and Gynecology
Medicolegal Consultant
Chairman, AMOGS Medicolegal
Committee (2018–2020)
Past President, Amravati Obstetrics and
Gynecology Society (2008-2009)
Amravati

Amit Upadhyay FNB (Reproductive Medicine) DNB FCPS DGO
Director and Consultant
Srijan Fertility and Women Care Center
Borivali, Mumbai
Consultant, Shreeji Hospital
Ghatkopar, Mumbai

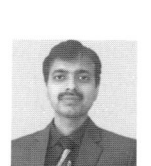

Amol P Pawar MD DGO
Associate Professor, Nowrosjee Wadia
Maternity Hospital, Mumbai

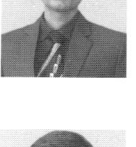

Arati Shah MBBS MS MICOG
Consultant Obstetrician and
Gynecologist, Pulse Clinic
Ahmedabad

Asha Advani MBBS DGO MD DPH DHA
Consultant Gynecologist
Special Office FWMCH, Mumbai

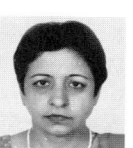

Asha Dalal MD DGO MAMS FICOG
Director Ob/Gyn. Sir HN Reliance
Foundation Hospital and Research
Centre, Mumbai
Former Professor and Head, Deaptment
of Ob/Gyn, TN Medical College and
BYL Nair Ch Hospital, Mumbai
President, AMOGS 2014–2016
National Editor of J of Ob/Gyn of India 2011–2014
UNICEF Expert in the field of PPTCT
Ex-Ad hoc Chairman of the Board of Studies, Mumbai
University

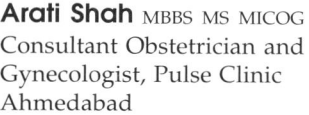

Ashok Shukla
DNB FCPS DGO MICOG LLB LLM
Consultant and Medical Director, Sai
Aashirwad Maternity and Nursing
Home, Honorary Consultant, Wockardt
Hospital, Mira Road
Honorary Consultant, Pandit Bhimsen Muncipal
Hospital, Bhayander
Chairperson, Medicolegal cell, IMA Maharashtra state
Co-Convenor, NoAH-Association of Medical
Consultants, Mumbai
Past President, IMA, Mirabhy branch
Ex-member, Managing Committee of MOGS

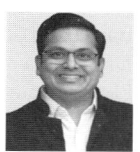

Ashwini Bhalerao Gandhi
MD DGO DFP FCPS DNB FICOG
Consultant Gynaecologist
PD Hinduja Hospital, Mumbai
Vice President, The Federation of Obst
and Gynec Societies of India (2013)
President, The Mumbai Obst and Gynec
Society (2012-2013)
Chairperson, Adolescent Health Committee of FOGSI
(2004–08)

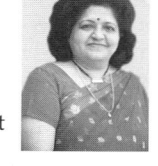

Atul Ganatra MD DGO
Obstetrician Gynecologist and
Gynecological Endoscopist
Dr RJ Ganatra's Nursing Home, Mumbai
Co-ordinator, Department of Gynec
Endoscopy, Fortis Hospitals, Mumbai
Consultant, Fertility and IVF Clinic
Jupiter Hospital, Thane

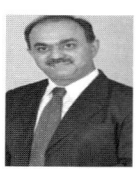

Balaji Jadhav
MD (Obst & Gyne), DHA (TISS)
Professor, Additional and Unit Head
HBT Medical College and Dr RN
Cooper Municipal General Hospital
Juhu, Mumbai

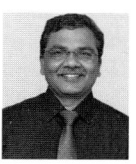

Bipin Pandit MD DGO DFP
Practicing Obstetrician and
Gynaecologist and
Director, Mukund Hospital
Hon. Gynaecologist at Dr LH
Hiranandani Hospital, Powai
Hon. Gynaecologist at Seven Hills Hospital, Marol
Past Hon Gynaecologist at
Dr RN Cooper Hospital, Irla
Hon. Gynaecologist at L and
T Welfare Center, Andheri, Mumbai

CN Aditi MBBS
Member, Menstrual Hygiene
Management Consortium, Tamil Nadu
Director, Aditi Hospital, Trichy

Charmila Ayyavoo
MD DGO DFP FICOG PGDCR
Director, Aditi Hospital and Parvathy
Ayyavoo Fertility Centre, Trichy
Consultant, Southern Railway Hospital
Trichy
Hon. Consultant Maruthi Hospital, Trichy
Teaching Faculty, J and J Community College, Trichy

Deepika Nandanwar Sadawarte
MD Community Medicine DNB Social and
Preventive Medicine
Assistant Professor
Department of Community Medicine
Seth GS Medical College and KEM
Hospital, Mumbai

Devki Potwar MS DNEB DGO DRM
Consultant Obstetrician and
Gynaecologist, Laparoscopic Surgeon
and Infertility Specialist, Breach
Candy Hospital, Saifee Hospital
Babies and Us—Fertility and IVF Centre
Opera House, Mumbai

Gajanan Velhal MD
Professor and Head
Department of Community Medicine
Seth GS Medical College and KEM
Hospital
Parel, Mumbai

Girish Nilkanth Kumthekar
MD (Ob & Gy) LLB (Spl) Dip. Reproductive Med
(Germany)
Consulting Obstetrician and Gynecologist
Infertility Specialist
Medicolegal Consultant
Asst Professor (Contract), Dr VM Govt Med Col, Solapur
Navjeevan Fertility and IVF Center
Hon. Consultant, Ashwini Sahakari Rugnalaya

Gorakh G Mandrupkar
MB DGO FCPS FICOG PGDMLS
Consultant in Reproductive
Endocrinology
Joint Secretary FOGSI (2014)

Hitesha Ramnani
DNB (OBGY) FIRM (ICOG)
Clinical Associate
Corion Fertility Clinic, Andheri, Mumbai

Hrishikesh D Pai
MD FCPS FICOG MSc (USA)
Gynecologist and Head, IVF Unit
Lilavati Hospital
Scientific Director, Bloom IVF, Mumbai

Jayashree Mondkar MD DCH
Dean, Professor and Head (Retd)
Department of Neonatology
Lokmanya Tilak Municipal Medical
College and General Hospital, Mumbai

Kalika Joshi BHMS (Homeopath)
IVF Co-ordinator
Corion Fertility Clinic
Andheri, Mumbai

Kanchan Kumta MD DGO
Ex-Special Officer Family Welfare and
Mother Child Health, Mumbai
Consultant Gynaecologists, National
Urban Health Mission

Kaushal Kadam MD
Medical Director
Corion Fertility Clinic
Lokhandwala Road
Andheri, Mumbai

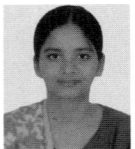
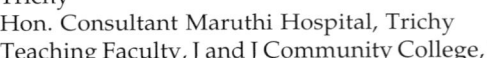
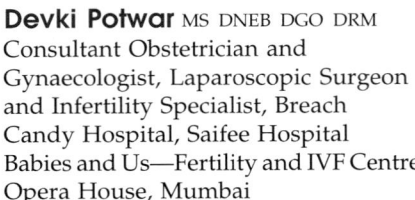
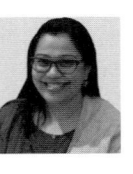
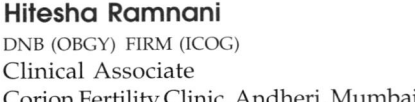
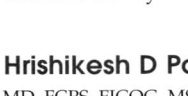
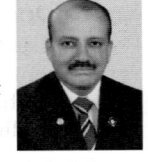
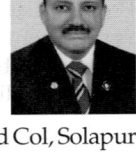
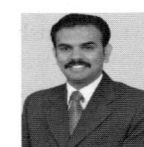
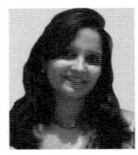
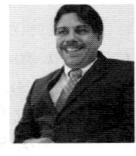
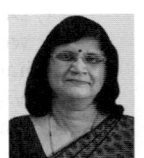
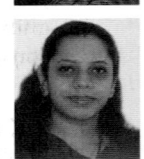
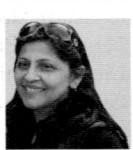
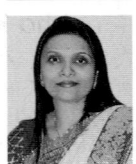

Contributors

Kusum Jashnanai MD
Professor and Head
Department of Pathology
BYL Nair Ch. Hospital and TN
Medical College, Mumbai

MC Patel MD
Gynaecologist and Medicolegal
Counsellor
Niru Maternity and Nursing Home
34, Manjushree Society
Ranna Park, Ghatlodia, Ahmedabad

Madhuri Patel MD DGO
Consultant Obstetrician and
Gynaecologist
Deputy Secretary General
The Federation of Obstetric and
Gynecological Societies of India

Mandakini Megh
MD DGO FICMCH FICMU FICOG
Chairperson ICOG-FOGSI
International Vice President, MWIA
Central Asia
Consulting Obstetrician and
Gynecologist
Director, Dr Megh's Gynaeo-care (a specialized clinic for women and adolescent girls)
Dean, Indian College of Medical Ultrasound (former); Vice President, FOGSI (2012-13)
Head, Cama and Albless Hospital (former); Deputy Director, Government of Maharashtra (former)
RCH, Family Welfare, World Bank, Maternal Health Consultant, UNICEF; Past President IFUMB

Mandar K Sadawarte
MD Community Medicine, DNB Social and Preventive Medicine
Assistant Professor
Department of Community Medicine
GGMC and JJ Group of Hospitals
Mumbai

Manisha Khare MD (Pathology)
Secretary, Anti-Ragging Committee
Professor and Head
Department of Pathology
HBT Medical College and Dr RN
Cooper Hospital, Mumbai

Manisha T Kundnani
MD FNB (Reprod Med) FNUS
Director and Consultant
Infertility Specialist
Fertility Square, The IVF Clinic
Malad
Chief Infertility Consultant
Wockhardt Hospital, Mira Road

Meenakshi Deshpande
MBBS MD (OBGYN)
Consulting Obstetrician Gynaecologist
High Risk Pregnancy Consultant
FOGSI Trainer-VAW Cell
(Violence against Women)

Meenakshi Rao MD DGO
Special Officr Incharge
Family Welfare Department
Municipal Corporation of Greater
Mumbai

Namrata Rajput
MS DNB DGO DRM (Germany)
Director and Consultant
Srijan Fertility and Women Care Center
Borivali, Mumbai
Consultant Shreeji Hospital
Ghatkopar, Mumbai

Nandita Palshetkar MD FCPS FICOG
Scientific Director, Bloom IVF
Professor of Gynecology
DY Patil Medical College
Navi Mumbai

Nikhil Datar MD DNB FCPS FICOG
LLB DGO
Consultant and Medical Director
Cloudnine Hospital, Mumbai
Partner Lifewave Hospital
Director, Yashada Maternity Nursing
Home

Nithya R Iyer MBBS MS (OBS-GYNAEC)
Consultant Gynaecologist
Life Wave Hospital
Mumbai

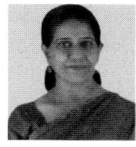
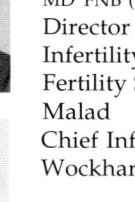
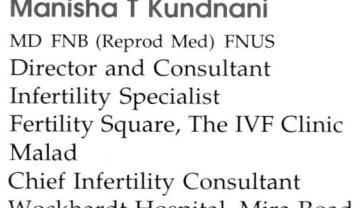
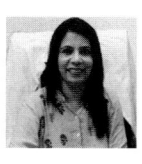
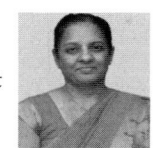
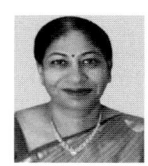
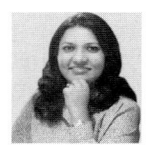
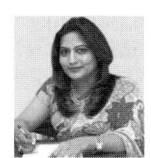
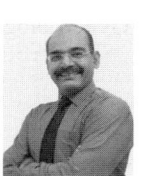
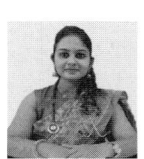

Pratik Tambe MD FICOG
Chairperson, FOGSI Endocrinology Committee (2017–2019)
Managing Council Member, MOGS
Managing Council Member, MSR, AMC, IAGE (2015–2018)
Mentor, MOGS Youth Council (2015–2018)

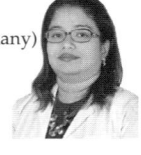

Preeti Yogesh Bhandari
MRCPI (Ireland), MS, DNB, MICOG, DRM (Germany)
Consultant Obstetrician and Gynecologist
Infertility Specialist
Ahalia Hospital, Abu Dhabi, United Arab Emirates (UAE)

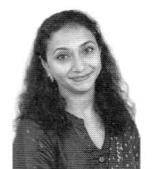

Preeti Deshpande
MS (OBGY) Consultant Obs and Gyn
Raheja-Fortis Hospital, Guru Nanak Hospital, Fellowship Infertility Advanced Endoscopic Training IRCAD (France), Mumbai

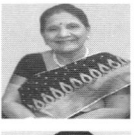

Pushpa Thorat MD MS DGO FICMCH
Ex-Deputy Director of Health Services
Ex. Maternal Health Consultant
UNICEF Consultant Gynae & Obst

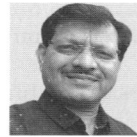

Rajashree Dayanand Katke
MD OBGY FICOG FMAS
Professor and Head, Department of OB and GY, SRTR Medical College Ambajogai, Ex-Professor, Grant Govt Medical College, Mumbai, Ex-Superintendent, Cama and Albless Hospital, Mumbai

Rajesh Darade
Director, Vaishnavi Hospital and Endoscopy Centre (PG Institute)
New Hope Test Tube Baby Center Latur, Maharashtra
Former Associate Professor and Head of Unit Department of Obstetrics and Gynecology Government Medical College, Latur
Member, Board of Studies and Faculty, MUHS, Nashik
Registrar CPS, Mumbai

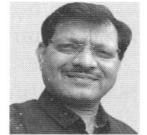

Rakhee Sahu MD DGO FCPS Diploma in endoscopy (Germany)
Consultant
Dr LH Hiranandani Hospital, Mumbai
Ex-Associate Professor, Nowrosjee Wadia Hospital, Mumbai
Member, Youth council, MOGS

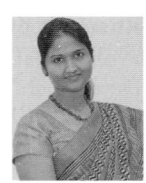

Rashmi Jalvee MS DGO DNB
Assistant Professor
Department of Obstetrics and Gynaecology
Dr RN Cooper Hospital
Mumbai, Maharashtra

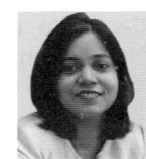

Reena J Wani
MD FRCOG FICOG DNBE DGO DFP FCPS
Professor (Addl) and Head
Department of Ostetrics and Gynaecology
HBT Medical College and Dr RN Cooper Municipal General Hospital
Ex-Professor (Addl), I/C Family Welfare Program
TN Medical College and BYL Nair Ch Hospital, Mumbai
Chairperson, FOGSI Perinatology Committee 2015–2017
Core Committee Member, FOGSI Violence Against Women Cell
Managing Committee Member, MOGS, UNESCO Bioethics
President, MBPC (Mumbai Breast Feeding Promotion Committee)
Section Editor, TIP; Peer Reviewer, JOGI

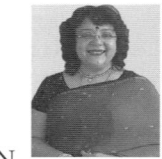

S Krishna Kumar MD FICOG
Consultant Obstetrician and Gynecologist
Kumar's Maternity and Surgical Nursing Home
Dombivli, Maharashtra

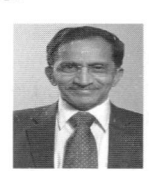

Sachin Mumbare MD (PSM)
Professor and Head, Department of Community Medicine
Ashwini Rural Medical College Hospital and Research Centre, Solapur

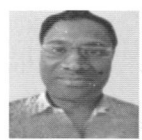

Contributors

Sampath Kumari
MD DGO FICOG FC Diab. FIME
Professor, Department of Ostetrics and Gynaecology
Madras Medical College
President, Board of Studies
Dr MGR Medical University
Member, Board of Studies—Meenakshi Medical University, Kanchipuram
Chairperson, FOGSI Adolescent Health Committee 2016–19
Member, ICOG Governing Council

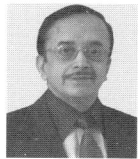

Sanjay Gupte
MD DGO FICOG LLB FRCOG
Director, Gupte Hospital and Centre for Research in Reproduction, Pune

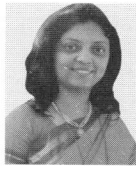

Sanuja Oke MBBS DGO MD DPH DHA
Assistant Consultant, Obstetrics and Gynaecology
Gupte Hospital and Centre for Research in Reproduction
Pune

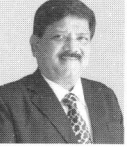

Shivkumar S Utture MS FICS (USA)
President
Maharashtra Medical Council
Executive Comm. Maharashtra Medical Council 2012–2017
Past President, IMA Mumbai Branch
CWC Member (IMA HQ)
Professor, Department of Surgery
Grant Medical College JJ Hospital

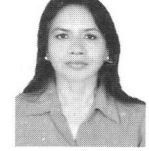

Shomita Biswas IFS
Member-Secretary
Maharashtra State Commission for Women, Mumbai

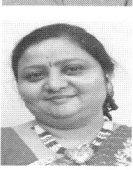

Shradda Agarwal DGO FICOG
Consultant, Gynecologist KC Hospital Palwal
Member, Breast Committee FOGSI
Founder, Palwal Obstetrics and Gynec-society

Shweta Khade MBBS DNB DGO
Assistant Professor
Lokmanya Tilak Municipal Medical College and General Hospital, Mumbai

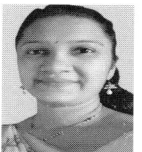

Sneha Shirodkar
Professor, Department of Obstetrics and Gynecology
TN Medical College and BYL Nair Charitable Hospital, Mumbai

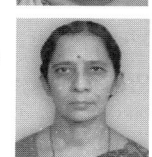

Suchitra Pandit MD DNB FRCOG (UK) FICOG DFP MNAMS B.Pharm
Senior Consultant, Obstetrician and Gynecologist, Kokilaben Dhirubhai Ambani Hospital and Research Hospital, Mumbai
President, FOGSI (2014-2015)
President, MOGS (2013-2014)
Vice President, FOGSI 2008-09
West Zone Coordinator-ISOPARB (2008–2011)
Secretary, Kishori Adolescent Empowerment project of FOGSI, Sion
ICDS, UNICEF for training of underprivileged girls from Dharavi; Chairperson, Young Talent Promotion Committee FOGSI (2003–07)

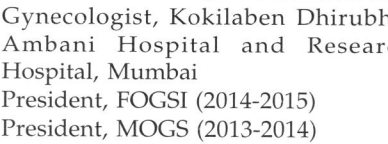

Swati Manerkar MD
Additional Professor
Department of Neonatology
Lokmanya Tilak Municipal Medical College and General Hospital, Mumbai

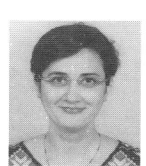

Vipin Checker MD DGO
Immediate Past President, AMC (Association of Medical Consultants)
Editor: *Medicolegal Manual For Police* (AMC Publication); Alternate CWC Member, IMA MS (2019-2020)
Ex-Vice President, IMA MS (2017-2018)
Regular CWC Member, IMA MS (2016–2018)

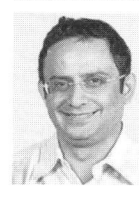

YS Nandanwar MD
Professor and Head, DY Patil Medical College, Nerul
PhD Guide and Medical Suptd, DY Patil Medical College, Nerul
Member, Ethics Committee NIRRH ICMR, Mumbai; Ex-Professor and Head, LTMMC Sion Hospital, Mumbai

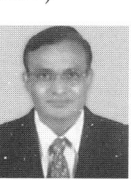

Contents

Message by CN Purandare	vi
Message by Shomita Biswas	vi
Foreword by Usha Saraiya	vii
Foreword by Alpesh Gandhi	viii
Preface to the Second Edition	ix
Preface to the First Edition	x
Contributors	xi

SECTION I: MTP AND PCPNDT ACT

1. Medical Termination of Pregnancy (MTP) Act—Rules and Regulations 3
 Mandakini Megh
2. MTP Act: Registration of Place and Maintenance of Records 12
 Gorakh G Mandrupkar
3. MTP Act—Need for Change 17
 Nikhil Datar and Nithya R Iyer
4. PCPNDT Act and Rules 23
 Mandakini Megh and Meenakshi Rao
5. PCPNDT Act: Practitioner's Perspective 36
 Atul Ganatra
6. An Update on POCSO Act and Challenges in Relation to MTP Act 44
 Ashok Shukla
7. Medicolegal Challenges in PCPNDT Act: Case Examples 49
 MC Patel
8. Recent Judgments and Legal Update 58
 Sanjay Gupte, Arati Shah and Sanuja Oke

SECTION II: OBSTETRIC CARE

9. Obstetrician's Responsibility: Maintenance of Records 71
 Reena J Wani
10. Recent Changes in Maternal Death Review 78
 Rajashree Dayanand Katke and Kanchan Kumta
11. Maternal Death Review: Facility-Based MDR 86
 Deepika Nandanwar Sadawarte, Mandar K Sadawarte and YS Nandanwar

12. Guidelines for Postmortem in Obstetric Deaths — 103
    Kusum Jashnanai
13. Maternal Deaths: Global Scenario and Practitioner's Perspective — 111
    Preeti Deshpande
14. Human Milk Banking in a Developing Country — 119
    Jayashree Mondkar and Swati Manerkar
15. Role of Paramedical Staff — 125
    Pushpa Thorat
16. Training of Medical and Paramedical Staff in Obstetric Care — 129
    Reena J Wani and Rashmi Jalvee

SECTION III: SURGICAL PROCEDURES and TL

17. National Guidelines for Female Sterilization and Male Sterilization — 135
    Asha Advani
18. National Guidelines for Mini-Lap Tubal Sterilization — 145
    Rashmi Jalvee and Reena J Wani
19. National Guidelines for Laparoscopic Tubal Ligation and Managing Its Complications — 156
    Madhuri Patel and Amol P Pawar
20. Criteria for Selection of Patients for Tubal Ligation — 179
    Devki Potwar and Asha Dalal
21. MTP and Tubal Ligations—Problems at Rural Areas of India — 185
    Gajanan Velhal and Sneha Shirodkar
22. Medicolegal Issues and Informed Consent Format in Sterilization Operation — 195
    Meenakshi Deshpande

Section IV: INFERTILITY PRACTICE

23. ICMR Guidelines and Practice of Infertility — 207
    S Krishna Kumar
24. Ethics in Infertility Practice — 217
    Preeti Bhandari
25. Surrogacy — 225
    Kaushal Kadam, Hitesha Ramnani and Kalika Joshi
26. Regulatory Aspects of Assisted Reproduction — 232
    Nandita Palshetkar, Hrishikesh D Pai and Manisha T Kundnani
27. Setting Up an IUI Clinic — 239
    Pratik Tambe and Shradda Agarwal

SECTION V: WOMEN RIGHTS

28. Protection and Safety Issues of Women and Children—　251
An Update on Various Acts and Laws
Alka Kuthe

29. Role of Women Commission in Domestic Violence　265
Mandakini Megh, Shomita Biswas and Preeti Deshpande

30. Policy Decisions for Women's Health　273
Rajesh Darade and Sachin Mumbare

31. National Health Mission Welfare Programs for Women　290
Suchitra Pandit and Rakhee Sahu

32. Janani Suraksha Yojana (JSY)　304
Balaji Jadhav and Shweta Khade

33. Adoption　313
Namrata Rajput and Amit Upadhyay

34. Government Policies Regarding Adolescent Reproductive Health　318
Ashwini Bhalerao Gandhi and Sampath Kumari

35. Lifestyle Modifications for Empowering Women　325
Charmila Ayyavoo and CN Aditi

36. Medical Councils and Doctors: Medical Ethics Training—　331
the Need of the Hour
Shivkumar S Utture

37. Domestic Violence Act　337
Reena J Wani and Preeti Deshpande

SECTION VI: RECENT UPDATES

38. Assault on Doctors and Remedies against the Same　349
Vipin Checker

39. Anti-ragging Rules and Regulations in the Medical Education System　357
in India
Manisha Khare

40. Biomedical Waste Management　364
Bipin Pandit and Vipin Checker

41. Clinical Establishment Act in Day-to-Day Practice　372
Girish Kumthekar

Index　377

Section 1

MTP and PCPNDT Act

1. Medical Termination of Pregnancy (MTP) Act—Rules and Regulations
2. MTP Act: Registration of Place and Maintenance of Records
3. MTP Act—Need for Change
4. PCPNDT Act and Rules
5. PCPNDT Act: Practitioner's Perspective
6. An Update on POCSO Act and Challenges in Relation to MTP Act
7. Medicolegal Challenges in PCPNDT Act: Case Examples
8. Recent Judgments and Legal Update

Chapter 1

Medical Termination of Pregnancy (MTP) Act— Rules and Regulations

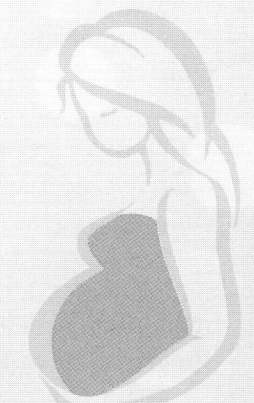

○ Mandakini Megh

The Medical Termination of Pregnancy (MTP) Act came into existence in India in 1971. As per this Act, MTP is the lawful abortion of a foetus and it empowers a woman to decide whether to continue her pregnancy or terminate it.

History

In India, the British enacted the Indian Penal Code in 1860 which declared induced abortions as illegal, the only exception being when abortion was induced to save the life of the woman.[1] Although this clause in the penal code was changed in Great Britain in 1967, India did not change it until 1971.[1] Countless women died attempting illegal abortions as a result of the penal code. The Medical Termination of Pregnancy Act, 1971 (MTP Act)[2] was enacted in India to reduce the mortality and morbidity associated with unsafe abortions. The Act was amended in 2002[3] and further on October 29, 2014, the Ministry of Health and Family Welfare released a draft of the MTP (Amendment) Bill 2014.[4]

MEDICAL TERMINATION OF PREGNANCY ACT[2-6]

The MTP Act enacted in 1971 and amended in 2002; the MTP Rules, 2003[5]; and the MTP Regulations, 2003 govern the provision of abortions of MTP in India. The MTP Act, and the Rules and Regulations framed thereunder provide an ambit under which legal abortion services can be provided up to 20 weeks of pregnancy.

The MTP Act provides details about the following aspects of abortion services:
- Conditions under which pregnancy may be terminated. [MTP Act: Section 3 (2)]
- Who can provide abortion services. [MTP Act: Section 2 (d) and Rule 4]

- Sites where abortion service can be provided. [MTP Act: Section 4]
- Documentation and records for abortion services. [Rule 5, Rule 9, Regulation 3, Regulation 4 (5), and Regulation 5]
- Punishments for violation of the MTP Act. [MTP Act: Section 5 (2), Section 5 (3) and Section 5 (4)]

Conditions under which a Pregnancy may be Terminated

The MTP Act allows for termination of pregnancy in case of:
- Continuation of pregnancy would involve risk to the life of pregnant woman or may cause grave injury to her physical or mental health
- Substantial risk that the child, if born, would be seriously handicapped due to physical or mental abnormalities
- Pregnancy is caused by rape (presumed to constitute grave injury to mental health)
- Pregnancy is caused due to failure of contraceptive in married woman or her husband (presumed to constitute grave injury to mental health).

Who can Provide Abortion Services

MTP can be legally provided only by a 'registered medical practitioner' (RMP)—a medical practitioner who possesses any recognised medical qualification as defined in Clause (h) of Section 2 of Indian Medical Council Act, 1956, whose name has been entered in a State Medical Register and who has one or more of the following experience or training in gynaecology and obstetrics (OBGY):

1. In the case of a medical practitioner, who was registered in a State Medical Register immediately before the commencement of the Act, with experience in the practice of OBGY for a period not less than three years.
2. In the case of a medical practitioner, who was registered in a State Medical Register after the commencement of the Act and
    a. Has completed six months of house surgery in OBGY; or
    b. Has experience in any hospital for a period of not less than one year in the practice of OBGY; or
    c. Holds a postgraduate degree or diploma in OBGY; or
    d. Has assisted an RMP in the performance of 25 cases of MTP of which at least five have been performed independently, in a hospital established or maintained by the Government, or a training institute approved for this purpose by the Government. This training will enable the RMP to do only first trimester terminations (up to 12 weeks of gestation).

When can Pregnancy be Terminated

Pregnancy can be terminated by 1 RMP up to 12 weeks of pregnancy and up to 20 weeks with the consent of 2 RMPs.

Sites where Abortion Service can be Provided

No termination of pregnancy shall be made in accordance with this Act at any place other than
   i. Hospital established or maintained by the Government or
  ii. A place approved by the Government or the District Level Committee (DLC) headed by the Chief Medical Officer (CMO) or District Health Officer (DHO).

No place shall be approved under Clause (ii)
- unless the Government is satisfied that termination of pregnancies may be done therein under safe and hygienic conditions; and.
- unless the following facilities are provided therein, namely
   – In case of first trimester (12 weeks of pregnancy): A gynaecology examination/labour table, resuscitation and sterilization equipment drugs and parental fluid, back-up facilities for treatment of shock and facilities for transportation; and
   – In case of second trimester (up to 20 weeks of pregnancy):
      a. Operation table and instruments for performing abdominal or gynaecological surgery
      b. Anaesthetic equipment, resuscitation equipment and sterilization equipment
      c. Drugs and parental fluids for emergency use, notified by Government of India from time to time

The certificate of approval by the DLC needs to be conspicuously displayed at the site to be easily visible to persons visiting the place.

MTP Act allows provision of medical methods of abortion (MMA) up to seven weeks of pregnancy at an unapproved site provided it has access/referral linkages to an MTP approved site. For the purpose of access, the RMP should display a certificate to this effect from the owner of the approved site.

In case of an emergency, any pregnancy may be terminated by an RMP to save the life of the woman at an unapproved place. Information about the same must be sent to the CMO the same day or latest the next working day.

The termination of pregnancy by a person who is not a RMP shall be an offence punishable with rigorous imprisonment for a term not be less than 2 years but which may extend to 7 years.

Whoever terminates any pregnancy in a place other than approved under the MTP Act shall be punishable with rigorous imprisonment for a term not less than 2 years but which may extend to 7 years.

Any person being owner of a place which is not approved under MTP Act shall be punishable with rigorous imprisonment for a term not be less than 2 years but which may extend to 7 years.

If a person wilfully contravenes or wilfully fails to comply with the requirements of any regulation made penalty of ₹1000.

Documentation and Records for Abortion Services

Form I—*Opinion form* for each MTP done must be duly filled with reason for termination and signature with date **within three hours of MTP.** Opinion of the second RMP in case of

2nd trimester abortions must also be recorded either at the time of admission or within three hours of MTP. **The column for indicating the reason for MTP must never be left blank.**

Form II—*Reporting format*—A monthly statement of all MTPs done must be sent to CMO on this format. This should include both surgical and medical methods of abortions (MMA).

Form III—*Admission register*—All MTPs conducted at the facility must be recorded in the admission register maintained at the facility for each calendar year. The register must be maintained for a period of five years from the last entry. Entries shall be made serially and a fresh serial shall be started at the start of each calendar year and the serial number of the particular year shall be distinguished from the serial number of other years by mentioning the year against the serial number. Admission Register is a confidential document and is not open to inspection by any person except under the authority of law.

Form C—*Consent form*—Consent of only the woman is required if she is of and above the age of 18 years. Consent from husband/parent/guardian is not required for seeking an abortion from a woman who is of or above 18 years of age and who is not mentally ill.

Only in case of a minor and/or a mentally ill woman of any age, her guardian's consent is required. Guardian under the MTP Act means a person having the care of a minor or a mentally ill person. This person does not necessarily have to be the legal guardian.

Additional documentation of age proof is not required in addition to Form C.

Form B—*Certificate of approval* for a 'private' place issued by the DLC chaired by the CMO shall be conspicuously displayed such that it is easily visible to visitors. All Government facilities are by default approved to provide Comprehensive Abortion Care services and therefore do not need a certificate of approval.

Medical Termination of Pregnancy (Amendment) Bill 2014[4]

On October 29, 2014 the Ministry of Health and Family Welfare (MOHFW) released a draft of the MTP (Amendment) Bill, which proposes to improve access to abortion and at the same time reduce women's dependency on healthcare providers during the process of seeking abortion.

- The bill proposes to replace the term "Registered medical practitioners" by the term "Registered healthcare providers" thus including vaids, hakims, Siddha practitioners, homeopaths as well as nurses and ANMs (auxiliary nurse midwives). The Bill thus proposes to train and allow non-allopathic and mid-level healthcare providers to perform abortions.
- It outlines the methods of abortion more clearly than the 1971 MTP Act, recognising medical termination of pregnancy as a separate and legal technique of abortion.
- First-trimester abortion will be considered a matter of woman's choice and a physician's opinion will no longer be required.
- A woman will require only one physician's opinion in the second trimester.
- The Amendment Bill also explicitly extends abortion care to unmarried women and aims at ensuring privacy for women seeking abortion.
- The gestational limit for abortion will be extended from 20 to 24 weeks and in addition, abortion will be provided for specific foetal anomalies after this period.
The amendment to the MTP Act is still pending.

MTP Amendment Bill 2019[7]

The ministry is in the process of finalizing the Medical Termination of Pregnancy (MTP) Draft Amendment Bill, 2019 which will allow the much needed relaxations on abortion services for a defined set of women. One category includes victims of sexual violence (rape and incest). They will be allowed to terminate their pregnancy beyond the fetal age of 20 weeks within 24 weeks. Another category includes abortion of foetuses certified by doctors to be "incompatible with life".

The amendment to the MTP Act is still pending and many women have been forced to move the Supreme Court for permission to end their pregnancies that are beyond the legal limit of 20 weeks, after the delay in the MTP Act amendment.

REFERENCES

1. Chandrasekhar S. India's Abortion Experience Denton, TX: University of North Texas Press, 1994.
2. The Medical Termination of Pregnancy Act, 1971. New Delhi: GoI; 1971[cited 2018 Sep 5]. Act No. 34 of 1971. Available from: http://tcw.nic.in/Acts/MTP-Act-1971.pdf
3. Ministry of Health and Family Welfare—Guidelines of MTP Act amended in 2002
4. Draft Medical Termination of Pregnancy (Amendment) Bill 2014. New Delhi: GoI; 29 October 2014. Available from: http://www.mohfw. nic.in
5. Ministry of Health and Family Welfare (Department of Family Welfare) Notification New Delhi. The 13th June 2003.
6. Ministry of Health and Family Welfare. Guidance: Ensuring Access to Safe Abortion and Addressing Gender Biased Sex Selection: February 2015.
7. https://m.tribuneindia.com/news/archive/news-detail-820796

ANNEXURE

Various Forms Under MTP Act 1971

FORM A

[See sub-rule (2) of rule 5]

Form of application for the approval of a place under Clause (b) of Section 4.

Category of approved place:

A. Pregnancy can be terminated up to 12 weeks
B. Pregnancy can be terminated up to 20 weeks
   1. Name of the place (in capital letters)
   2. Address in full
   3. Non-Governmental/Private/Nursing Home/Other Institutions
   4. State, if the following facilities are available at the place—Medical Termination of Pregnancy (MTP) Act—Rules and Regulations

CATEGORY A

   i. Gynaecological examination/labour table.
   ii. Resuscitation equipment
   iii. Sterilization equipment
   iv. Facilities for treatment of shock, including emergency drugs.
   v. Facilities for transportation, if required.

CATEGORY B

   i. An operation table and instruments for performance abdominal or gynaecological surgery.
   ii. Drugs and parental fluid in sufficient supply emergency cases
   iii. Anaesthetic equipment, resuscitation equipment and sterilisation equipment.

Place:

Date: Signature of the owner of the place

FORM B

[Refer sub-rule (6) of rule 5]

Certificate of approval

The place described below is hereby approved for the purpose of the Medical Termination of Pregnancy Act, 1971 (34 of 1971).

As read within up to .... weeks

Name of the place

Address and other descriptions

Name of the owner

Place:

Date: To the Government of the ....

FORM C
(See Rule 9)

I .... daughter/wife of .... aged about .... years of .... (here state the permanent address) at present residing at .... do hereby give my consent to be termination of my pregnancy at .... (State the name of place where the pregnancy is to be terminated).

Place:
Date:

Signature

(To be filled in by guardian where the woman is a mentally ill person or minor).

I .... son/daughter/wife of .... aged about .... years of .... at present residing at (permanent address) .... do hereby give my consent to the termination of my pregnancy of my ward .... who is a minor/lunatic at .... (place of termination of pregnancy).

Place:
Date:

Signature

FORM I
(See Regulation 3)

I .... (Name and qualifications of the Registered Medical Practitioner in block letters) .... (Full address of the Registered Medical Practitioner)

I .... (Name and qualifications of the Registered Medical Practitioner in block letters) .... (Full address of the Registered Medical Practitioner) hereby certify that *I/We/am/are of opinion, formed in good faith, that it is necessary to terminate the pregnancy of .... (Full name of pregnant woman in block letters) resident of .... (Full address of woman in block letters) for the reasons given below**.

I/We hereby give intimation that *I/We terminated the pregnancy of the woman referred to above who bears the serial No. .... in the Admission Register of the Hospital/approved place.

Place:
Date:

Signatures of Registered Medical Practitioners

*Strike out whichever is not applicable.
** of the reasons specified items (i) to (v) write the one which is appropriate:
  i. In order to save the life of the pregnant woman.
  ii. In order to prevent grave injury to the physical or mental health of the pregnant woman.
  iii. In view of the substantial risk that if the child was born it would suffer from such physical or mental abnormalities as to be seriously handicapped.

iv. As the pregnancy is alleged by pregnant woman to have been caused by rape.
v. As the pregnancy has occurred as a result of failure of any contraceptive device or methods used by married woman or her husband for the purpose of limiting the number of children.

Note: Account may be taken of the pregnant woman's actual or reasonably foreseeable environment in determining whether the continuance of a pregnancy would involve a grave injury to her physical or mental health.

Place:
Date:

Signature of the Registered Medical Practitioner

FORM II

[See Regulation 4 (5)]

1. Name of the State ....
2. Name of Hospital/approved place ....
3. Duration of pregnancy (give total no. only)
   a. Up to 12 weeks ....
   b. Between 12 and 20 weeks ....
4. Religions of women:
   a. Hindu
   b. Muslim
   c. Christian
   d. Others
   e. Total
5. Termination with acceptance of contraception:
   a. Sterilisation
   b. IUD
6. Reasons for termination (give total number under each sub-head):
   a. Danger to life of the pregnant woman.
   b. Grave injury to the physical health of the pregnant woman.
   c. Grave injury to the mental health of the pregnant woman.
   d. Pregnancy caused by rape.
   e. Substantial risk that if the child was born, it would suffer from such physical or mental abnormalities as to be seriously handicapped.
   f. Failure of any contraceptive device or method.

Signature of the Officer In-charge with date

FORM III

(See Regulation 5)

ADMISSION REGISTER

(To be destroyed on the expiry of five years from the dated of the last entry in the Register)

1	2	3	4	5	6	7
S. no.	Date of admission	Name of patient	Wife/ daughter of	Age	Religion	Address

8	9	10	11	12	13	14
Duration of pregnancy	Reason on which pregnancy terminated	Date of termination of pregnancy	Date of discharge of patient	Result and remarks	Name of registered medical practitioner(s) by whom the opinion is formed	Name of registered medical practitioner(s) by whom pregnancy terminated

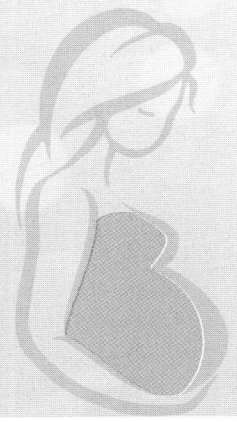

Chapter 2

MTP Act: Registration of Place and Maintenance of Records

○ Gorakh G Mandrupkar

Introduction

In India, we have a very liberal and proactive law for medical termination of pregnancy. Abortion is not considered as a basic right of an Indian woman but getting access to safe abortion under this law is definitely considered to be the basic right of every Indian woman.

Certain licenses for registration of place as well as certain norms for records and documentations are given by this law, which are mandatory.

Place where Pregnancy may be Terminated

"No termination of pregnancy shall be made in accordance with this Act at any place other than
a. A hospital established or maintained by Government, or
b. A place for the time being approved for the purpose of this Act by Government or a District Level Committee constituted by that Government with the Chief Medical Officer or District Health Officer as the Chairperson of the said Committee: Provided that the District Level Committee shall consist of not less than three and not more than five members including the Chairperson, as the Government may specify from time to time."

Approval of Place

For this, we have to refer the Rule 5 of this Act which states that:
1. No place shall be approved:
   a. Unless the Government is satisfied that termination of pregnancies may be done therein under safe and hygienic conditions; and

b. Unless the following facilities are provided therein

In case of first trimester (up to 12 weeks of pregnancy)
- A gynecology examination/labor table
- Resuscitation and sterilization equipment
- Drugs and parental fluid
- Back up facilities for treatment of shock
- Facilities for transportation

In case of second trimester (from 12 to 20 weeks of pregnancy)
- Along with the above all...
- Operation table
- Instruments for performing abdominal or gynecological surgery
- Anesthesia equipment
- Resuscitation equipment
- Sterilization equipment
- Drugs and parental fluids for emergency use, notified by Government of India from time to time.

How to Apply?

Every application for the approval of a place shall be in Form A and shall be addressed to the chief medical officer of the district (district civil surgeon/MOHFW of corporation).

The place shall be inspected within 2 months of receiving the application and certificate of approval may be issued within the next 2 months, or in case any deficiency has been noted, within 2 months of the deficiency having been rectified by the applicant.

The chief medical officer of the district, after inspection of place, and if satisfied after such verification, enquiry or inspection, that termination of pregnancies may be done under safe and hygienic conditions, at the place, recommend the approval of such place to the committee.

The district level committee (DLC)* may after considering the application and the recommendations of the chief medical officer of the district approve such place and issue a certificate of approval in Form B.

The certificate of approval issued by the committee shall be conspicuously displayed at the place to be easily visible to persons visiting the place.

{* District level committee: Composition and tenure: One member of the district level committee shall be gynecologist/surgeon/anesthesiologist and other members from the local medical profession, non-governmental organizations, and panchayat raj institution of the district: Provided that one of the members of committee shall be a woman. Tenure of the committee shall be for two calendar years and the tenure of the non-government members shall not be more than two terms.}

Who can Perform MTP?

As per the Rule 4 of this Act,
a. A registered medical practitioner[#], registered in a State Medical Register immediately before the commencement of the Act (i.e. before 1971), experienced in the practice of gynecology and obstetrics for a period of not less than three years.

b. A registered medical practitioner,
   i. Who has completed six months of house surgency in gynecology and obstetrics; or
   ii. Unless the following facilities are provided therein, if he had experience at any hospital for a period of not less than one year in the practice of obstetrics and gynecology; or
c. If he has assisted a registered medical practitioner in the performance of twenty-five cases of medical termination of pregnancy of which at least five have been performed independently, in a hospital established or maintained, or a training institute approved for this purpose by the Government.
d. In case of a medical practitioner who has been registered in a State Medical Register and who holds a postgraduate degree or diploma in gynecology and obstetrics, the experience or training gained during the course of such degree or diploma.

{Training under sub-rule c would enable to do only 1st Trimester (up to 12 weeks) terminations. For the terminations from 12–20 weeks, experience or training under sub-rules: a, b and d shall apply.}

(#"Registered medical practitioner" means a medical practitioner who possesses any recognized medical qualification as defined in Clause (h) of Section 2 of the Indian Medical Council Act, 1956, whose name has been entered in a State Medical Register and who has such experience or training in gynecology and obstetrics as may be prescribed by rules made under this Act.)

Maintenance of Records

1. Form C: Consent form

   Before doing MTP (medical/surgical), consent should be obtained in the Form C from a woman undergoing MTP who is above 18 years with sound mental health.

   When she is minor (below age 18), consent must be obtained from legal guardian.

2. Form I (One): Form of certifying opinion or opinions

   Every registered medical practitioner who terminates any pregnancy shall, within three hours from the termination of the pregnancy, certify such termination in Form I.

   Up to 12 weeks of pregnancy opinion of one registered medical practitioner and from 12 to 20 weeks of gestation, opinion of two registered medical practitioners is taken.

Custody of Forms: Regulation 04

1. Form C and Form I together shall be placed in an envelope which shall be sealed by the registered medical practitioner.
2. On every envelope there shall be noted the serial number assigned to the pregnant woman in the admission register (Form III) and the name and address of the registered medical practitioner or practitioners by whom the pregnancy was terminated and such envelope shall be marked "Secret".
3. Every envelope shall be sent immediately after the termination of the pregnancy to the head of the hospital or owner of the approved place where the pregnancy was terminated.
4. On receipt of the envelope, the head of the hospital or owner of the approved place shall arrange to keep the same in safe custody.

5. Every head of the hospital or owner of the approved place shall send to the district chief medical officer, in Form II a monthly statement of cases where medical termination of pregnancy has been done.
6. Where the pregnancy is not terminated in an approved place or hospital for life-saving indication, every envelope shall be sent by registered post to the chief medical officer of the district on the same day on which the pregnancy was terminated or on the next working day following the day on which the pregnancy was terminated.

Maintenance of Admission Register (FORM III): Regulation 05

1. Every head of the hospital or owner of the approved place shall maintain a register in Form III for recording therein the details of the admissions of women for the termination of their pregnancies and keep such register for a period of five years from the end of the calendar year it relates to.
2. The entries in the Admission Register shall be made serially and a fresh serial shall be started at the commencement of each calendar year and the serial number of the particular year shall be distinguished from the serial number of other years by mentioning the year against the serial number, for example, Serial Number 5 of 2018 and Serial Number 5 of 2019 shall be mentioned as 5/2018 and 5/2019.
3. Admission Register shall be a secret document and the information contained therein as to the name and other particulars of the pregnant woman shall not be disclosed to any person.

Admission Register not to be Open to Inspection: Regulation 06

"Admission Register shall be kept in the safe custody of the head of the hospital or owner of the approved place, or by any person authorized by such head or owner and shall not be open for inspection by any person except under the authority of law: First class magistrate/district civil surgeon/MOHFW of corporation/or designated officer by district chief medical officer.

Provided that the registered medical practitioner on the application of an employed woman whose pregnancy has been terminated, grant a certificate for the purpose of enabling her to obtain leave from her employer: Provided further that any such employer shall not disclose this information to any other person.

Entries in Other Registers Maintained in Hospital or Approved Place: Regulation 07

In other hospital records like OPD case-sheet, operation theatre register, follow-up card or any other document or register other than the admission register, reference to the pregnant woman undergoing MTP shall be made therein by the serial number assigned to the woman in the admission register and not by her name.

Destruction of Admission Register and Other Papers: Regulation 08

Every admission register shall be destroyed on the expiry of a period of five years from the date of the last entry in that register and other papers on the expiry of a period of three years from the date of the termination of the pregnancy concerned provided no medicolegal case is going on.

In that case save as otherwise directed by the Chief Secretary to the union territory administration or for in relation to any proceeding pending before him, as directed by a District Judge or a Magistrate of the first class.

Frequently Asked Questions

1. Does a specific doctor only can perform MTP in said premises?
   No.
   Form B gives approval to place and not to specific practitioner or anesthesiologist though their names are written mistakenly on certificate. Any registered medical practitioner defined under this Act can perform MTP at any such approved hospital provided he/she follows the rules of maintenance of record keeping (MTP Act regulation 04).
2. Can any medical officer check admission register during inspection of hospital?
   Only district civil surgeon/MOHFW of corporation/or designated officer for inspection by these officers with written order can ask for admission register for inspection.
   (MTP Act regulation 06)
3. Can a doctor/head of institute handover record to police for investigations?
   No, not directly.
   Investigating authorities have to write to district civil surgeon/MOHFW of corporation about the said record. With written permission from these authorities, copy of necessary record should be handed over to police.
4. Is there any linkage between PCPNDT and MTP law?
   No. Not at all.
   PCPNDT law is for prevention of sex selection and regulation of technologies and techniques related to it.
   MTP law is for legalizing and promoting safe abortion services.
   The implementing authorities of both the laws are same, so many a times wrongly both of these laws are mixed together.

BIBLIOGRAPHY

MTP Act: Bare Act Book. GOI, 34 of 1971 (2003 amended)

Chapter 3

MTP Act—Need for Change

○ Nikhil Datar ○ Nithya R Iyer

Abortion is not a pure medical or a legal issue. It has many facets ranging from ethics to morality to religion. In the ancient days abortion was considered as a sin and an action against God. However, circumstances have always made women practice some form of birth control and/or abortion for centuries. The concept of abortion has generated intense moral, ethical, political and legal debates since long. Abortion is not merely a techno-medical issue but "the fulcrum of a much broader ideological struggle in which the very meanings of the family, the state, motherhood and young women's sexuality are contested".

In India, attitudes and practices have changed significantly with education and empowerment of women. Abortion in India has been legal since 1971. The Act was amended in 2002. The MTP Act is in need of one more amendment in the interest of women's rights.

BACKGROUND OF THE MTP ACT IN INDIA

Before 1971

The Indian Penal Code 1860 (IPC), which is the basic criminal law of the country, keeping in view with the religious, moral, social and ethical background of the Indian community, has made "induced abortion" a criminal offence under Sections 312 to 316 of IPC 1860.[1]

The IPC states that "whoever voluntarily causes a woman with a child to miscarry shall—if such a miscarriage be not caused in good faith for the purpose of saving life of the woman, be punished with imprisonment of either description for a term which may extend to 3 years or with a fine or with both and if the woman be 'quick' with child shall be punished either with a term which may be extended up to 7 years and shall be liable to fine."[1]

Thus, 'induced abortion' is an offence under two circumstances.
1. When the woman is 'with child' (as soon as gestation begins), or
2. When she is 'quick with child' (as soon as quickening is felt by mother)

Countless women died attempting illegal abortions as a result of the penal code, and it was a combination of this and the growing population that made the country reconsider its initial stance.[1] In 1964, the Central Family Planning Board of the Government of India met and formed a committee designed to examine the subject of abortion from medical, legal, social, and moral standpoints.[1] The Abortion Study Committee, led by the Health Minister of the State of Maharashtra, Mr Shantilal Shah, spent two years studying the issue, and submitted a report with its suggestions in December 1966.[1] This report considered the penal code to be too restrictive and recommended that the law related to abortions be relaxed.

1971 and Beyond

The Medical Termination of Pregnancy (MTP) Act, was enacted by the Indian Parliament in the year 1971 with the intention to reduce avoidable wastage of women's life.[2] The MTP Act came into effect from 1 April 1972 and was amended in the years 1975 and 2002.

When it was introduced, it was a great achievement for women's health. Nearly 30 years later, the law and associated rules and regulations are considered "overtly medicalised" and "bureaucratic", and as such, not oriented toward women's right to access safe and legal abortion services.

CURRENT SCENARIO

In last 40 years, medical science has evolved significantly. With the advent of ultrasound it is possible to diagnose abnormalities in the fetus in the womb and give an accurate prognosis to the woman. The methods of inducing abortions have evolved significantly making late terminations relatively far safer. However, the law has not kept pace with these medical advances.

The author challenged the provisions of the MTP Act by filling a case "Dr Nikhil Datar and others Vs Government of India" on behalf of one of his patients who carried a 24 weeks severely abnormal fetus and wished to terminate her pregnancy. This was the first case in the history of Indian judiciary on this issue.

Till now, the author has helped nearly 100 women who wished to terminate their pregnancies which were advanced beyond 20 weeks because of severe fetal abnormality or when they were as a result of rape. The author has helped them pro bono to seek judicial intervention at various High Courts and the Supreme Court of India. The courts, after analysing the issues on case to case basis, have allowed almost all these women to undergo termination of pregnancy even though the gestation was advanced beyond 20 weeks. **It must be noted that the MTP Act is not yet amended. Till then, the only remedy available is to approach the High Court.**

PITFALLS IN THE INDIAN MTP ACT

1. A woman's right to abortion is not 'unconditional'. In other words, a woman cannot demand for an abortion without any reasons. According to the MTP Act, Section 3(2)(b): Pregnancy can be terminated only if:
   - There is a substantial risk that if the child were born, it would suffer from such physical or mental abnormalities as to be seriously handicapped.

- The continuance of the pregnancy would involve a risk to the life of the pregnant woman or of grave injury to her physical or mental health.

Thus, MTP Act, 1971 does not give unconditional right to a woman to terminate her own pregnancy. The complete decision depends on the medical practitioner, who in "good faith" can approve termination of pregnancy.

A provider dependant law, however liberal it may be, can become 'restrictive' under different socio-political and religious compulsions, without the alteration of even a single word.

Thus, the IPC and the MTP Act infringes the right to privacy, right to health and right to dignity which is guaranteed by Article 21 (right to life and right to personal liberty).[3]

2. India is not against abortions, it does not believe in the "pro-life" ideology. MTP. Act, 1971 in its Sections 3, 2(2) states that "MTP can be performed where there is 'substantial risk' that if the child were born, it would suffer from such physical or mental abnormalities as to be seriously handicapped". But this is allowed only till 20 weeks. However, no explanation for the arbitrary limit of 20 weeks period is found in the Shantilal Shah Committee report (1966) as well as in parliamentary discussions.

In India, there is no official pronouncement of age of viability. The clarity on concept of when to call a termination of pregnancy an 'abortion' and when to call it a 'delivery' is not there.

It is important to note that there is no specific quantification available as how to measure the 'substantiality' of a particular handicap. In the Shantilal Shah Committee Report, Dr HL Shivpuri had stated that "The word 'substantial risk' is very vague ... it is open to different interpretations by courts of law and may lead to endless trouble for doctor concerned. Efforts should have been made to better define the risks". But unfortunately this controversial term still stands undefined. The doctors can only give the statistical prognosis regarding any handicap but not individualistic prognosis.

With the advent of newer technologies, an accurate prenatal diagnosis can be given to the patient. Many abnormalities can be detected before 20 weeks but cardiac, gastrointestinal anomalies may not get detected below 20 weeks. Typically, results of amniocentesis get available after 20 weeks. In rural India, we are fighting for access to healthcare. Women may not be able to seek medical services before 20 weeks. In such a situation, will it be fair to diagnose an anomaly, give a grave prognosis and still compel a woman to continue the pregnancy against her wish?

FIGO Committee for The Study of Ethical Aspects of Human Reproduction and Women's Health[4] agreed that a woman carrying a severely malformed fetus had the ethical right to have her pregnancy terminated. The qualification 'severe' is used in this context to indicate malformations that are either potentially lethal or whose nature is such that even with medical treatment, they are likely, in the view of the parents and their medical advisors, to result in unacceptable mental and/or physical disability." Also late termination has medically became very safe and it is being used when there is a risk to mother's life or in cases of fetal death in the womb.

3. The Nuffield Council on Bioethics[5] is funded jointly by the Medical Research Council, the Nuffield Foundation and the Welcome Trust and it consists of health economist, disability

commissioner, anthropologist, reputed doctors from fields of obstetrics, neonatology, lawyers, ethicist, rights activists.

While discussing the critical care decisions in fetal and neonatal medicine, the council came up with the following conclusions:

- "We regard the moment of birth, which is straightforward to identify, and usually represents a significant threshold in potential viability, as the significant moral and legal point of transition for judgements about preserving life—working party.
- When the baby's life results in a level of irremediable suffering, there is no ethical obligation to act in order to preserve that life—working party.
- It would be wrong to force a woman to behave rightly by submitting to medical or surgical interventions to benefit a foetus against her will."

4. Unlike other countries where the law is titled as "Abortion Act", it is titled as "Medical termination of pregnancy Act" in India. Probably, in 1971, the parliament was not keen on using the word "abortion" directly to avoid socio-political implications. Under the Act, the term "Termination of pregnancy" is not defined. Plain reading of the term implies that any procedure that terminates the pregnant status of the woman is termination of pregnancy. It means that irrespective of the fetal status, alive or dead, any procedure that separates the products of conception from the uterus is MTP. Thus, missed miscarriage or even induction of labour done for severe growth restriction could also be construed to fall under this definition. On the other hand, the term abortion has a specific and clear meaning. The word is defined as "any procedure that causes or hastens the process of fetal death." This clarity will also help to solve the ethical question while dealing with late terminations beyond 20 weeks. At this point of time, there is no clarity on how to deal with the live fetus after late termination. In most of the countries like UK, which allow late terminations, it is a norm to do intrauterine feticide and ensure that dead fetus is born when late abortion is done. In India, we are completely unclear on this issue.

5. As per the MTP Act, the rules are laid down by the Central Government and it empowers the state and district governments to make regulations. This adds layers of bureaucratic procedures, leading to unnecessary administrative barriers. Thus, the general spirit of state regulations appears to be 'controlling' than 'facilitating' abortion services.

6. The MTP Act covers those pregnancies which occur out of failure of contraception, but this clause is applicable only to married couples. Hence, illegal abortions are the only resource for the most vulnerable women in need—the unmarried, the adolescent girls, separated and single women.

7. The regulatory processes as mentioned in the MTP Act and regulations should have equitable and transparent policies to be applied to both private and public sectors. There is an assumption that public health institutions, by the virtue of being in the public sector, have a regulatory process built within them.

8. Amended MTP Rule mandates the district committee to inspect the facility seeking registration within two months of receiving the application. However, it does not specify measures or redressal mechanism if the certification procedures are not completed within the stipulated time frame.

9. Section 4 of the MTP Regulations states that detailed record and reporting procedures are to be followed while maintaining confidentiality of the abortion seeker. As per the regulations, the name of the patient undergoing the MTP should not be mentioned anywhere else except the admission register and consent form. It is expected to seal both the forms in an envelope. Since the name is to be kept secret, how does one address the woman? How does one confirm her identity according to the WHO's safe surgery checklist? How does one give discharge card or bill? How does one fill up online reporting form without name being mentioned? These practical questions need to be addressed clearly.
10. Under the "Drug and Cosmetics Act" it is expected to maintain a separate register of scheduled drugs. Since mifepristone and misoprostol come under this category, a separate register is needed to be maintained along with the details of the usage. This is again contradictory to the above mentioned provisions of the MTP Act.
11. **The PCPNDT Act and the MTP Act:** Though the aim of both these acts are very distinct, there have been attempts to link the two laws with the intention of preventing sex-selective abortion. But it is necessary to understand that the two laws are not contradictory or conflicting but can easily coexist.
12. Code of Medical Ethics specifies that before performing an operation, the physician should obtain in writing the consent from the husband or wife, parent or guardian in the case of minor, or the patient, himself as the case may be. In an operation which may result in sterility the consent of both husband and wife is needed. No act of *in vitro* fertilization or artificial insemination shall be undertaken without the informed consent of the female patient and her spouse as well as the donor. Such consent shall be obtained in writing only after the patient is provided, at her own level of comprehension, with sufficient information about the purpose, methods, risks, inconveniences, disappointments of the procedure and possible risks and hazards. But in case a woman wants to abort such a conception, as per the MTP Act, she can get an MTP performed without the consent of her husband. Thus, in this manner the MTP Act also conflicts the Code of Medical Ethics.
13. **MTP Act and POCSO Act:** According to POCSO Act, only a woman above the age of 18 years can consent for act of sex. It means that any sexual act done by a minor is considered as "without consent" and amounts to rape. When a girl below the age of 18 seeks medical help for termination of pregnancy, the doctor mandatorily needs to inform the police. This puts the privacy of the woman, which is given paramount importance under the MTP Act, at stake. Since most of the young girls would rather not want to inform the police, they are again not left with a choice but to undergo illegal terminations in the hands of the quacks, risking their lives.

CONCLUSION

The MTP Act needs major amendments in three sectors.
- Rights of abortion of a woman must be respected and recognized.
- Especially for substantial foetal anomalies, termination must be allowed irrespective of gestational age.
- The conflicting legal positions under other laws such as IPC, code of medical ethics need to be resolved at once.

The author had challenged the provisions of the MTP Act in the High Court of Bombay in 2008 for one of his patients. He is still pursuing the special leave petition at the Supreme Court of India. In the recent past, the National Commission for women have recommended amendments to the law.[6]

The report of the committee of Mr Naresh Dayal and NK Ganguly is not yet acted upon by the Government.[7] The gynaecologists from the country are also the second victims of this lopsided law. They need to wake up and start collecting meticulous data particularly on severe anomalies reported beyond 20 weeks of pregnancy. This will go a long way in establishing that this is a public health hazard. Unless this is not demonstrated, the law will not change for the better.

REFERENCES

1. S. Chandrashekhar. *India's Abortion Experience*. Denton: University of North Texas Press, 1994.
2. "India". UN. Retrieved 30 March 2014.
3. Upendra Baxi. *Abortion and the law in India*. New Delhi: s.n., 1986-87
4. Recommendations on Ethical Issues in Obstetrics and Gynecology by the FIGO Committee for the Study of Ethical Aspects of Human Reproduction". October 2009.
5. http://www.nuffieldbioethics.org/sites/default/files/CCD%20web%20version%2022%20June%2007%20(updated).pdf
6. http://timesofindia.indiatimes.com/india/Allow-abortions-up-to-24-weeks-national-womens-panel-says/articleshow/18313104.cms
7. http://www.hindustantimes.com/india-news/niketa-effect-govt-to-review-abortion-laws/article1-335780.aspx

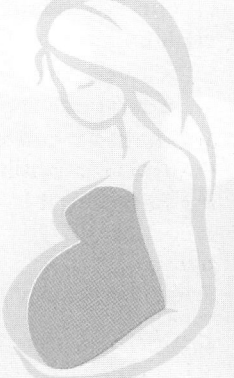

Chapter 4

PCPNDT Act and Rules

○ Mandakini Megh ○ Meenakshi Rao

INTRODUCTION

"It is no exaggeration to call this gendercide. Women are missing in their millions—aborted, killed, neglected to death."

—The Economist, Leaders, Gendercide, March 6th, 2010.

The practice of sex selective abortion (or social sex selection) has been a critical influencer of skewed sex ratios. It has, therefore, been sought to be legally regulated or termed illegal in some countries of the world, and India is one of them. There is a little doubt that strong socio-cultural and religious biases and a preference for sons in some communities have shaped societal attitudes in favour of the son.[1]

As members of a profession which has a privileged status and has bestowed on us a position of honour, it is our ethical responsibility to ensure that no one from our profession indulges in unethical and unlawful practices. The Pre-natal Diagnostic Techniques Act, 1994 and its subsequent amendment in 2003 as the Pre-conception and Prenatal Diagnostic Techniques (Prohibition of Sex Selection) Act (PCPNDT Act) were not brought into force because common people were resorting to sex selection, but because the medical fraternity made it possible and easy for them to do so.

The child sex ratio is calculated as the number of girls per 1000 boys in the 0–6 years age group. In India, the ratio has shown a sharp decline from 976 girls to 1000 boys in 1961 to 927 as per the 2001 census.[2] The declining child sex ratio has its roots in the practice of sex selection. In certain parts of the country, there are less than 800 girls for every 1000 boys. The child sex ratio is a powerful indicator of the social health of any society.

The adverse child sex ratio can severely impact the delicate equilibrium of nature and destroy our moral and social fabric. Contrary to what many believe, lesser number of girls in a society will not enhance their status. Instead, this could lead to increased violence against women, rape, abduction, trafficking and onset of practices such as polyandry (many men marrying one woman).

The law has its own place but has been hampered by difficulties in implementation and societal apathy. Efforts are being made to effectively implement the law.

Sex selection is not only about technology. At the heart of the matter is the low status of women in society and the deep-rooted prejudices they face through their life. Consequently, what we see is discrimination and neglect of the girl child, which could be in terms of inadequate nutrition, denial or limited access to education and health, child labour and domestic violence. At its worst, it translates into one of the most repugnant form of violence against women: Sex selection.

The Commonly used Techniques for Sex Selection

Pre-conception Techniques

- Pre-implantation genetic diagnosis
- Sperm sorting and sperm separation

Prenatal Diagnostic Techniques (PNDT)

Developed in the 1970s, PND through techniques such as ultrasound scanning and amniocentesis followed by sex selective abortion, remains the most common method of sex selection practiced around the world for the last three decades.

- Amniocentesis
- Chorion villus biopsy
- Sonography
- NIPT

Other Methods

- Diet
- Ayurvedic therapies

Background

Amniocentesis was first introduced in India in 1975 by the All India Institute of Medical Sciences (AIIMS), New Delhi, for detecting congenital deformities in a fetus. By the mid-1980s, it was being largely misused to determine the sex of the unborn child and to carry out sex selective abortions—with the girl child as the obvious target in Maharashtra, Punjab and Haryana. The practice soon spread to the rest of the country.

In 1988, the state of Maharashtra became the first in the country to ban prenatal sex determination through the enactment of the *Maharashtra Regulation of Prenatal Diagnostics Techniques Act*. At the national level the *Prenatal Diagnostic Techniques (Regulation and Prevention of Misuse) Act* (PNDT Act) was enacted on September 20, 1994.

The 1994, Act provided for the "regulation of the use of prenatal diagnostic techniques for the purpose of detecting genetic or metabolic disorders, chromosomal abnormalities or certain congenital malformations or sex-linked disorders and for the prevention of misuse of such techniques for the purpose of pre-natal sex determination leading to female feticide and for matters connected therewith or incidental thereto." Except under certain specific conditions, no individual or genetic counselling center or genetic laboratory or genetic clinic shall conduct or allow the conduct in its facility of, prenatal diagnostic techniques including ultrasonography for the purpose of determining the sex of the fetus; and "no person conducting prenatal diagnostic procedures shall communicate to the pregnant woman concerned or her relatives the sex of the fetus by words, signs or in any other manner."

The Act provides for the constitution of a *Central Supervisory Board (CSB)* whose function is mainly advisory, to review and monitor implementation of the Act and for the appointment of *Appropriate Authorities* (AAs) in States and Union territories to enforce the law and penalize defaulters and *Advisory Committees* (ACs) to aid and advise the AAs.

Provisions under the Act

Important Sections of the Act

Section 5 deals with the prohibition of communicating the sex of the fetus. Misuse of PCPNDT even by a qualified person, solely for sex-determination and in conditions not falling under the exceptions under the Act.

Section 6 deals with prohibition of determination of sex. Sex selection which would include any technique, procedure, test, administration, prescription or provision of anything, before or after conception, for the purpose of ensuring or increasing the probability of birth of male child. This would include even Ayurvedic pills or any alternative therapy claiming to be effective for this purpose.

Section 18 deals with registration of genetic counseling centers (GCC), genetic laboratories (GL) or genetic clinics (GC).

Section 22 deals with prohibition of advertisement relating to pre-conception and prenatal determination of sex and punishment for contravention. Issue, publication or circulation of any advertisement of facilities or any means of selecting or determining sex of the fetus before or after conception. The advertisement may be in any form: Notice, circular, label, wrapper or any other document, advertisement through internet (any search engine) or any other media in electronic or print form, and also includes any visible representation made by means of any hoarding, wall-painting, signal, light, sound, and smoke or gas.

Section 29 deals with maintenance of records by genetic counseling centers, genetic laboratories or genetic clinics. Every genetic counseling centre, genetic laboratory, genetic clinic, ultrasound clinic and imaging centre is required to maintain a register showing the names and addresses of the men or women given genetic counseling, subjected to prenatal diagnostic procedures or tests, the names of their spouses or fathers and the date on which they first reported for such counseling, procedure or test.

Rule 3B deals with sale of ultrasound machines/imaging machines. No organization including a commercial organization or a person, including manufacturer, importer, dealer or supplier of ultrasound machines/imaging machines or any other equipment, capable of detecting sex of fetus, shall sell, distribute, supply, rent, allow or authorize the use of any such machine or equipment in any manner, whether on payment or otherwise to any GCC, GL, genetic clinic, ultrasound clinic or imaging centre or a person not registered under the Act.

Amendments

The Prenatal Diagnostic Techniques (Regulation and Prevention of Misuse) Act, 1994 has since been amended with effect from 14.2.2003 following a public interest litigation (PIL) filed in 2000 and the findings revealed by the census 2001.

Amendments to the Act Mainly Cover to

1. Bring the technique of pre-conception sex selection within the ambit of this Act so as to prevent the use of such technologies which significantly contribute to the declining sex ratio.
2. Bring the use of ultrasound machines within the purview of this Act more explicitly so as to curb their misuse for detection and disclosure of sex of the fetus lest it should lead to female feticide.
3. Further empower the CSB for monitoring the implementation of the Act.
4. Introduce state level supervisory board for monitoring and reviewing the implementation of the Act in states/UTs.
5. Constitute a multi-member state appropriate authority (AA) for better implementation and monitoring of the Act in the states.
6. Make punishments prescribed under the Act more stringent so as to serve as deterrent for minimizing violations of the Act.
7. Empower the AAs with the powers of Civil Court for search, seizure and sealing the machines, equipment and records of the violators of law including sealing of premises and commissioning of witnesses.
8. Making mandatory the maintenance of proper records in respect of the use of ultrasound machines and other equipment capable of detection of sex of fetus and also in respect of tests and procedures leading to pre-conception selection of sex.
9. Regulate the sale of ultrasound machines only to the bodies registered under the Act.
10. Prescribes punishments for contravention of its provisions—imprisonment up to three years and a fine up to 10000.

Based on the amendments made to the Act, the Rules framed thereunder have also been amended under the amended rules.
1. **A provision for appeal has been made:** Any person having grievance against the sub-district level AA can make an appeal to the district level AA within 30 days of the order of subdistrict, similarly for grievance against the district level AA, an appeal can be made to the state/UT level AA within 30 days of the order of the district level AA. Appeal can be made to the central government against the order of the central appropriate authority and to state government against the state appropriate authority

2. **23 indications, prescribed by ICMR**, have been included in the PNDT Rules for which ultrasound scanning can be conducted during pregnancy for the well-being of the pregnant woman and her fetus.
3. Forms have been simplified. **Consent** is required only in case of **invasive techniques.**
4. For non-invasive techniques like ultrasonography, the medical professional is required to make a declaration on each report of ultrasonography/image scanning, certifying that he/she has neither detected nor disclosed the sex of the fetus to anybody. Before undergoing such test, the pregnant woman has to declare that she does not want to know the sex of the fetus.[3]

MINISTRY OF HEALTH AND FAMILY WELFARE NOTIFICATION
New Delhi, the 31st January, 2014
Amendment Rules, 2014

1. In the Pre-conception and Pre-natal Diagnostic Techniques (Prohibition of Sex Selection) Rules, 1996, for Form F, the following Form shall be substituted: [See Proviso to Section 4(3), Rule 9(4) and Rule 10(1A)]

FORM FOR MAINTENANCE OF RECORD IN CASE OF PRENATAL DIAGNOSTIC TEST/ PROCEDURE BY GENETIC CLINIC/ULTRASOUND CLINIC/IMAGING CENTRE

Section A: To be filled in for all Diagnostic Procedures/Tests

1. Name and complete address of Genetic Clinic/Ultrasound Clinic/Imaging Centre: _____
2. Registration No. (Under PCPNDT Act, 1994) _____
3. Patient's name _____ Age _____
4. Total number of living children: _____
    a. Number of living sons with age of each living son (in years or months): _____
    b. Number of living daughters with age of each living daughter (in years or months): _____
5. Husband's/Wife's/Father's/Mother's Name: _____
6. Full postal address of the patient with contact number, if any: _____

7. a. Referred by (full name and address of Doctor(s)/Genetic Counseling Centre): _____

    (Referral slips to be preserved carefully with Form F)
    b. Self-referral by Gynaecologist/Radiologist/Registered Medical Practitioner conducting the diagnostic procedures: _____

(Referral note with indications and case papers of the patient to be preserved with Form F) (Self-referral does not mean a client coming to a clinic and requesting for the test or the relative/s requesting for the test of a pregnant woman)

8. Last menstrual period or weeks of pregnancy: _____

Section B: To be filled in for performing non-invasive diagnostic procedures/tests only

9. Name of the doctor performing the procedure/s: _____
10. Indication/s for diagnosis procedure: _____
    (specify with reference to the request made in the referral slip or in a self-referral note) Ultrasonography prenatal diagnosis during pregnancy should only be performed when indicated. The following is the representative list of indications for ultrasound during pregnancy. (Put a "Tick" against the appropriate indication/s for ultrasound).
    i. To diagnose intrauterine and/or ectopic pregnancy and confirm viability.
    ii. Estimation of gestational age (dating).
    iii. Detection of number of fetuses and their chorionicity.
    iv. Suspected pregnancy with IUCD *in situ* or suspected pregnancy following contraceptive failure/MTP failure.
    v. Vaginal bleeding/leaking.
    vi. Follow-up of cases of abortion.
    vii. Assessment of cervical canal and diameter of internal os.
    viii. Discrepancy between uterine size and period of amenorrhea.
    ix. Any suspected adnexal or uterine pathology/abnormality.
    x. Detection of chromosomal abnormalities, fetal structural defects and other abnormalities and their follow-up.
    xi. To evaluate fetal presentation and position.
    xii. Assessment of liquor amnii.
    xiii. Preterm labor/preterm premature rupture of membranes.
    xiv. Evaluation of placental position, thickness, grading and abnormalities (placenta praevia, retroplacental hemorrhage, abnormal adherence, etc.).
    xv. Evaluation of umbilical cord—presentation, insertion, nuchal encirclement, number of vessels and presence of true knot.
    xvi. Evaluation of previous caesarean section scars.
    xvii. Evaluation of fetal growth parameters, fetal weight and fetal well-being.
    xviii. Color flow mapping and duplex Doppler studies.
    xix. Ultrasound-guided procedures such as medical termination of pregnancy, external cephalic version, etc. and their follow-up.
    xx. Adjunct to diagnostic and therapeutic invasive interventions such as chorionic villus sampling (CVS), amniocenteses, fetal blood sampling, fetal skin biopsy, amnio-infusion, intrauterine infusion, placement of shunts, etc.
    xxi. Observation of intrapartum events.
    xxii. Medical/surgical conditions complicating pregnancy.
    xxiii. Research/scientific studies in recognized institutions.

11. Procedures carried out (non-invasive) (put a "Tick" on the appropriate procedure)
    i. Ultrasound (important note: Ultrasound is not indicated/advised/performed to determine the sex of fetus except for diagnosis of sex-linked diseases such as Duchenne muscular dystrophy, hemophilia A, B, etc.)
    ii. Any other (specify): _____
12. Date on which declaration of the pregnant woman/person was obtained: _____
13. Date on which procedures carried out: _____
14. Result of the non-invasive procedure carried out (report in brief of the test including ultrasound carried out): _____
15. The result of prenatal diagnostic procedures was conveyed to _____ on_____
16. Any indication for MTP as per the abnormality detected in the diagnostic procedures/tests: _____

Date:
Place:
         Name, Signature and Registration Number with Seal of the Gynaecologist/
Radiologist/Registered Medical Practitioner Place: Performing diagnostic procedure/s

Section C: To be filled for performing invasive procedures/tests only
17. Name of the doctor/s performing the procedure/s: _____
18. History of genetic/medical disease in the family (specify): _____
    Basis of diagnosis ("Tick" on appropriate basis of diagnosis):
    a. Clinical
    b. Bio-chemical
    c. Cytogenetic
    d. Others (e.g. radiological, ultrasonography, etc. specify)
19. Indication/s for the diagnosis procedure ("Tick" on appropriate indication/s):
    A. Previous child/children with:
        i. Chromosomal disorders
        ii. Metabolic disorders
        iii. Congenital anomaly
        iv. Mental disability
        v. Haemoglobinopathy
        vi. Sex-linked disorders
        vii. Single gene disorder
        viii. Any other (specify)
    B. Advanced maternal age (35 years)
    C. Mother/father/sibling has genetic disease (specify)
    D. Other (specify): _____
20. Date on which consent of the pregnant woman/person was obtained in Form G prescribed in PCPNDT Act, 1994: _____

21. Invasive procedures carried out ("Tick" on appropriate indication/s)
    i. Amniocentesis
    ii. Chorionic villi aspiration
    iii. Fetal biopsy
    iv. Cordocentesis
    v. Any other (specify)
22. Any complication/s of invasive procedure (specify): _____
_____
23. Additional tests recommended (please mention if applicable)
    i. Chromosomal studies
    ii. Biochemical studies
    iii. Molecular studies
    iv. Pre-implantation gender diagnosis
    v. Any other (specify)
24. Result of the procedures/tests carried out (report in brief of the invasive tests/procedures carried out): _____
25. Date on which procedures carried out: _____
26. The result of prenatal diagnostic procedures was conveyed to _____ on _____
27. Any indication for MTP as per the abnormality detected in the diagnostic procedures/tests: _____

Date:
Place
        Name, Signature and Registration Number with Seal of the Gynaecologist/Radiologist/Registered Medical Practitioner performing Diagnostic Procedure/s

Section D: Declaration

DECLARATION OF THE PERSON UNDERGOING PRENATAL DIAGNOSTIC TEST/PROCEDURE

I, Mrs/Mr _____ declare that by undergoing _____ Prenatal Diagnostic Test/Procedure. I do not want to know the sex of my foetus.

Date: Signature/thumb impression of the person undergoing the Prenatal Diagnostic Test/Procedure
In case of thumb impression:
Identified by (Name) _____ Age: _____ Sex: _____
Relation (if any): _____ Address and Contact No.: _____
_____
Signature of a person attesting thumb impression: _____
Date: _____

DECLARATION OF DOCTOR/PERSON CONDUCTING PRENATAL DIAGNOSTIC PROCEDURE/TEST

I, _____ (name of the person conducting ultrasonography/image scanning) declare that while conducting ultrasonography/image scanning on Ms/Mr _____ _____ (name of the pregnant woman or the person undergoing pre-natal diagnostic procedure/test), I have neither detected nor disclosed the sex of her fetus to anybody in any manner.

Signature: _____

Date: _____

Name in Capitals, Registration Number with Seal of the Gynaecologist/ Radiologist/Registered Medical Practitioner conducting diagnostic procedure

Registration and Qualification Requirements for Places and Professionals

Genetic counseling centre (GCC): An institute, hospital, nursing home, or any other place by whatever name called which provides genetic counseling to patients. A genetic counseling centre should be under a medical geneticist or a gynecologist/pediatrician having 6 months experience or 4 weeks training in genetic counseling.

Genetic clinic (GC): Any clinic, institute, hospital, nursing home, or any other place by whatever name called which is used for conducting pre-natal diagnostic procedures. Genetic clinic will also include each and every mobile genetic clinic. For a genetic clinic, the gynecologist should have adequate experience in prenatal diagnostic procedures, i.e. should have performed at least 20 procedures in chorionic villi aspirations per vagina or per abdomen, chorionic villi biopsy, amniocentesis, cordocentesis, fetoscopy, fetal skin or organ biopsy or fetal blood sampling, etc. under supervision of an experienced gynecologist in these fields. A registered medical practitioner (who possesses any recognized medical qualification as defined in the Indian Medical Council Act, 1956 and whose name has been entered in a State Medical Register) practicing in a genetic clinic should have a postgraduate degree or diploma or six months training duly imparted in the manner prescribed in the "PCPNDT (Prohibition of sex selection), (six months training Rules) 2014" or one year experience in sonography or image scanning or a medical geneticist.

Genetic laboratory (GL): Any laboratory and includes a place where facilities are provided for conducting analysis or tests of samples received from genetic clinic for pre-natal diagnostic test.

Qualification and Training in Ultrasonography for MBBS Doctors (www.med-edu.in)

1. "Principle rules" means the Pre-conception and Pre-natal Diagnostic Techniques (Prohibition of Sex Selection) Rules, 1996.
2. "Six months training" means the training imparted under these rules.

3. Nomenclature of the six months training in ultrasonography. The six months training imparted under these rules shall be known as "the Fundamentals in abdominopelvic ultrasonography: Level one for MBBS Doctors".
4. Period of the training. The period of training for obtaining a certificate of training shall be 300 clock hours.
5. Components of the six months training curriculum.
   1. The major components of the training curriculum shall be:
      a. Theory based knowledge to equip registered medical practitioners with the knowledge, professional skills, attitudes and clinical competencies;
      b. Skill-based knowledge; and
      c. Log book and assessment.
   2. The comprehensive syllabus for the said six months training is as specified in Schedule I.
   3. The details related to log book and assessment are as specified in Schedule II.
6. Eligibility for training: Any registered medical practitioner shall be eligible for undertaking the said six months training. Registered medical practitioners who are already registered for conducting ultrasonography in a genetic clinic or ultrasound clinic or imaging centre on the basis of one year experience or six months training are required to clear a competency based evaluation for the purpose of renewal of registration.
7. Fee structure for the training:
   a. The training fee for conducting the six months training shall not exceed ₹20,000/-
   b. For registered medical practitioners who are already registered for conducting ultra sonography in a genetic clinic or ultrasound clinic or imaging centre and require to clear a competency based evaluation, the fee shall not exceed ₹10,000/-.
   c. Fee structure or waiver thereof for in service registered medical practitioners shall be decided by the respective centers.
8. Competency based evaluation shall be held as per Schedule II after six months training is completed.
9. Validity of the training certificate: Certification of training obtained from any state shall be applicable for the purposes of registration under Act in all states.
   (Prohibition of Sex Selection) Act and Rules, a Handbook of Pre-conception and Prenatal Diagnostic Techniques Act and Rules with Amendments published by Ministry of Health, Government of India has made available (please refer the website for details www.pndt.nic.in)

Requirements of Record-keeping by GCC, GC and GL

Under Section 9 of the PCPNDT Rules, 1996, every GCC, GL, GC shall send a complete report in respect of all pre-conception or pregnancy related procedures/techniques/tests conducted by them in respect of each month by 5th day of the following month to the concerned appropriate authority and keep the record of Form F with them for two years. It is pertinent to mention that every sonologist is required to fill Form F before conducting an ultrasound on a pregnant mother. The form has 19 questions including the reason for conducting the sonography, along with patient details.

As per the Act, the following records are to be maintained by any GCC, GC or GL, under the Act

- Form D, i.e. the form regarding maintenance of records by GCC Form E, i.e. the form for maintenance of records by GL
- Form F, i.e. the form for maintenance of record in respect of the pregnant woman by GL/ultrasound clinic/imaging centre, including declaration of the pregnant woman and doctors
- Form G, i.e. the form of consent for invasive techniques

Checklist for Registration of a Genetic Clinic, Counseling Centre, USG Centre, Imaging Centre

1. Application—Form A (two copies)
2. Affidavit containing undertakings from owners that they shall not conduct any test or procedure for selection of sex before or after conception and they will not disclose the sex of the fetus to anybody. They shall prominently display a notice saying they do not conduct such tests[4]
3. Particulars about fee paid ₹25000 for any one type of service, ₹35000 for a combination thereof (by demand draft in favor of AA)[5]
4. Site plan of place
5. If a society/trust: Registration certificate from Competent Authority and a copy of Rules and Regulations/Board Resolution.
6. Quotation/proforma invoice for sonography machine from authorized dealer/manufacturer (if relevant) with company PNDT Certificate.
7. Certified photostat copy/copies of educational qualifications and MMC registration of the person operating the machine (wherever applicable)
8. Certified photostat copy/copies of training/experience certificate of the person operating the machine (wherever applicable)
9. In case of a nursing home, registration under the Nursing Home Act
10. Any other additional documents/papers as considered necessary by appropriate authorities[6]

What should the Scan Centers do under the Act?

Display

Registration certificate, PNDT board and pamphlets

Records

Mandatory records for GCC, GL, USG clinic and imaging center
1. Register showing in serial order
    - Name and Addresses of men or women given genetic counseling and/or subjected to prenatal diagnostic procedure or test.
    - Names of their spouses or fathers; and
    - Date on which they first reported for such counseling.
2. GCC—maintenance of record as per Form D.

3. GL—maintenance of records as per Form E.
4. GC—maintenance of record as per Form F

Form D/E/F under the Rules

The scan centre shall send consolidated report statutorily by 5th for the previous month to the AA or any officer so authorized.

Other Kinds of Records

- Case records
- Forms of consent
- Laboratory results
- Microscopic pictures
- Sonographic plates or slides
- Recommendations and letters.

The referrals notes of the doctor recommending scan and a declaration from the pregnant mother regarding her non-interest in knowing the sex of the fetus is a must for every case.

For how long do the records have to be maintained?

All records should be maintained for at least two years[7] after any prenatal diagnostic technique has been performed on a pregnant woman. However, if there is any legal proceeding pending in the Court of Law, then these records should not be destroyed till the proceedings have been disposed off.[8] In case the records are maintained on a computer or any other electronic equipment, a printed copy of the record is to be taken and preserved after authentication by the person responsible for such a record.[9] Records at all reasonable times are to be made available for inspection to the AA or a person authorized by the AA.[10]

Punishments for the Offences

An offence under this law is

Cognizable: A police officer may arrest the offender without warrant,

Non-bailable: Getting bail is not the right of the accused. The courts have discretion to grant bail.

Non-compoundable: Parties to the case cannot settle the case out of court and decide not to prosecute (Sec 27).

The punishments for offences involving sex selection or sex determination and non-maintenance of records (violation of Sections 5 and 6 of Act) are:

- Imprisonment of up to 3 years (5 years in case of subsequent offence) and fine of ₹10,000 ('fifty thousand in case of subsequent offence). However, this does not apply to any woman who was compelled by anyone to undergo such diagnostic techniques or such selection.
- Name of the registered medical practitioner shall be reported by the appropriate authority to the State Medical Council concerned for taking necessary action including suspension of the registration if the charges are framed by the Court and till the case is disposed of, and

on conviction, for removal of his name from the register of the Council for a period of five years for the first offence, and permanently for the subsequent offence.
- If any person seeks aid for sex selection or for conducting prenatal diagnostic technique on any pregnant other than those specified in Subsection (2) of Section 4, he shall be punishable with imprisonment up to three years and with fine up to fifty thousand rupees for the first offence and for any subsequent offence with imprisonment up to five years and with fine up to one lakh rupees.

For registration related offences, the appropriate authority (AA) may:
- Suspend or cancel the registration, as per the magnitude of the violation.
- During the period of suspension of registration, the equipment will be sealed and signed and kept with the owner.
- After cancellation of the registration, the equipment has to be sealed and seized.

For non-registration, 5 times the registration fee may be charged as penalty and an undertaking shall have to be furnished as per the PNDT Rules.

For violation of Section 22 of PNDT Act 1994[12] (any advertisement related offences) the prescribed punishment is imprisonment which may extend to 3 years; and fine which may extend to ₹10,000. For other offences, the prescribed punishment is: Imprisonment which may extend to 3 months or with fine which may extend to ₹1,000 for first offence and additional fine up to ₹500 per day may be levied for the period of contravention for subsequent offence.

If a company violates the PCPNDT Act, then the person in charge of the organization is liable for punishment.

CONCLUSION

Along with the enforcement of law, what is needed is a mindset change. Each one of us counts. Each one of us has a role to play—as parents, siblings, family members and friends. And as professionals, whether teachers, doctors, lawyers, judges, administrators, law enforcement personnel, elected representatives, journalists, writers, artists . . .

REFERENCES

1. Centre for Youth and Development Activities. Reflections against the campaign under sex selection and exploring ways forward, 2007.
2. Census 2001, Office of the Registrar General and Census Commissioner, Ministry of Home Affairs, India, 2001.
3. Rule 10(1A)
4. Rule 4
5. Rule
6. Requirements for Form A and supporting documents see Rules 4(1) and 8(1)
7. Sec 29(1)
8. Provision to Sec 29 (1) to be read with Rule 9(6)
9. Rule 9(7)
10. Section 29(2)
11. www.pndt.nic.in.
12. Section 22
13. www.med-edu.in

Chapter 5

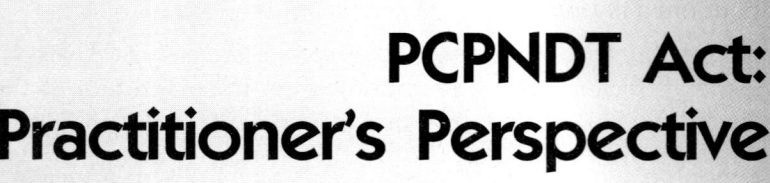

PCPNDT Act: Practitioner's Perspective

○ Atul Ganatra

The Prenatal Diagnostic Techniques Act of 1994 and its subsequent amendment in 2003 as the Pre-conception and Prenatal Diagnostic Techniques (prohibition of sex selection) Act (PCPNDT Act) was brought into force to stop female feticide.

As members of the gynaecological fraternity and as responsible citizens and members of society, it is our duty to not indulge in unethical and unlawful practices. We, as gynaecologists, have to prove a point here, not only to the society but also to the authorities that USG is used not only a diagnostic tool but also as a life-saving investigation in many cases.

It has been observed that many of our colleagues are not well-versed with the PCPNDT Act, which can get them into unnecessary trouble with the authorities. We do not intend to print the whole Act but just to present the basic requirements in a simplified manner. In the first part of this series, we have made a list of do's and don'ts, which will make it easier for our members to follow the legal PCPNDT Act.

- Understanding the social aspect
- Understanding the PCPNDT Act
- Record keeping is must
- No harm in a few formalities like Form F and monthly report.
- All of us have to obey the law of land
- Pledge to eradicate the menace of female feticide from our society
- Try to get the actual culprits behind the bars

Do's

- Registration of the clinic is mandatory. Only one registration per clinic is required (even if there is more than one machine). Details of all machines and all gynaecologists (along with copies of their certificates) should be submitted.

- Portability of sonography machine not allowed.
- Copy of the registration certificate must be displayed—one near the USG machine and another in the waiting room.
- Signage, in English and in the local language, must be displayed, indicating that fetal sex is not disclosed in the clinic.
- Ensure that the number of machines and the gynaecologists attached to the clinic have been mentioned in the registration certificate or on a separate sheet by the appropriate authorities (AA).
- Form F must be filled in completely and without any delay as soon as the patient's USG is done. The signed consent of the patient as well as the gynaecologist's signature are a must. Form G is only for invasive procedures.
- A monthly report should be submitted to the AA regularly, before the 5th of every month. A copy of the same, with the signature of the AA acknowledging receipt, must be preserved
- All copies of Form F and monthly reports should be preserved for 2 years. The referral letters from doctors should also be preserved.
- PCPNDT Act booklet must be available in the waiting room.
- The AA must be informed, in writing, about changes in any machine or radiologist. A copy of the same, with the signature of the AA, should be preserved.
- If a locum radiologist is appointed, the AA must be informed in advance (with the details of the locum radiologist's registration and Medical Council registration certificate).
- Be cooperative if and when the AA visits your clinic to examine the records.

Don'ts
- Do not disclose the sex of the child to anyone—under any pressure or in any circumstances.
- Do not start a USG clinic without PCPNDT registration.
- Do not visit any clinic or hospital for USG unless it is registered for PCPNDT, even if it is for non-obstetric reasons (exception can be made when it is for a very urgent/life-threatening case, but this has to be proved by documentation).
- Registration certificates are non-transferable. Do not give your degree certificate to anyone or any place unless you are visiting it regularly.
- Do not give an experience certificate to anyone.
- Do not get scared by anyone if you are following all the rules as per the PCPNDT law.
- Do not allow anyone to check your records unless the person is accompanied by the AA or legally authorized by AA.
- Do not hesitate to ask for an ID before allowing any person to search your records.
- NGOs on their own can neither instruct you nor can they check your records.

GREY AREAS
Copy of Form F to be given to patients: Who can answer—two versions.
- Preserving of films.
- Preserving of reports.

AREAS OF CONCERN

- Lack of proper knowledge on the part of appropriate authority (AA).
- Non-uniform implementation of the Act as per the understanding of AAs.
- Making of laws by AAs—Maharashtra, Gujarat.
- No time/intention mainly in case of registrations
- New/renewals—advance notice never given by AAs as per CSB minutes.
- Adamant AAs.
- No proper co-ordination between Center/State/District.
- Nobody cares/listens at Government level.

REGISTRATION

What is Registered?

- Centre/USG machine/Sonologist/Place, etc.
- The answer is that it is the place (clinic or center or hospital or nursing home) where ultrasound is performed.
- No separate registration is required for a number of machines at the same place.

Procedure of Registration

- Application in duplicate (Form 'A') to the CMO of District or any other Medical Officer constituted as an appropriate authority.
- Every application should be accompanied by an affidavit containing an undertaking that the Clinic/Centre shall not conduct a test or procedure for selection or detection of sex of the fetus.
- Undertaking that you will prominently display a notice for the same.
- ₹ 25,000, for ultrasound clinic/imaging centre; ₹ 35,000/- for any combination of genetic lab/clinic

Procedure of Certification

- Application will be scrutinized by appropriate authority regarding fulfillment of requirements under the Act.
- Enquiry by the AA includes an inspection of the premises after giving due notice to applicant
- After AA is satisfied, the application will be placed before the Advisory Committee which then shall scrutinize the application and advise the AA.
- AA after considering the advice will grant certificate of registration in duplicate.
- It is mandatory to display the certificate of registration
- Certificate is non-transferable

Rejection of Application for Registration

- If after enquiry and after giving an opportunity of hearing to the applicant and after taking advise from the Advisory Committee, the Appropriate Authority has come to a conclusion

that the applicant has not complied with the requirements of the Act, then the said application will be rejected.
- The reasons for the rejection shall be given in writing and as specified in Form C appended to the Rules under PNDT Act.
- The rejection of registration shall be communicated to the applicant within 90 days from the date of the receipt of the registration.

Cancellation or Suspension of Registration

- Appropriate authority can at any time either on its own or on a complaint by anyone can issue a show cause notice to the genetic counselling centre, genetic laboratory or genetic clinic, ultrasound clinic or imaging centre as to why its registration should not be cancelled or suspended for breach of any of the provisions of the PNDT Act or the Rules. The reasons for every such notice should be mentioned in the notice itself.
- Thereafter the clinic, laboratory or center must be given an opportunity to defend itself against the charges. After giving the center, laboratory or clinic a reasonable opportunity of being heard and after taking into account the advice given by the Advisory Committee, the appropriate authority may either suspend the registration of such a place or cancel the registration depending upon the gravity of the charge.
- Action can be taken by the Appropriate Authority irrespective of any criminal action that will be taken against such a place.
- In certain exceptional cases like in the case of public interest, the appropriate authority may suspend or cancel registration without issuing a show cause notice. However, the reasons for waiving show cause notice have to be given in written.

Provision of Appeal

- Any *genetic counselling center, genetic laboratory* or *genetic clinic* may appeal against an order of cancellation or suspension of registration within 30 days of the order of cancellation or suspension. The appeal may be made to:
  1. The appropriate authority at the district level if the order is passed by the appropriate authority at sub-district level.
  2. The appropriate authority at the State/UT level if the order is passed by the appropriate authority at district level.
- Each appeal shall be disposed of by the district appropriate authority or by the state/UT appropriate authority, as the case may be, within 60 days of its receipt. The appeal shall be made to the central government if the order is passed by the central appropriate authority.
- The appeal shall be made to the state government if the order is passed by the state appropriate authority.

Renewal of Registration

- Every certificate of registration shall be valid for a period of five years since its issuance.
- Thirty days before the date of expiry of the certificate of registration, a fresh application for a certificate of registration should be made.

- The application for renewal must be made in duplicate in the prescribed Form A (same as the one prescribed for obtaining the first registration certificate) to the appropriate authority.
- The appropriate authority shall acknowledge the receipt of the application in the acknowledgement slip provided at the bottom of Form A on the very same day if personally delivered, otherwise on the next day by post.
- Along with the application for renewal of certificate, registration fees of half of what was initially payable will be paid depending upon whether it is for a *genetic counselling center, genetic laboratory* or *genetic clinic*, ultrasound clinic or imaging center or for a joint facility.
- After the receipt of the application, the appropriate authority will hold an enquiry including an inspection of the premises after giving due notice into whether the applicant has fulfilled all the requirements necessary under the Act. The appropriate authority will also give the applicant a hearing.
- After conducting the enquiry and hearing, if the appropriate authority finds everything satisfactory, then it will place the application before the Advisory Committee for its scrutiny.
- Thereafter having regard to the advice of the Advisory Committee, the appropriate authority will renew the certificate of registration in the prescribed Form B (same as the one prescribed for the first registration certificate) for a further period of 5 years starting from the date of expiry of the old certificate.
- On the receipt of the renewed certificate of registration in duplicate, the two copies of the earlier certificates will have to be surrendered immediately to the appropriate authority.
- One copy of the renewed certificate has to be displayed in a conspicuous place of the center, laboratory or clinic.
- If the appropriate authority fails to renew the certificate of registration within 90 days of its receiving the application for renewal, it will amount to automatic renewal or deemed renewal.

Rejection of Application of Renewal
- After conducting an enquiry into the application for renewal, after hearing the applicant and after taking the advice of the Advisory Committee, if the appropriate authority finds that the applicant has not complied with the requirements of the Act, then, the appropriate authority can reject the application for renewal.
- Every order of rejection will contain reasons for rejection and it will be communicated in the prescribed Form C49 (same as the one prescribed for the initial rejection).
- Once the applicant receives the communication of rejection, the applicant must immediately surrender both the copies of the earlier certificate of registration.
- In case the appropriate authority fails to communicate its rejection to the applicant within 90 days of receiving the application for renewal, then it amounts to automatic renewal or deemed renewal.

FORM A
[See Rule 4(1) and 8(1)]
(To be submitted in duplicate with supporting documents as enclosures)
Form application for registration for renewal of registration of a genetic counselling centre/ genetic laboratory/genetic clinic/ultrasound clinic/imaging centre

ACKNOWLEDGEMENT
[See Rule 4(2) and 8(1)]

The application in Form A in duplicate for grant*/renewal* of registration of Genetic Counselling Centre/Genetic Laboratory/Genetic Clinic/Ultrasound Clinic/Imaging Centre by .... (Name and address of applicant) has been received by the appropriate authority .... on (date).

*The list of enclosures attached to the application in Form A has been verified with the enclosure submitted and found to be correct or
*On verification it is found that the following documents mentioned in the list of enclosures are not actually enclosed.

ORIGINAL/DUPLICATE FOR DISPLAY

FORM B
[See Rule 6(2), 6(5) and 8(2)]
Certificate of Registration (To be issued in duplicate)

FORM C
[See Rule 6(3), 6(5) and 8(3)]
Form for Rejection of Application for Grant/Renewal of Registration

FORM D
[See Rule 9(2)]
Form for Maintanance of Records by the Genetic Counselling Centre

FORM E
[See Rule 9(3)]
Form for Maintenance of Records by Genetic Laboratory

FORM H
[See Rule 9(5)]
Form for maintenance of permanent record of applications for grant/rejection of registration under the Prenatal Diagnostic Techniques (regulation and prevention of misuse) Act, 1994.

FORM F (refer to Chapter 4)

See Provision to Section 4(3), Rule 9(4) and Rule 10(1A)

Form for Maintenance of Record in Respect of the Pregnant Woman
By
Genetic Clinic/Ultrasound Clinic/Imaging Centre

FORM G

(See Rule 10)

Form of Consent

(For invasive techniques)

I .... wife/daughter of .... Age .... years residing at .... hereby state that I have been explained fully the probable side effects and after effects of the prenatal diagnostic procedures wish to undergo the pre-implantation/prenatal diagnostic technique/test/procedures in my own interest to find out the possibility of any abnormality (i.e. disease/deformity/disorder) in the child I am carrying.

I undertake not to terminate the pregnancy if the prenatal procedure/technique/test conducted show the absence of disease/deformity/disorder.

I understand that the sex of the fetus will not be disclosed to me.

I understand that breach of this undertaking will make me liable to penalty as prescribed in the prenatal Diagnostic Technique (Regulation and Prevention of Misuse) Act, 1994 (57 of 1994) and Rules framed Thereunder.

Date: _____

Signature of the pregnant woman

I have explained the contents of the above to the patient and her companion (Name ....

.... Address

.... Relationship .... in a language she/they understand

Name, Signature and Registration number of Gynaecologist

Date: .... Medical Geneticist Radiologist/Paediatrician/Director of the Clinic/Centre/Laboratory

Name of the Ultrasound Clinic/Imaging Centre   **Reg.No:**

Complete report in respect of pre-conception or pregnancy related procedures/techniques/tests

S.No	Date	Name of patient Husband/father	Age	Reg.No	Address	Ref. by	Length of preg.	Indication	No. of children with sex	Nature of proc.	Particulars of doctor	Report	Was MTP adv.

Source: www.ncpcr.gov.in PCPNDT Act 1994

Chapter 6

An Update on POCSO Act and Challenges in Relation to MTP Act

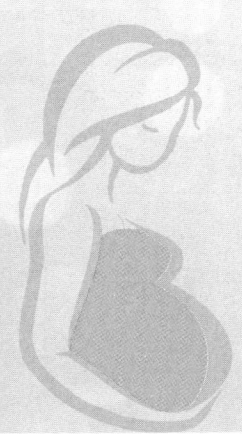

○ Ashok Shukla

The Protection of Children from Sexual Offences Act, 2012, is an enactment to provide for protection of children (any person below eighteen years of age) from the offences of sexual assault, sexual harassment and pornography with due regard for safeguarding the interest and well-being of the child at every stage of the judicial process. It also incorporates child-friendly procedures for reporting, recording of evidence, investigation and trial of offences and provision for establishment of Special Courts for speedy trial of such offences to help the survivor speedy justice.

World Health Organization estimates that globally some 40 million children aged 0–14 years suffer from some form of abuse and neglect requiring health and social care.

The Act defines a child as any person below eighteen years of age, and regards the best interests and welfare of the child as matter of paramount importance at every stage, to ensure the healthy physical, emotional, intellectual and social development of the child. The Act is gender neutral. In POCSO Act, the term sexual assault is used instead of rape. If grave harm is caused to the victim or if the offence is committed by a person in authority, the offence is termed "aggravated" offence.

How to Assess Age of a Child Victim/Survivor?
- Age of victim has to be determined in the same manner as is being done in respect of a person who is accused of an offence;
- Age has to be determined in terms of Section 94 of Juvenile Justice Act;
- The Court has first to look for the available certificates;

- The Court has to rely on first preference certificate irrespective of availability of other certificate;
- The Court cannot doubt the first preference certificate on the ground that other certificates are showing some different age;
- Medical opinion can be sought for only if all priority certificates are found to be not available;
- Medical opinion does not provide the exact age;
- Sufficient margin (say two years) on either side has to be given in respect of medical opinion;
- Range of age in medical opinion upon margin being given will leave room for doubts;
- Benefit of doubt has to go in favour of the accused and therefore, the upper age of medical opinion has to be accepted by the court in respect of age of victim.

Salient Features of POCSO 2012

Section	Provision
S.3	**Penetrative Sexual Assault:** Insertion, penetration, manipulation with the penis, any body part, or any object into the vagina, mouth, urethra or anus of a child.
S.5	**Aggravated Penetrative Sexual Assault:** 'Person in authority' and/or if additional harm and injury is committed.
S.7	**Sexual Assault:** Touching a child with sexual intent (non-penetrative) (touching vagina, penis, anus, breast or any body part of a child).
S.9	**Aggravated Sexual Assault:** 'Person in authority' and/or if additional harm and injury is committed.
S.11	**Sexual Harassment:** Word, sound, gesture, exhibiting any body part, showing pornography with sexual intent. Making a child exhibit any body part, stalking the child, threatening the use of pornographic media
S.13 and S.15	**Pornography:** Use of a child for pornographic purposes. Storing pornographic media of a child for commercial use.
S.19–21	**Mandatory Reporting:** S.19 (1) any person who has knowledge of sexual offence committed or likely to be committed on a child S.20 management and staff of media, hotels, lodges, hospitals, clubs, studios and photographic facilities S.21 Failure to report or record is punishable S.21 (3) However, a child who fails to report not punished.

All offences under the POCSO Act are considered as grave offences. Hence they are non-bailable and cognisable and the trial is to be conducted by the Court of Sessions.

Punishment for Offences for Using Child for Pornographic Purposes

Offence	POCSO Act, 2012	2019 Bill
Use of child for pornographic purposes	Maximum: 5 years	Minimum: 5 years
Use of child for pornographic purposes resulting in penetrative sexual assault	Minimum: 10 years	Minimum: 10 years (in case of child below 16 years: 20 years)
	Maximum: Life imprisonment	Maximum: Life imprisonment
Use of child for pornographic purposes resulting in aggravated penetrative sexual assault	Life imprisonment	Minimum: 20 years Maximum: Life imprisonment, or death.
Use of child for pornographic purposes resulting in sexual assault	Minimum: Six years Maximum: Eight years	Minimum: Three years Maximum: Five years
Use of child for pornographic purposes resulting in aggravated sexual assault	Minimum: Eight years Maximum: 10 years	Minimum: Five years Maximum: Seven years

The Protection of Children from Sexual Offences (Amendment) Bill, 2019 was introduced in Rajya Sabha by the Minister of Women and Child Development, Ms. Smriti Zubin Irani, on July 18, 2019. The Bill amends the Protection of Children from Sexual Offences Act, 2012. It was passed in Lok Sabha on 1st August 2019.

The amendments were aimed at establishing clarity regarding the aspects of child abuse and punishment thereof, hence amendments in Sections 2, 4, 5, 6, 9, 14, 15, 34, 42 and 45 of the POCSO Act 2012 were made.

Sections 4, 5 and 6 was amended to provide option of stringent punishment, including death penalty, for committing sexual assault and aggravated penetrative sexual assault crime on a child to protect the children from sexual abuse.

Sections 14 and 15 of the POCSO Act 2012 was to address the menace of child pornography. It was proposed to levy fine for not destroying or deleting or reporting the pornographic material involving a child with an intention to share or transmit it.

Role of Attending Physician under POCSO Act

1. It is mandatory for attending physician to provide such information to the Special Juvenile Police Unit (SJPU) or to the local police as the case may be under Section 20 and failure to report shall be punished with imprisonment of either description which may extend to six months or with fine or with both under Section 21.
2. Medical examination of a child (Section 27): The medical examination of the child in respect of whom any offence has been committed shall be conducted in accordance with [Section 164A] of Code of Criminal Procedure, 1973 (2 of 1974) not waiting for FIR or complaint to be registered. In case the victim is a girl child, the medical examination shall be conducted by a woman doctor in presence of the parent of the child or any other person whom the

child reposes trust or confidence or in absence of any relative then examination should be conducted in presence of woman nominated by the head of the medical institution.
3. Emergency Medical Care Rule 5, POCSO Rules 2012: Emergency medical care shall be rendered in such a manner as to protect the privacy of the child, and in presence of the parent or guardian or any other person in whom the child has trust and confidence without demanding any legal or magisterial requisition or other documentation as a pre-requisite to rendering such care. The registered medical practitioner rendering emergency medical care shall provide treatment to all injuries, treatment for exposure to STD including prophylaxis, treatment for exposure to HIV including prophylaxis for HIV, possible pregnancy and emergency contraception as well as if need arises, then psychological consultation can be referred for.

CHALLENGES OF POCSO ACT IN RELATION TO MTP ACT

The Medical Termination of Pregnancy (MTP) Act 1971—a law that was considered ahead of its times—legalized abortion in India up to 20 weeks of pregnancy, based on certain conditions and when provided by a registered medical practitioner at a registered medical facility.

The main intention of the Act was easy access for safe legal abortion.

The Medical Termination of Pregnancy Regulations, 1975 state that the admission register of MTP shall be a secret document and the information contained therein as to the name and other particulars of the pregnant woman shall not be disclosed to any person. The consent forms would be kept in separate envelope with marking as SECRET on the envelope.

The POCSO Act requires medical providers to report any case of underage pregnancy (below 18 years of age) as a case of sexual assault/abuse. In accordance with International Child Protection Standards, the Act provides for mandatory reporting of sexual offences and it casts legal duty upon any person who has knowledge or a suspicion that a child has been sexually abused. POCSO unfortunately criminalises consensual adolescent sexual activity. Minor girl under POCSO Act is considered unable to give consent for sexual intercourse hence irrespective of marital status mandatory reporting has to be done by medical provider to the local police authority. Madras High Court has suggested amendments to POCSO Act over consensual sex after 16 years of age.

MTP Act Section 8 guarantees protection for providers who act in good faith. In less than 18 years pregnant patient, it becomes the legal duty for the medical providers to follow all legal requirements under both MTP and the POCSO Act.

ISSUES TO BE KEPT IN MIND DURING TERMINATION OF PREGNANY IN A CHILD (<18 YEARS)

1. Mandatory reporting to the local police or special juvenile police unit or child protection committee.
2. POCSO Act only mentions reporting and not investigating by the medical provider or lodging FIR. So the medical provider can go ahead with the treatment and does not require to wait for the authorities to take action and may proceed with the termination of the pregnancy in line with the provisions of the MTP Act after maintaining the detailed case records.

3. Consent for termination: As here the child being a minor, consent becomes invalid and hence guardian's consent would be required for MTP. The MTP Act defines Guardian as a person having the care of the minor person. This means any adult (above age of 18 years) who has the care of the minor girl could be *de facto* guardian and could consent to an abortion on her behalf.
4. Rape is a legal ground for terminating a pregnancy under Section 3 of the MTP Act and the limit in the Act is up to 20 weeks. It is important to provide medical care at the earliest and on the other side legal proceedings can continue.
5. Products of conception: MTP Act Section 8 guarantees protection for providers who act in good faith so providers who dispose of the products of conception due to inadequate facilities, etc. should be protected from prosecution. Since pregnancy in a minor girl is termed rape, therefore under Section 201, the products of conception might be the evidence of the offence.

CONCLUSION

Some more amendments would be required in both MTP Act regarding the duration of pregnancy as many times pregnancy is detected late; and in POCSO Act where the age of consent for sexual activity is 18 years causing many young women above 16 years of age in consensual sexual relationship getting diverted to quacks for termination of pregnancy endangering their life and obstructing the easy access to safe abortion what she had before POCSO Act. But till the government considers these factors and make appropriate amendments, all medical service providers have to fulfil all the requirements and legal obligations of both MTP Act and POCSO Act.

BIBLIOGRAPHY

1. Age Determination of a Victim By: Rakesh Kumar Singh Latestlaws.com
2. Increasing Access to Comprehensive Abortion Care: An Initiative of Federation of Obstetric and Gynecological Societies of India & Global Health Strategies, Dr. Mandakini Megh and Dr. Atul Ganatra.
3. Ipas Development Foundation (IDF) in close collaboration with CHLET—Centre of Health Law, Ethics, and Technology Jindal Global Law School 2017, Authors: MS Kerry, MC Broom, MS Dipika Jain and MS Medha Gandhi.
4. Legal Provisions Concerning Sexual Violence against Women and Children in India Special Service and Features (27 January, 2015 15:35 IST) Press Information Bureau, Government of India.
5. Regional Committee for Africa, 54 (2011). Child sexual abuse: a silent health emergency: Report of the Regional Director.
6. The Medical termination of Pregnancy Act 1971.
7. The Protection of Children from Sexual Offences Act 2012.

Chapter 7

Medicolegal Challenges in PCPNDT Act: Case Examples

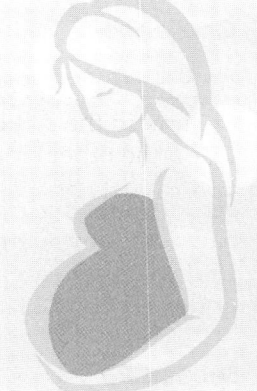

○ MC Patel

In the population censes of 1971, 1981 and 1991, serious gender imbalance between 0 and 6 years of male children to female children was noticed. To check gender imbalance, Pre-Natal Diagnostic Technique (Regulation and Prevention of misuse) Act was enacted in 1994. In spite of the PNDT Act 1994, there was no improvement in the figures in census of 2001. On the contrary, further gender imbalance was noticed making the issue more of social worry.

It was noticed that ratio of 0–6 years of male to female children in India was 1000:945 in 1991 and 1000:927 in 2001. Public interest litigation was filed by NGOs before the Supreme court for better implementation of the Act to check gender imbalance. So, further amendments were made in 2002 and 2003 and pre-conceptional sex selection was added and the Act is known as The Pre-conception and Pre-natal Diagnostic Techniques (Prohibition of Sex Selection)—PCPNDT Act. From time to time, further amendments were added in sections and rules in 2011, 2012, 2013, 2014, etc, for better implementation of the Act.

AIMS

- Prohibition of pre-natal determination and/or communication of the sex of the foetus.
- Prohibition of pre-conceptional sex selection.
- Prohibition of any advertisement by any person and/or organisation and/or institution regarding facilities of pre-natal sex determination and/or pre-conceptional sex selection.
- Any centre, managing antenatal patients, must be registered under this Act either as a genetic counselling centre, genetic laboratory, genetic clinic and/or ultrasound clinic/imaging centre.
- No centre can function without registration (Section 18)
- All these centres are regulated under PNDT Act.

Punishment under PCPNDT Act

Any offence under this Act shall be *cognizable, non-bailable and non-compoundable.*

Challenge 1

As the offence is non-bailable, if appropriate authority has involved the police, police can make an arrest and only court can grant bail.

It has happened in many cases especially when team from Rajasthan has raided for search and seizure. In Gujarat, doctors from Modasa, Himmatnagar, Panchmahal, Banaskantha were arrested and the lower court rejected bail. The High Court of Rajasthan, Jodhpur bench granted bail and they were out of custody. Doctors remained in jail for approximately 5 days to 15 days. There are provisions for punishment for contravention of any provision of this Act under Sections 23 and 25.

Section 23

Provision of punishment for person giving the aids:
- For first conviction: Imprisonment of up to 3 years and fine of up to ₹10,000.
- Any subsequent conviction: Imprisonment of up to 5 years and fine of up to ₹50,000.
- Name of registered medical practitioner (RMP) shall be reported by appropriate authority to State Medical Council for necessary action including suspension of registration, if charges are framed.

Challenge 2

- Merely on framing the charge sheet, appropriate authorities can write to the Medical Council of the respective state to take necessary action including suspension of registration.
- There is provision that on conviction of a doctor, his name can be removed from Register of Council for 5 years in case of first offence; and permanently for the subsequent offence.

This is not fair as the offense is yet to be proved.

In one instance in Ganganagar, Rajasthan, the appropriate authority filed a case in court of First Class Magistrate against 18 doctors on a single ground that during inspection of their respective clinic, the doctors were found without aprons and name plates and charge sheet was framed. The appropriate authority wrote to Medical Council of Rajasthan to take necessary action including suspension of registration. In response, Medical Council registration of all eighteen doctors was suspended. Of course, the ruling was challenged in the High Court of Rajasthan, which ruled in favour of the doctors that merely on framing of charge sheet, such kind of action cannot be taken.

Provision for punishment for person seeking the aids:

For first conviction: Imprisonment up to 3 years and fine up to Rs. 50,000.

Any subsequent conviction: Imprisonment up to 5 years and fine up to Rs. 1 Lakh.

Husband and relatives of the pregnant woman undergoing prenatal diagnostic technique for the purpose of sex determination shall be presumed to have compelled the woman to undergo the same unless the contrary is proved. Provision of the Act shall not apply to the woman who was compelled to undergo such technique.

The provision also applies to pre-conceptional sex selection.

Challenge 3

Very few or almost negligible cases has been filed against patient or relatives seeking aids for prenatal sex determination and/or pre-conceptional sex selection.

In our society, there is a wrong belief that cases can only be filed against doctors doing sonography. If cases are filed against patients or relatives seeking sex determination or pre-conceptional sex selection, then there will be a fear in society and demand for sex determination or pre-conceptional sex selection will be reduced. After all, this is type of demand and supply. If there is no demand, there will be no supply.

Section 25

Contravention of any provisions or any rules for which no penalty has been elsewhere provided in this Act:
- There will be punishment of imprisonment up to 3 months or fine up to Rs. 1000 or both.
- Continuing contravention, additional Rs. 500 for everyday during which such contravention continues after conviction for the first such contravention.

Under Section 4(3) of the Act

Any deficiency or inaccuracy found in record shall amount to contravention of provisions of Section 5 or Section 6 of the Act unless contrary is proved by the person conducting antenatal ultrasonography.

Thus, any deficiency or inaccuracy in record may invite litigation, sealing of ultrasound machine and suspension or cancellation of registration of PCPNDT.

Challenge 4

Maximum cases filed against the doctors are on the grounds of inaccuracy or deficiency of records or of not preserving records properly.

Therefore, persons doing sonography are under obligation to maintain records properly as per the provision of the Act. The doctors should remember that prevention is always better than cure and ignorance of the law cannot be an excuse.

Registration of Certificate

- Registration of the centre is mandatory either as genetic counselling centre, genetic laboratory, genetic clinic and/or ultrasonography centre/imaging centre.
- **No centre can function without registration**
- One cannot buy, install or use USG machine for antenatal sonography unless the centre is registered and details of the sonography machine/s are intimated to the authority.
- As such, there is registration of place and not the person or the machine

- Only details of persons working in the centre (name, qualifications with Medical Council registration number) and machines installed (make, model, manufacturer) are to be provided
- However, many appropriate authorities insist separate registration for each machine with registration fees which is wrong interpretation by appropriate authority.

One copy of Form B is to be displayed at a conspicuous place at the place of business [Rule 6(2)]

Challenge 5

In certificate of registration, details of sonography machine is to be included.

In many cases, ground of the case is 'there was no detail of sonography machine in form B, i.e. Certificate of Registration'. If there is change in sonography machine (buy/sell), it is to be intimated to appropriate authority. Certificate of registration should also be sent to appropriate authority for necessary change.

Renewal of Registration of certificate: One should apply for renewal 30 days before the date of expiry of Certificate of Registration [Rule 8(1)]

Deemed Renewal [Rule 8(6)]: In event of failure of the appropriate authority to renew the Certificate of Registration or to communicate within a period of **90 days** from the date of receipt of application for renewal of registration, the certificate of registration shall be deemed to have been renewed.

Challenge 6

For renewal of registration, one may apply before 30 days of expiry.

Provision of deemed renewal only applies if there is no communication from appropriate authority in regards to either renewal or rejection within 90 days. Thus, if the appropriate authority does not take any decision, then after 30 days any registered centre stands unregistered.

Maintenance and Preservation of Records [Rule (9)]

- A doctor is bound to produce records when asked by the appropriate authority and the Court and if he does not, adverse inference might be drawn.
- Good record is good defence, poor record is poor defence and no record is no defence.
    - It is mandatory to duly fill and sign prescribed forms:
    - Form D for Genetic Counselling Centre [R9(2)]
    - Form E for Genetic Laboratory [R9(3)]
    - Form F for Genetic Clinic/Ultrasonography Centre/ Imaging Science Centre [R9(4)]
    - Form G for Invasive Procedures [R 10(1)] with declaration from patient duly signed.
    - Form H: Appropriate authority shall maintain a permanent record of applications for grant of renewal of certificate of registration. Letter of intimation of every change of employee, place, address and equipment installed. [R9(5)]

You can send specimen for investigation to registered genetic laboratory only. Genetic laboratory can receive specimen from registered centre only. It shall not be necessary for genetic laboratory to obtain a fresh consent if consent is taken by genetic clinic.

Challenge 7

Cases filed against doctors are on the grounds that signature of patient on declaration form is not taken or doctors doing sonography have not signed the declaration.

It is mandatory for the patient undergoing the sonography and the person doing the sonography to sign the declaration.

Declaration of patient is mandatory for any ultrasound or invasive procedure irrespective of the gestational age as under

"I, Ms. .... declare that by undergoing ultrasonography/image scanning, etc, I do not want to know the sex of my foetus"

Signature/Thumb Impression of pregnant woman
Thumb impression is to be identified by proper person
Copy should be given to pregnant woman

Declaration of person doing the sonography is also mandatory on Form F or G (as per case) and on report of sonography/imaging scanning as under:

"I, Dr. .... declare that while conducting ultrasonography/image scanning on Ms. ...., I have neither detected nor disclosed the sex of her foetus to anybody in any manner."

Signature

Form should be filled up in duplicate
- One copy to be kept for office record [R 9(4)]
- One copy to be sent to the Appropriate Authority every month before 5th of next month. [R 9(8)]

Challenge 8

Records can be preserved in any media but a copy of the record shall be taken and will be authenticated by person responsible for such record.

Thus, even after preserving record in any media, hard copy is required.

Preservation of Records

- One can preserve records on computer or any electronic equipment [Rule 9(7)] but printed copy of records shall be taken and preserved after authentication by a person responsible for such records
- Records are to be preserved for two years from the date of completion to date of counselling, prenatal diagnostic procedure or prenatal diagnostic test.
- In event of any legal proceeding, records should be preserved till the final disposal of case or for two years whichever is later.

Submission of Records
One copy of respective form is to be submitted to appropriate authority every month before 5th of next month **[Rule 9(8)].**

Online Submission
In some states, authorities insist on submitting respective forms online in a given prescribed period.

Online Submission of Nil Report
In some states, authorities insist on submitting 'NIL' report within a stipulated time, if there is no sonography during the respective month.

Challenge 9
In some states, the appropriate authority insists on to maintain register with all the details of form F.
There is no provision to support this demand as per the Act.

Register [Rule 9(1)]
Register having four columns should be maintained, i.e.
1. Sr. No
2. Name and Address of the woman and the relative given genetic counselling, subjected to prenatal diagnostic procedure or pre-natal diagnostic tests
3. Name of spouse/father and
4. Date on which they first reported for such counseling, procedure or test

Challenge 10
Consent of patient:
- Written consent of pregnant woman is mandatory, if one does ultrasound examination or invasive procedure irrespective of gestational age.
- One copy should be given to pregnant woman

Referral Chits/Letters
- If patient is referred from outside, referral letter is to be preserved with respective form
- If it is self reference, then copy of case paper is also to be preserved with referral chit with indication/s (made by person advising ultrasound examination) with respective form

Intimation of change [Rule (13)] of employee, place, address, equipment installed to be intimated at least 30 days in advance of the expected date of such change by person in whose name registration is.

Non-use of Machine

- If the ultrasonography machine is not working, it is for repairs, permanent non-use or is given back to company, the appropriate authority must be intimated.
- If it is permanent non-use, machine can be disposed off (demolished) in presence of appropriate authority or his representative.

Doctor Visiting as a Sonologist [Rule 3(3)]

Every Medical Practitioner qualified under the Act to conduct ultrasonography in a genetic clinic/ultrasound clinic/imaging centre shall be permitted to be registered with a maximum of **TWO** such Clinics/Centers **within a district.**

The consulting hours for such medical practitioner shall be clearly specified by each clinic/centre.

Public Information (Rule 17)

1. Every genetic counselling centre, genetic laboratory, genetic clinic, ultrasound clinic and imaging centre shall prominently display on its premises a notice in English and in the local language or languages that *"Disclosure of the sex of foetus is prohibited under law"* for the information of the public, e.g.

> **NIRU MATERNITY AND NURSING HOME**
> 34, Manjushree Society Ranna Park,
> Ghatlodia. Amdavad 380061
> ANTE natal Sex Determimation is Punishable Offence
> Sex Determination is Not Done Here

2. *Copy of Act:* At least one copy, each of the Act and the rules shall be available on the premises of every genetic counseling centre, genetic laboratory, genetic clinic, ultrasound clinic and imaging centre and shall be made available to the client *on demand for persual.*
It should be available in English and preferably in the local language.

Rule 18(8)

Display his/her name and designation prominently on the dress worn by him/her to avoid litigation which had happened in Ganganagar, Rajasthan.

Section 30

Under the provision of this section, appropriate authority or the person designated by appropriate authority suomotu or on complaint may visit the Centre for inspection, search and seizure of documents and/or sonography machine (as per Rule 12 of the Act), if he has reason to believe that centre is violating provisions of the Act.

Section 20

Under the provision of this section, appropriate authority may suspend or cancel the registration after due procedure, i.e. notice, giving opportunity of being heard or without notice, in public interest, can proceed for suspension but reasons are to be recorded in writing.

Thus, under provisions of the Act, appropriate authority has power to proceed accordingly.

Important Points
- Always co-operate with the authority whenever they visit clinic for inspection
- Never panic or get excited
- Be careful before giving any signature or commission of offence on inspection
- Take time to consult your medical legal advisor, if required
- If your ultrasonography machine is sealed, keep records of all papers with valid signature of the government authority in file and select an intelligent medicolegal lawyer.
- Always reply show cause notice within the time given by appropriate authority as prescribed in notice (e.g. 7 to 10 days)

Remedies
When are they required?
- Notice issued
- Court case filed
- Sonography machine sealed
- Registration of centre suspended/cancelled

Appeal under Section 21 Rule 19 of the Act
- Aggrieved person may prefer appeal within 30 days
- If it is preferred after 30 days, the appropriate authority may condone the delay on satisfaction of the sufficient cause of delay.
- If one is aggrieved by the decision of subdistrict appropriate authority, he can prefer appeal before district appropriate authority
- If one is aggrieved by the decision of district appropriate authority, he can prefer appeal before state/UT level appropriate authority.
- Similarly, appeal can be referred to state government for decision of state appropriate authority and central government for decision of central appropriate authority.
- Each appeal shall be disposed off by the district appropriate authority or by the state/union territory appropriate authority, as the case may be, within 60 days of its receipt. [Rule 19 (3)].

Challenge 11
Usually, the appellate authority does not dispose off the appeal within 60 days.

Judicial Remedies

One can prefer appeal before Judicial Magistrate first class or Metropolitan Magistrate or Sessions Court or High Court or Supreme Court in succession as the case may be.

What FOGSI does?

- Harassment of FOGSIans by appropriate authority in some cases due to wrong interpretation of the provisions of the Act has come to the notice of FOGSI.
- FOGSI is always on toes to be helpful and to guide members in any given situation. There is a PCPNDT cell in FOGSI to take care of these issues.
- Regular meetings of cell are held to discuss problems of members related to PCPNDT Act.
- Regular CMEs and workshops are organised through member societies to update members and make them vigilant to not end up in litigation and if required, then solutions to get rid of them.

FOGSI preferred a writ petition before the Supreme Court with a panel of learned advocates headed by Soly Sorabjee and Shyam Diwan (both learned and senior advocates in Supreme Court). The main objective was to convince the Supreme Court that clerical errors were not synonymous with sex determination.

The following points were requested:
1. There should be graded punishment.
2. Punishment could not be equal for sex determination and inaccuracy in record
3. There should not be criminal complaints for inaccuracy of record keeping
4. There should not be action on appeal by Appropriate Authority by the Medical Council merely on framing of charge and before conviction.
5. Renewal of registration should not be withheld merely on grounds of pending case against member.

However, FOGSI was unlucky. The Supreme Court did not allow the appeal.

Take Home Message

- Please do not get involved in pre-natal sex determination or pre-conceptional sex selection.
- Comply with the provisions of the Act to avoid litigation under PC PNDT Act.

Have a litigation free practice!!!!

BIBLIOGRAPHY

www.ncpcr.gov.in PC PNDT Act 1994

Chapter 8

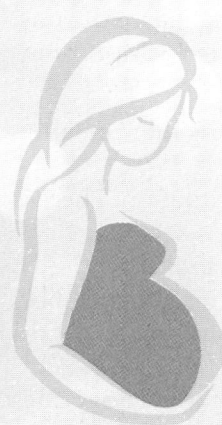

Recent Judgments and Legal Update

○ Sanjay Gupte ○ Arati Shah ○ Sanuja Oke

Landmark judgments by the Supreme Court are important to medical practitioners in day-to-day practice as they form the case law. As far as Indian judiciary is concerned, there are two types of laws:
1. *Statutory laws:* These are the laws actually enacted by the parliament.
2. *Case laws:* These are the decisions by Supreme Court which become binding on all the lower courts.

As far as hospitals and medical practitioners are concerned, there are more than 100 statutory laws pertaining to our profession.
- Laws governing commissioning of hospital
- Laws governing qualification/practice and conduct of professionals
- Laws governing sale, storage of drugs and safe medication
- Laws governing management of patients
- Laws governing environment safety
- Laws governing the medicolegal aspects
- Laws governing professional training and research
- Laws governing safety of patients, public and staff within the hospital premises
- Laws governing the business aspects

As far as medical practice in India is concerned, significant case law started with the case in 1969. Interestingly, in this case, one doctor sued another doctor and pursued the matter till the Supreme Court. This case was as follows:

Dr Laxman Balkrishna Joshi v/s Dr Trimbak Bapu Godbole and Another (1968)[1]

A patient, who was the son of Dr Godbole, suffered from fracture of the femur. The accused doctor while putting the leg in plaster used manual traction and used excessive force during traction, with the help of three other men although such traction is never done under Morphine alone but should have been done under proper general anesthesia. This led to severe shock causing the death of the boy. On these facts, the Supreme Court held that the doctor was liable to pay damages to the parents of the boy.

This case laid down certain legal principles to define medical negligence which are still rightly followed by the Indian courts till this day.

These principles were:
- A person who holds himself out ready to give medical advice and treatment impliedly holds forth that he is possessed of skill and knowledge for the purpose.
- Such a person when consulted by a patient owes certain duties, namely a duty of care deciding whether to undertake the case, a duty of care in deciding what treatment to give, and a duty of care in the administration of the treatment. **A breach of any these duties** gives a right of action of negligence against him.
- The medical practitioner has discretion in choosing the treatment, which he proposes to give to the patient, and such discretion is wider in case of emergency, but he must exercise a reasonable degree of care according to the circumstances of each case.

The second case which totally altered the medicolegal scenario was as follows:

Indian Medical Association versus VP Shantha and Others (1996)[2]

This landmark judgment decided that service rendered by medical professionals comes under Section 2(1)(0) of the Act and hence the Consumer Protection Act was applied to the medical practitioners.

It defined conditions such as
- Who is a consumer?
- What is negligence?
- What is deficiency in service?
- What are the patent conditions under which medical practitioners can be held responsible, e.g.
  - Removal of the wrong limb;
  - Performance of an operation on the wrong patient;
  - Giving injection of a drug to which a patient is allergic without looking into the out-patient card containing the warning;
  - Use of wrong gas during the course of an anesthetic, etc.

Interestingly, this decision had enumerated the above conditions where the Consumer Protection Act should be applied and also explicitly mentioned that complex medical situations should be sent to the civil courts! However, in the following years, these directions have been modified by the further decisions.

The third important case for medical practitioners was as follows.

Poonam Verma versus Ashwin Patel and Others (1996)[3]

This significant case was decided in 1996. This was regarding cross pathy practice. Here, a homeopath doctor treated a patient with allopathic drugs; though the treatment given was not actually wrong, the court decided that a doctor who has a qualification in Ayurvedic or Homeopathic medicine will be liable if he prescribes Allopathic treatment which may or may not cause any harm and the court defined this as a negligence 'per se' meaning thereby that even if no actual harm occurs, it will still be held as negligence.

The professional may be held liable for negligence on the ground that he was not possessed of the requisite skill which he professes to have.

Again, as the days passed, this directive also stands modified in the actual practice.

The next landmark judgment is by NCDRC.

Sarwat Ali Khan versus Prof R Gogi and Others (1997)[4]

There are camps of cataract operations. In one such camp, 52 cataract operations were performed between 26th and 28th September 1995 in an Eye Hospital. 14 patients lost their vision in the operated eye because of infection. An enquiry revealed that in the operation theatre two autoclaves were not working properly. The courts decided that the onus was on doctors. They should have checked all these sterilization processes and equipment. This equipment is absolutely necessary to carry out sterilization of instruments, cotton, pads, linen, etc., and the damage occurred because of its absence in actual working condition. The doctors were held liable. This is a very important decision as though normally doctors do not carry out the sterilization process, they are vicariously held responsible.

Dr Sr Louie and Another versus Smt Kannolil Pathumma and Another (1992)[5]

An interesting case of Dr Louie, an MD from Germany, Freiburg, a German Degree which is equivalent to an MBBS degree in India. In India, she practiced Obstetrics and Gynecology. When the case went to the courts, the National Consumer Commission held that Dr Louie showed herself as an MD although she was only MD by German qualification. She was guilty of negligence in treating a woman and her baby who died during delivery. In this case, there was failure of vacuum application, and the baby was delivered in an asphyxiated condition. The courts held her guilty for misrepresentation of her skills.

Pt Parmanand Katara versus Union of India and Others[6]

In this case, the courts decided about emergency medical care which should and has to be given by all the doctors whenever emergency cases are brought to them. In this case, an accident victim was sent from one hospital to another and finally succumbed. The doctors and hospital were reluctant to take this case as the hospitals and doctors did not want to get involved in the police proceedings which they perceived as being hazardous as it was going to be a Medicolegal case. So, the Supreme Court decided that treatment must be given by any hospital where the patient goes to at that particular moment to save the life of the patient.

The facts of this case were as follows.

The petitioner referred to a report published in the newspaper "The Hindustan Times" in which it was mentioned that a scooterist was knocked down by a speeding car. On seeing the profusely bleeding scooterist, a pedestrian picked up the injured and took him to the nearest hospital. The doctors refused to attend the patient and told the man that he should take the patient to another hospital located 20 kilometers away authorized to handle medicolegal cases. The injured was then taken to that hospital but by the time he could reach, the victim succumbed to his injuries.

Importantly in this decision, the courts had also directed the police to respect the medical profession and cause minimal hassles to the doctors and hospital in such cases.

Spring Medows Hospital and Another versus Harjol Ahluwalia through KS Ahluwalia (1998)[7]

This case decided the 'vicarious' liability so called on the doctor. A minor child was admitted by his parents to a nursing home as he had fever. The doctor diagnosed typhoid fever and gave medicines for typhoid fever. A nurse asked the father of the patient to get injection Chloroquine instead of Chloromycetine which was to be administered. The nurse administered the injection to the patient who immediately collapsed and suffered brain damage. The National Commission held the doctor negligent in performing his duty as instead of administering the injection himself, he permitted the nurse to give the injection. He did not check the injection to be given. Both the doctor and nurse were held negligent and the hospital was also held liable as it was decided that the hospital will be held liable for the employees if they commit wrong and the doctors will be vicariously held liable if they do not supervise the action which is to be supervised by them.

Sethuraman Subramaniam Iyer versus Triveni Nursing Home and Another (1998)[8]

In another significant case, a small operation was being carried out on the nasal septum under local anesthesia. Unfortunately, the patient had cardiac arrest and died on the table. In this case decided by National Consumer Forum in 1998, the forum rightly said that the bad outcome doesn't always mean negligence by the doctor. All the necessary precautions and effective measures to resuscitate the patient were taken and that's why the doctor was not held negligent and the complaint was dismissed. The State Commission relied on the affidavits of four doctors who opined that there was no negligence. The complainant had not given any expert evidence to support his allegation. But, as we will discuss later, the scenario has changed in later cases.

State of Punjab versus Shiv Ram (2005)[9]—Failure of Sterilization

Decision in this case came as a great relief to gynecologists. We, gynecologists, are worried about sterilization failure. This can happen in spite of all due care and when failure happened in cases before this particular one, doctors were held liable for the failure.

This case finally decided and Supreme Court said the failure of sterilization is always a possibility and the surgeon cannot be held liable if it fails, unless, a patent negligence was proved (like by laparoscopy) in blocking the tubes.

The decision stated that—merely because woman having undergone sterilization operation became pregnant and delivered child, the operating surgeon or his employer cannot be held liable for compensation on account of unwanted pregnancy. Claim is sustainable only if there was negligence on part of surgeon in performing surgery or surgeon assured 100% exclusion of pregnancy after surgery.

In spite of having undergone sterilization operation, if couple opts for bearing the child, it ceases to be unwanted child—compensation for maintenance and for upbringing of such child cannot be claimed.

CONSENT FOR SURGERY

The matter of consent is extremely important for any medical practitioner in day-to-day practice.

Supreme Court of India has come out with very important judgment in case of **Samira Kohli versus Dr Manchanda.**[10]

An endometrosis case was taken up for laparoscopy and when the problem was seen to be very severe the doctor came out to obtain consent from patient's mother for hysterectomy and went ahead and did the hysterectomy surgery which was objected to later by the patient. Because rightly she was not mentally ready for such major surgery, which was not discussed with her beforehand. Even though it was in the interest of the patient herself, Supreme Court decided and put down certain principles which are very important. Firstly, the Supreme Court decided that consent must be **"real and valid"** which means that the patient has to have **capacity and competence** to give the consent. A patient under anesthesia does not have capacity to give consent. One should also bear in mind that a patient who is in pain may not be having capacity to give consent.

The patient must be given adequate information and this adequate information means
- Nature and procedure of the treatment, its purpose, benefits and effect
- Alternatives if any available
- An outline of the substantial risks; and
- Adverse consequences of refusing treatment.

All this should be included and informed to the patient before the consent. One good point the Supreme Court mentioned here was that this information may be given by a doctor or a member of his/her team and this is helpful as the assistant doctor involved in treatment may be able to give this information and that should be taken as valid.

The Court further said that there is no need to explain remote or theoretical risks involved, like in every case, one doesn't have to emphasize on cardiac arrest which may scare the patient and patient may not want to undergo even an indicated surgery. An important point in this decision was that **consent given only for a diagnostic procedure cannot be considered as consent for the therapeutic treatment.** The fact that an unauthorized additional surgery is beneficial to the patient, or it would save considerable time and expense to the patient or would relieve the patient from pain and suffering in future, are no grounds of defense. **The only exception to this rule is where the additional procedure though unauthorized is for a lifesaving procedure.** When one is anticipating such a problem, the solution is to discuss these possibilities and then to go ahead if that possibility arises later.

Jacob Mathew versus Respondents: State of Punjab and Others (2005)[11]

Guidelines for prosecuting medical professionals under the criminal law.
The courts said that
- Cases of doctors (surgeons and physicians) being subjected to criminal prosecution are on an increase.
- Sometimes, such prosecutions are filed by private complainants and sometimes by police based on FIR lodged and cognizance taken. The investigating officer and the private complainant cannot always be assumed to have knowledge of medical science so as to determine whether the act of the accused medical professional amounts to rash or negligent act within the domain of criminal law under Section 304-A of IPC.
- A private complaint may not be entertained unless the complainant has produced opinion given by another competent doctor to support the charge of rashness or negligence on the part of the accused doctor. The investigating officer should, before proceeding against the doctor accused of rash or negligent act or omission, obtain an independent and competent medical opinion preferably from a doctor in government service qualified in that branch of medical practice who is expected to give an impartial and unbiased opinion.
- A doctor accused of rashness or negligence, may not be arrested in a routine manner (simply because a charge has been leveled against him) unless his arrest is necessary for furthering the investigation, for collecting evidence or on a suspicion that the doctor would not make himself available to face prosecution unless arrested.

LOCUM ARRANGEMENT

Nabhan Farhan Sah versus Dr Latha Sharma (2007)[12]

This is about the common scenario where the doctor sometimes has to make a locum arrangement. Here the baby was in NICU and the doctor had to leave town. He made arrangement for adequate care of the baby by keeping a locum doctor who was equivalent before leaving town. The relatives blamed this argument when baby died and alleged it as negligence by the doctor, but the courts said this cannot be called as negligence as adequate locum arrangements were made by the doctor.

The next two cases deal with the matter of compensation for negligence. Before the below cases, the courts followed the "multiplier method" which was based on the method followed in road traffic accident so far. That means, whatever was the income of the patient, was multiplied by the life expectancy and accordingly, the compensation was calculated. Here, for the first case, the Supreme Court enunciated the principle of 'Restitutio in integrum.'

The facts of the case were:

Delivery of premature baby took place with birth weight of 1250 gm at Egmore, Chennai Govt hospital. Baby suffered blindness (ROP) due to 100% oxygen. Baby was not screened between 2–4 weeks as was mandatory. The doctors were held liable and the Supreme Court declared that the principle of awarding compensation that can be safely relied on is 'restitutio in integrum.' The said principle provides that a person entitled to damages should, as nearly as possible, get that sum of money which would put him in the same position as he would have been if he had not sustained the wrong. Compensation of Rs. 1,38,00,000/- was awarded.

Balram Prasad versus Kunal Saha (2013)[13]

The same principle was used in the famous Kolkata case and this probably stands as the highest compensation awarded in a medicolegal case in Indian courts. Here, in similar situation, it was decided that Dr Kunal Saha's wife succumbed due to alleged negligence by the doctors and the courts decided held the doctors liable and decided compensation of Rs. 6,08,00,550/- with 6% interest amounting to 13 crores. The take home message is if doctors are involved in high risk practice, they have to think of insurance and sometimes the premium may be very high because the compensations methods have definitely changed.

Nizam Institute of Medical Sciences versus Prasanth S Dhananka and Others (2009)[14]

This case decided two things. Here, 20 years old student had to undergo spinal tumor surgery which was in the grey zone of cardiothoracic and neurological surgery. The cardiothoracic surgeon operated on him and did not take help of neurosurgeon during surgery and the patient suffered from paraplegia. The court objected to this cross speciality practice, the compensation was calculated by the Restitution in integrum method and the doctors had to pay a big compensation.

Now, we will come to the case which we had referred to previously as a cardiac arrest case in which it was decided that if adequate measures were taken to resuscitate the patient after the cardiac arrest, then the doctor was not held liable. But in this below case, the courts have taken a different view of 'Res ipsa loquitur'.

Shyam Sunder versus State of Rajasthan (1974)[15]

This was a case of cardiac arrest on the table. The courts applied the principle of 'Res ipsa loquitur'. The normal rule is that "it is for the plaintiff to prove negligence", but, in some cases, considerable hardship is caused to the plaintiff as the true cause of the accident is not known to him, but is solely within the knowledge of the defendant who caused it (e.g. as the cardiac arrest occurred inside the operation theatre where patient has no access).

This case forms the basis of the present thinking of the courts.

Now we come to final two very important judgments decided by the Supreme Court itself. The first case was as follows.

Kusum Sharma and Others versus Batra Hospital and Medical Research (2010)[16]

In this case, the petitioner's husband had an adrenal mass which was removed by surgeon with "anterior" approach. There can be two approaches for this surgery: Anterior approach and posterior approach. The surgeon, while using the anterior approach, had difficulty and the pancreas were injured inadvertently and eventually a fistula developed. In spite of a lot of efforts to save the patient, the patient succumbed.

Both the parties had experts arguing for and against the approach that was used and so the court and none other than the very eminent Justice Dalveer Bhandari went into this case in detail and has given the decision. I think the principles that the court came up with are historic principles and I believe that they are going to stay with us for a long time.

The Supreme Court said that,

On scrutiny of the leading cases of medical negligence in our country, some basic principles emerge in dealing with cases of medical negligence. While deciding whether the medical professional is guilty of medical negligence, following well-known principles must be kept in view:

i. Negligence is the breach of a duty exercised by omission to do something which a reasonable man, guided by those considerations which ordinarily regulate the conduct of human affairs, would do, or doing something which a prudent and reasonable man would not do.

This is the so called 'Bolam' principle,[17] which is recognized all over the world.

ii. Negligence is an essential ingredient of the offence. The negligence, to be established by the prosecution, must be culpable or gross and not negligence merely based upon an error of judgment.

iii. The medical professional is expected to bring a reasonable degree of skill and knowledge and must exercise a reasonable degree of care. Neither the very highest nor a very low degree of care and competence judged in the light of the particular circumstance of each case is what the law requires.

iv. A medical practitioner would be liable only where his conduct fell below that of the standard of a reasonably competent practitioner in his field.

v. In the realm of diagnosis and treatment, there is scope for genuine difference of opinion and one professional doctor is clearly not negligent merely because his conclusion differs from that of another professional doctor.

vi. The medical professional is often called upon to adopt a procedure which involves higher element of risk, but which he honestly believes as providing greater chances of success for the patient rather than a procedure involving lesser risk but higher chances of failure. Just because a professional looking at the gravity of illness has taken higher element of risk to redeem the patient out of his/her suffering and did not yield the desired result may not amount to negligence.

vii. Negligence cannot be attributed to a doctor so long as he performs his duties with reasonable skill and competence. Merely because the doctor chooses one course of action in preference to the other one available, he would not be liable if the course of action chosen by him was acceptable to the medical profession.

viii. It would not be conducive to the efficiency of the medical profession if no doctor could administer medicine without a halter round his neck.

ix. It is our bounden duty and obligation of the civil society to ensure that the medical professionals are not unnecessarily harassed or humiliated so that they can perform their professional duties without fear and apprehension.

x. The medical practitioners at times also have to be saved from such a class of complainants who use criminal process as a tool for pressurizing the medical professionals/hospitals, particularly private hospitals or clinics, for extracting uncalled for compensation. Such malicious proceedings deserve to be discarded.

xi. The medical professionals are entitled to get protection so long as they perform their duties with reasonable skill and competence and in the interest of the patients. The interest and welfare of the patients have to be paramount for the medical professionals.

The above principles enunciated by the justice have a great historic significance in defining the medical negligence in India.

However, even after the above almost doctrinal judgment, the next case has paved the way for paradigm change in the court's thinking.

Arunkumar Manglik vs Chirayu Health and Medicare Pvt Ltd (2019)[18]

This case was apparently of dengue fever. Patient eventually died because of hemorrhagic complications due to low platelet count and leucopenia. The treatment administered was supported as correct by number of experts.

The discussion and dissection of law of medical negligence happened and a lot of evidence for and against what should have been done was given by the experts.

In this judgment, the Supreme Court commented on the Bolam case as: A doctor is not guilty of negligence if he has acted in accordance with a practice accepted as proper by a responsible body of medical men skilled in that particular art. The "Bolam test" has been the subject of academic debate and evaluation all over world now. So far as there was support from other medical practitioners, the doctor was not held liable. Among scholars, the Bolam test has been criticized on the ground that it fails to make the distinction between the ordinary skilled doctor and the reasonably competent doctor. But now, House of Lords have decided Bolitho test.[19] House of Lords: The use of these adjectives—responsible, reasonable and respectable—all show that the court has to be satisfied that the exponents of the body of opinion relied upon can demonstrate that such opinion has a logical basis.

Even if the body which decides is a medical body of experts, the court will definitely have to go in the details of how this was decided, there was no bias, they applied proper mind to the situation at hand before accepting the opinion as being responsible, reasonable or respectable. The judge will need to be satisfied that, in forming their views, the experts have directed their minds to the question of comparative risks and benefits and have reached a defensible conclusion on the matter."

This is very important: Any practice guideline of any professional body will be blindly accepted. It has to be a kind of guideline where the doctors have really applied their mind and worked in the details.

The court also committed that in adopting a standard of care, Indian courts must be conscious of the fact that a large number of hospitals and medical units in our country, especially in rural areas, do not have access to latest technology and medical equipment."

In conclusion, these landmark cases guide us towards the correct practice. They not only define the medical negligence but also reassure us that reasonable and standard care is what the courts expect from a medical practitioner. Hence, we need not be unduly stressed while consciously treating our patients. However, the latest judgment indicates that, the courts are moving from "Bolam Test" to the "Bolitho Test" where the judiciary retains the prerogative on deciding what reasonable and standard care is.

REFERENCES

1. Laxman Balkrishna Joshi vs Trimbak Bapu Godbole And Anr on 2 May 1968, Equivalent citations: 1969 AIR 128, 1969 SCR (1) 206.
2. Indian Medical Association vs VP Shantha and Ors on 13 November 1995, Equivalent citations: 1996 AIR 550, 1995 SCC (6) 651.
3. Poonam Verma vs Ashwin Patel and Ors on 10 May 1996, Equivalent citations: 1996 AIR 2111, 1996 SCC (4) 332.
4. Sarwat Ali Khan vs Prof R Gogi and others Original Petition No.181 of 1997, decided on 18.7.2007 by the National Consumer Commission.
5. Louie And Anr. vs Kannolil Pathumma And Anr. on 16 November 1992, National Consumer Disputes Redressal.
6. Pt. Parmanand Kataravs Union of India and Ors on 28 August 1989, Equivalent citations: 1989 AIR 2039, 1989 SCR (3) 997.
7. Supreme Court of India, M/S. Spring Meadows Hospital and Anr vs Harjol Ahluwalia Through, KS Ahluwalia and Another [(1998) 4 SCC 39].
8. Sethuraman Subramaniam Iyer vs Triveni Nursing Home and Another (1998), National Consumer Disputes Redressal Commission NCDRC.
9. Supreme Court of India, State of Punjab vs Shiv Ram and Ors on 25 August 2005.
10. Samira Kohli V/s Dr Manchanda Case No. CA 1949 of 1004 decided on 16th January 2008.
11. 2005 AIR SCW 3685 (From: Punjab and Haryana) RC Lahoti, CJI, CK Mathur and PK Balasubramanyan, JJ, Criminal Appeal Nos. 144-145 of 2004 D/5-8-2005. Appellant: Jacob Mathew Vs Respondents: State of Punjab and others
12. Nabhan Farhan Sah vs Latha Sharma (Dr.) (2007) June, Karnataka State Consumer Disputes Redressal Commission.
13. Balram Prasad vs Kunal Saha and Ors, 24 October 2013 Supreme Court of India (Civil Case).
14. Supreme Court of India 14 May 2009, Nizam Institute of Medical Sciences vs Prasanth S Dhananka and Ors. (2009).
15. Shyam Sunder and Others vs The State of Rajasthan on 12 March 1974 Equivalent citations: 1974 AIR 890, 1974 SCR (3) 549.
16. Supreme Court of India, Kusum Sharma and Ors vs Batra Hospital and Med. Research on 10 February 2010, Justice: Dalveer Bhandari.
17. Bolam vs Friern Health Management Committee. [1957] 1 W.L.R. 582 (QB).
18. Supreme Court of India, Arunkumar Manglik vs Chirayu Health and Medicare Pvt Ltd (9 Jan 2019) Judgment by Justice Dhananjay Chandrachud.
19. Bolitho v City and Hackney Health Authority 1997.

Section II

Obstetric Care

9. Obstetrician's Responsibility: Maintenance of Records
10. Recent Changes in Maternal Death Review
11. Maternal Death Review: Facility-Based MDR
12. Guidelines for Postmortem In Obstetric Deaths
13. Maternal Deaths: Global Scenario and Practitioners Perspective
14. Human Milk Banking in a Developing Country
15. Role of Paramedical Staff
16. Training of Medical and Paramedical Staff in Obstetric Care

Chapter 9

Obstetrician's Responsibility: Maintenance of Records

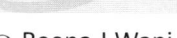

○ Reena J Wani

Documentation is the best defense you can produce, this is illustrated beautifully by the story of an eminent lawyer who had gone off for a vacation when the case he was to argue came up for hearing, his assistant was told to handle things, saying "My books will speak for themselves…" and he was proven right. Meticulous record-keeping, annotation of the day's proceedings and telephone conversations, and documentation of dialogues with concerned parties helped them to win the case!

As obstetricians we shoulder the responsibility of two clients—mother and unborn fetus. We have to ensure that things go as nature planned, with "Watchful Expectancy and Patient Observation" (pun intended) being the hallmark of a good obstetrician. However it has often been said that the most dangerous journey one can undertake in life is probably the journey through the maternal birth canal where many variables can change the outcome. Hence in fact the trend to higher CS rates for what is labelled as a "high-risk" or "precious" pregnancy. However, merely doing a cesarean section is not a guarantee that all will go well, hence there are many issues to be considered when we speak of outcomes in obstetric practice and hence maintenance of records is our responsibility.

Moliere had aptly said—"It is not just what you do, but what you do not do, for which you are accountable". After a woman becomes pregnant, in developing countries it may be a death sentence for her. Past President of FIGO Mahmoud Fathalla had remarked a few decades ago that women are dying not because of diseases we cannot treat but because Governments and countries are yet to take a decision that their lives are worth saving, this has been changing but still holds true.

Labour, birth and the immediate postnatal period is the most dangerous time for mothers and their newborn babies, and there is more that medical professionals need to do to help reduce mortality rates around the world, said then FIGO President Professor Sir Sabaratnam

Arulkumaran in his plenary lecture in March at the 2014 RCOG World Congress in Hyderabad, India. According to UN statistics there has been a decline in maternal mortality rates of 47 per cent since 1990 with Eastern and Southern Asia recording a decline of almost two-thirds. He mentioned that while maternal mortality ratios vary greatly between the developed and developing world, the main causes of maternal mortality remain the same, just on different scales.[1]

However, in addition to this RCOG has stressed the importance of data recording. The accurate recording of data, particularly serious incidents and adverse health outcomes, is a simple task that can be overlooked in busy birth settings but is hugely important to prevent maternal mortality in all countries. For example, the establishment of confidential enquiries into maternal deaths in the UK has been very successful in improving outcomes and reducing deaths by highlighting deficiencies in care.

For better health outcomes for mothers and their babies, there needs to be a two-pronged approach to making labour safer. As medical professionals we need to address the deficiencies within our organisational structures as well as improve our clinical standards through research and training. One will not work without the other. The availability of statistics and maternity dashboards, particularly in regard to serious incident reporting, is vital in all birth settings. This provides us with valuable information on where we need to improve as units and where our time and money can be spent more effectively.[1]

Maternal Death Review was started in Maharashtra State as per Government resolution dated 28/5/2010. As per guidelines it was expected that every death whether in institution or at community level, be reported and reviewed.[2] This move has promoted the need for proper record-keeping and has motivated many institutes to streamline the reporting and recording systems.

Maternity care is particularly susceptible to risk and, in England, the safety of maternity services has been the subject of recent inquiries and reviews. The National Health Service Litigation Authority (NHSLA) has developed a separate assessment scheme for maternity units, encompassing a wide range of standards. While maternity care is widely recognised as high-risk specialty, risk management is also pertinent to gynaecological practice.[3] Each unit should have a list of reporting incidents (trigger list) for maternity and gynaecology such as undiagnosed breech, unplanned return to theatre, birth trauma, faulty equipment, etc.[4]

What we need to remember is that when things do not go as planned, or unforeseen complications occur, proper documentation of the sequence of events can help us to see what could be done better next time, and also be useful in case any litigation ensues. The trend is now towards defensive practice, but we must be clear that anything done with the patient's best interests in mind will not be held against us. Hence accurate record-keeping and involvement of peers and seniors is recommended. It's been said that communicate, document your communication and involve the management/ authorities when you feel there may be a problem. This is called "Clinical Risk Management".

To optimise the reporting of incidents, staff should be aware and motivated. Avoid blame games and keep objective of improving care as the focus. Feedback drives motivation. Feedback does not stop at periodic summaries of reported incidents. It is more important to report what changes have been implemented and what demonstrable benefits have resulted from reported incidents.

Patient safety has always been a prime concern of the clinician. What has changed in the last decade is the way in which this important aspect of healthcare has been managed. In UK, the current approach to patient safety has been informed by risk management principles developed in the spheres of psychology, aviation and high reliability organizations. These principles must be applied at strategic and operational levels, by the clinical unit as a whole and by individual practitioners; they should be at the core of undergraduate, postgraduate and lifelong learning.[4]

"Res Ipsa Loquitar"

Events, things or facts speak for themselves—certain situations like a mop left behind in the abdomen, mismatched blood transfusion or wrong side operated are an invitation for litigation. To err is human, to forgive Divine, it has been said. However in medical practice the margin for error is very small, especially in our branch. Criminal prosecution of doctors has been described under most compelling circumstances, when negligence is proved beyond doubt. We should remember that simple lack of care, error of judgement, accident is not proof of negligence.

The judgement of Jacob Matthew v/s State of Punjab in Supreme Court of India (Para 3) gave three important rights to doctors. Firstly that police cannot proceed against a doctor accused of medical negligence without obtaining a suitable medical opinion, preferably from a doctor in the Government service. Second, criminal courts will also have to follow the exercise of getting a medical opinion before entertaining a private complaint against a doctor. Thirdly, the police cannot arrest a doctor accused of negligence in a routine manner.[5]

In our state, it has now become additional duty of the obstetrician to report "near-miss cases" to collect information of seriously ill pregnant mothers who have been saved who could have otherwise died. Operational definitions of near-miss as per WHO Guidelines are to be used and reporting done followed by review to help reduce maternal deaths due to these causes.[6,7]

The records to be maintained may vary as per the events/complications. For example, in case of postpartum haemorrhage, the amount of bleeding should be assessed and charted. It has been found that underestimation of blood loss and delay in replacing blood volume are the major factors leading to adverse outcomes. Hence having a standard drill and protocol for documentation side by side with treatment can possibly prevent poor outcome (Refer Chapter 13 for details). We cannot play God, we can play the best role to save lives in "the golden hour" of action.

The second patient we as obstetricians need to consider is the fetus. Litigations regarding poor fetal outcome and issues of mental handicap are now becoming more common, especially in the Western world. Common claims categories have included birth asphyxia, brachial plexus injury, wrongful birth and so on. Many analyses have been done but most of them identify problems, not solutions. Crucially the distinction between what, how and why is often unclear. For example, hypoxic brain injury is what happened, the failure to identify an abnormal fetal heart rate pattern is how it probably occurred but often missing is why a glaring abnormality was not recognised as such.[8]

For fetal monitoring in low resource settings a chart of intermittent fetal heart rate monitoring should be maintained by doctors, midwives and staff nurses on paper in addition to maternal parameters.

In better resource settings an "admission test" by electronic fetal monitoring in labour is useful. If normal then further intermittent fetal monitoring charts may be adequate for low risk patients.

Hence, the obstetricians' responsibility in correct and complete documentation and maintaining records takes a dual role, for both maternal and fetal outcomes. Although it has been said "in hindsight vision is 20-20" and it is very easy to point out faults post-hoc, having proper documentation will be a plus point in dealing with such situations.

The basic questions addressed include:
1. Risk identification as to what could go wrong
2. Risk analysis as to what is the chance it could go wrong
3. Risk treatment to minimize the chance of it happening or mitigate damage
4. Risk control as to what we can learn from things that go wrong

The key objective is to transform the prevailing culture of blame into a culture of safety and openness. Its remit is to look at systems rather than individuals. It aims at disseminating safety alerts and facilitates development of solutions to identified risks.

Patient safety incidents and near miss incidents can be reported to an anonymous data base. The aim is not a punitive action but accountability. Additionally it is important to report changes implemented and demonstrable benefits.

Improving maternal health is of WHO's key priorities. During United Nations General Assembly 2015 in New York, United Nations Secretary General Ban Ki-moon launched the global strategy for women's, children's and adolescents' health, 2016–2030. The strategy is a road map for post 2015 agenda as described by the sustainable development goals and seeks to end all preventable deaths of women, children and adolescents.[9,10]

Incident reporting and documentation will definitely be a step forward for these projects for staff training and to ensure support for health system.

Surveillance Systems and Data Maintenance

A review article has beautifully summarized the value of surveillance systems within the National Health System (NHS) in UK.[11]

It points out how the various methods in place, even if using standard formats can serve different purposes such as:
- Monitoring disease trends
- Clinical audit and evaluation, for example, the reduction in maternal deaths due to thromboembolism occurred after the release of the RCOG guidelines for thromboprophylaxis
- As a research tool, evidence-based data from records can be used to generate consensus on optimal management of rare diseases in which certain interventions may be of benefit, like AFE (amniotic fluid embolism) or certain congenital anomalies
- Resource Planning: For future clinical care, service provision and policies. For example, analysis of patient demographics and cesarean section (CS) trends showed that nearly one-

third increase in unplanned CS between 1980-2005 was directly attributable to women delaying the start of their families to later age.

Recordkeeping

As discussed above, we see the importance of accurate and meticulous documentation in many aspects of obstetric practice.

Let us now look at some core issues involved in any maternity unit which include the following.

Confidentiality of Records

Format of indoor papers or discharge cards should be standardized with "Private" or "Confidential" written on top.

Electronic records to have passwords for access.

Written discharges with details to be handed over to patient only. The importance of this was highlighted years ago by the case of Mrs V, seropositive mother who was discharged from a public hospital and the relatives found the card mentioning "HIV positive" which led her to be ostracized and removed from the home. Since then despite universal access to HIV screening in pregnancy under NACO/ MDACS protocols, there are strict guidelines on how reporting is to be done and disclosed.

Disclosure: To the hospital authority in-charge, never to third party. In case of death or serious disability claims, the hospital can handover copy of records only to the legal heir after proper identification and through proper channel.

Maintenance of records: Each hospital has its own guidelines but what is commonly done is

Outpatient records: 3 years

Indoor papers: 5 years

Medicolegal cases: Till case is settled

It is advisable to destroy/dispose of old registers and records after public notices in 2 national newspapers.

In MCGM institutes Medical Record Office (MRO): Patient held records are the norm for outpatient departments, however, we generate almost 50,000 indoor records annually. 10 years record maintained for these but for special groups (e.g. neurosurgery, psychiatry) for 15 years and for medicolegal cases indefinitely!! There is a move to HMIS (Hospital Management Information Systems) in the Municipal Corporation of Greater Mumbai (MCGM) in the past few years, which will facilitate record keeping but the current issues regarding volumes of data, personnel requirements and logistics involved are being sorted out.

Suggestions for Better Recordkeeping

- Computerization, bar-coding
- Trained staff, periodic checking, files to be maintained
- Avoid diagnosis and treatment on phone, no prescription without patient
- Complete records, no erasure/overwriting/obliteration

- No abbreviations—if used, should be standard and acceptable
- Legally adequate consent forms as per local government guidelines
- Proper operative notes in case of operative births (caesareans, vacuum, forceps), to be checked and signed by concerned senior consultant
- In case of complications necessitating additional procedures (e.g. obstetric hysterectomy, bowel injury) complete documentation of separate additional informed consent and notations from other staff/additional persons called in.

Reducing Medicolegal Problems: Strategies

Immediate: Simply remember A B C D

Appropriate choice of case, procedure, medication
Be prepared, back-up in case of high-risk situations particularly
Communication is the key to avoid anxiety, anger and litigation in many situations
Documentation of what happened and what measures were taken

Long-term: This is what will help in getting changes in the system

Standard protocols
Timely referral
Training/education

Key Points for Clinical Practice

- Consent
- Counsel the patient
- Complications are not all preventable
- Caution, call for help
- Care to maintain records, standards of care
- Consider the options for follow-up

Hence, to improve outcomes in obstetrics, regardless of where you are working or what is the healthcare situation, simple steps like careful following of protocols, meticulous record-keeping and periodic audits of past events can improve the result. In case things do not go well, clinical risk management with reporting of incidents can assist the obstetrician to have better outcomes the next time around. Choice is finally up to us to make the changes in practice for meticulous record-keeping!!

REFERENCES

1. RCOG Release 2014: FIGO President discusses how to make labour safer for women worldwide
2. Addl Director, State Family Welfare Bureau, Pune, No.SFWB/ RCH/CBMDR/ report/ file 24B/ D-10B/ 41177-220/ 2012
3. National Health Service Litigation Authority. Clinical Negligence Scheme for Trusts, Maternity. Clinical Risk Management Standards. London: NHLA; 2009 [www.nhsla.com/RiskManagement].
4. Improving Patient Safety: Risk Management for Maternity and Gynaecology. RCOG Clinical Governance Advice No. 2, Sept 2009.

5. Arrest of doctors for medical negligence-Now, impossible in India. 1MLCD (Suppl 9) Jacob Matthew v/s State of Punjab. In: Supplement 1. Medical Law Cases-For Doctors. Wolters Kluwer Medknow Publications. www.mlcd.in
6. Addl Director, State Family Welfare Bureau, Pune, No.SFWB/RCH/NM Cases/file 24B/D-10B/ 41126-77/2012
7. WHO Maternal Death and near-miss classifications. Pattison R, Lale S et al, on behalf of the WHO Working Group on Maternal Mortality and Morbidity Classifications. Bull World Health Organ. 2009 October; 87(10): 734.
8. Fox R, Yelland A, Draycott T. Analysis of legal claims—informing litigation systems and quality improvement. BJOG 2014; 121:6–10.
9. www.downtoearth.org.in
10. www.who.int/news-room/fact-sheets/detail/maternal-mortality
11. Culshaw N, Pasupathy D, Kyle P. The value of obstetric surveillance systems within the National Health System. The Obstetrician and Gynecologist 2013; 15: 85-9. http://onlinetog.org

Chapter 10

Recent Changes in Maternal Death Review

○ Rajashree Dayanand Katke ○ Kanchan Kumta

In the era of Sustainable Development Goals, India is committed to reduce its maternal mortality ratio to less than 70 per one lakh live births by 2030.

An important strategy that was adopted in the Reproductive and Child Health Program in 2010 was the Maternal Death Review. Analysis of the progress so far has brought to light certain gaps; the key gaps being:
1. Less than 50% of the estimated maternal deaths in India get reported under the health management information systems
2. While the institutional mechanisms for reviews have been established, the capacity to undertake quality reviews at various levels are weak.
3. The translation of key findings into action, in other words, the 'mechanism of response' has lagged behind.

These gaps have prompted the paradigm shift towards Maternal Death Surveillance and Response (MDSR), which focuses on taking action on information obtained from every maternal death so as to prevent further maternal deaths.

The new guidelines on MDSR were released by Ministry of Health and Family Welfare in 2017. A component of confidential review has been incorporated in the guidelines.
- MDSR is a continuous cycle of identification, notification and review of maternal deaths followed by actions to improve quality of care and prevent future deaths.
- Confidential review (CR): Multi-disciplinary anonymous investigation into all or a sample of maternal deaths, to critically observe the line of management adopted in instances of maternal morbidities and mortalities, and to identify the avoidable or remediable factors associated with them, so that the same could be corrected in the future.
- Under the Millennium Development Goal (MDG) 5, the target for India was to reduce Maternal Mortality Ratio (MMR) by three quarters between 1990 and 2015. Maternal

Mortality ratio (MMR) in India in the year 1990 was 556, which meant approximately 1.4 lakh women dying every year. The target for India was hence estimated at 139 per 1,00,000 live births by the year 2015. Globally, MMR at that time was 385, which translated into about 5.32 lakh women dying every year. As per the latest report of the Registrar General of India, Sample Registration System, Maternal Mortality ratio (MMR) of India was 167 per 100,000 live births in the period 2011–13. In terms of numbers, this translates into approximately 44,000 maternal deaths in India (303,000 maternal deaths during the same period globally). Despite one-third reduction, India remains one of the major contributors to maternal deaths in the world. For every death, there are many more who suffer varying degrees of morbid conditions.

Maternal death is a notifiable event. Classifying an event or disease as notifiable means it must be reported to the authorities within 24 hours (Form 1) and followed up by a more thorough report of medical causes and contributing factors.

Notification should be systematic including absence of cases (to be entered as zero).

"Whose faces are behind the numbers? What were their stories? What were their dreams? They left behind children and families. They also left behind clues as to why their lives ended so early".

Maternal mortality is disastrous news for the society, family, newborn and the obstetrician. Yet, we, the care providers to these apparently healthy women carrying another life within them are dumbfounded by the clinical conditions arising due to the pregnancy or the effects of the pregnancy. The rapid uprising of a condition and the worsening of commonly occurring benign conditions—pre-eclampsia, haemorrhage, etc., necessitates that all obstetricians are well-versed with the physiological changes and should be able to not only provide the best of obstetric care to the mother and the newborn but also perform or assist in performance of life-saving procedures.

- Maternal death—death of a woman while pregnant or within 42 days of termination of pregnancy, irrespective of the duration and site of the pregnancy, from any cause related to or aggravated by the pregnancy or its management but not from accidental or incidental causes.
- Maternal mortality ratio (MMR)—ratio of the number of maternal deaths during a given time period per 100,000 live births during the same time period. MMR is used as a measure of the quality of a healthcare system.
- Maternal mortality varies greatly across the regions, due to variations in underlying access to emergency obstetric care, antenatal care, anaemia rates among women, education levels of women, and other factors. Approximately 65–75% of the total estimated maternal deaths in India occur in a handful of states—Bihar, Madhya Pradesh, Rajasthan, Uttar Pradesh and Assam; all these states are part of the 18 high focus states under National Health Mission
- Uttar Pradesh alone contributes to more than 30% of the maternal deaths in India.
- The first and foremost step of the Maternal Death Review process is preparing a line list of all the maternal deaths in the area following which facility and/or community based maternal death reviews are to be undertaken. Currently, approximately 50% of the estimated maternal deaths across the country are being reported by states/UTs.

- Most importantly, states must focus on strengthening the Civil Registration System (CRS). States which have around 90% registration of deaths must focus on improving the registration to 100%. Mechanisms must be introduced for triangulation of data reported under the CRS and the data reported by the health department with the ultimate aim of strengthening the CRS such that it proves to be a single, reliable and robust source of data for maternal deaths in the state as this data can be extrapolated to calculate the maternal mortality ratio especially for small states/UTs where MMR is unavailable from the sample registration system.
- All maternal deaths reported will be investigated, irrespective of the place of death, i.e. at home, in facility or in transit; area of death, i.e. rural or urban. Maternal death review process will be undertaken at two levels:
  - Community level (community-based MDSR)
  - Facility level (facility-based MDSR)

Community-based MDSR is a method of identifying personal, family or community factors that may have contributed to the death by interviewing people such as family members or neighbours who are knowledgeable about the events leading to the death. Interview is done by using a verbal autopsy format (Form 5)

Pregnancy surveillance through MCTS/RCH portal, if strengthened, would improve reporting of maternal deaths. All maternal deaths must ultimately get reported through CRS.

Facility-based MDSR

Facility-based maternal death reviews are undertaken with the objective of improving the quality of services and responsiveness of the facility in the emergency situations by assessing the details of services provided with the help of format filled from the case sheet and by interviewing the close family members if needed. It is a process of learning lessons from the events of the past to prevent similar incidents in future. FBMDSR will be taken up for all Government teaching hospitals, referral hospitals and secondary level hospitals under other departments like Corporation, Railway, ESIC, etc., district hospital, sub-district and CHCs conducting more than 1000 deliveries/year. If regulatory mechanisms exist, states would instruct private tertiary care institutions to undertake maternal death reviews.

Pregnancy surveillance through MCTS/RCH portal, if strengthened, would improve community-based MDSR must also be conducted for all maternal deaths that take place in healthcare facilities. The district MDSR Committee must collate the findings of both facility as well as community-based reviews to draw a comprehensive understanding on the cause of maternal death and initiate appropriate corrective measures through CRS.

Classification of Cause of Death

Appropriate assessment and classification of cause of death is critical to maternal death reviews. A key area of concern is that an analysis of the data on maternal death reviews submitted by states/UTs in the health management information system for 2015-16 shows that more than 60% of the maternal deaths have been classified as others. Medical officers/facility nodal officers for MDSR must thus ensure that maternal deaths are appropriately classified to enable programme managers and district/state level authorities to take the necessary corrective actions based on the findings of the maternal death reviews.

As per the report of RGI in 2001–03, haemorrhage (38%), hypertensive disorders (5%), sepsis (11%), abortion (8%), obstructed labour (5%) and other conditions (34%) are the major causes of maternal mortality in India. In view of the fact that no further reports are available from the RGI, the following is an analysis of data available in MDSR software for 2015-16 to help program managers/medical officers understand the common causes of maternal deaths in our country.

It may, however, be noted that the list and percentages are only indicative and vary substantially across states depending on their MMR. Postpartum haemorrhage, antepartum haemorrhage and hypertensive disorders of pregnancy together continue to contribute to more than 30% of the total maternal deaths. Thromboembolism (4–5%), sepsis (3–4%), abortion (3–4%) and obstructed labour (around 2%) are other key direct obstetric causes of maternal death. Apart from these, *severe anaemia (25%)*, hepatic disorders (4%), respiratory disorders (2–3%), infectious diseases of liver (2–3%), congenital heart disease (1–2%), cardiomyopathy (1–2%), renal disorders (1–2%) and malaria (1%)/ tuberculosis (1%) are the key indirect obstetric causes of maternal deaths. Non-obstetric surgical causes account for nearly 3.5% of the maternal deaths. Strategies for reduction of MMR are to be designed based on the analysis of the cause of death and it is thus crucial that adequate attention is given to identification of cause of death.

It is recommended that maternal deaths must be classified on the basis of ICD-10. Action-oriented review mechanisms are the key to health systems improvement. Reviewing the MDSR data and using it for improved planning and instituting corrective measures is the most important aspect of the maternal death review.

While a biological complication is assigned as a cause of death, in fact most maternal deaths result from a chain of events that include many social, cultural and medical factors. Some of these can be prevented by taking action at one or more of the links in the chain of events that result in death, with a focus on the three delays in a mother receiving care for a complication. Social and cultural factors that may contribute to delay include:

a. First delay—decision-making process, not recognizing or understanding the danger signs, using traditional home care or informal service providers. Low education and poverty could aggravate this.
b. Second delay—lack of transport, poor roads, long commute to the nearest health facility, or delay in organizing funds if they have to pay for it.
c. Third delay—lack of medicines, blood, consumables, skilled manpower, etc., at the health facility.

Analysis involves circumstances of each death, identification of avoidable factors and action to improve care at all levels of the health system, from home to hospital.

Many of the findings will reflect upon the strength and functioning of the public healthcare delivery system.

Two types of data are generated from MDSR analysis—quantitative and qualitative (Table 10.1)

Qualitative analysis provides deep insight into the maternal death and suggests the program officers at block and district levels and service providers at each facility where maternal death

Table 10.1: Data analysis

Quantitative indicators, e.g.		Qualitative indicators, e.g.
Process indicators	Programme indicators	
a. Number of maternal deaths reported vs apprehended deaths	a. Place of delivery	a. Identification of complications during ANC
b. Number of maternal deaths investigated in district	b. Place of death	b. Care provided in the referred facilities
	c. Out of pocket expenditure	c. Money spent in seeking care
c. Number of facilities conducting FBMDSR	d. Number of cases received three antenatal check ups	d. Delay in identification of danger signs and decision making
d. % of maternal deaths reviewed by death review committee	e. Number of cases received PNC	e. Delay in reaching at appropriate facility
e. % of maternal deaths reviewed by DQAC	f. Mode of transport used and time taken to reach the facility	f. Delay in initiating treatment at the health facility

has happened, to take immediate corrective actions. Quantitative indicators are required to have a glimpse on implementation of the maternal death review system/program in the district/state. The quantitative indicators also provide information on whether the issue identified by qualitative analysis in a particular block or district is a general issue for the state that requires a policy change or not.

Qualitative data is generated from the case studies. Each case investigated at community and facility levels together completes the case and gives in-depth understanding of circumstances which lead to death. The data available at each level of maternal death review is different and this will define the type of analysis possible at those levels.

Analysis of Maternal Deaths Investigated

Analysis should be holistic (which captures the big picture), focused (only events directly contributing to death is discussed), normative (care provided is compared with standards/ GOI guidelines) and synthetic (groups problems into general categories).

Action Planning

Adopting a 'one size fits all' approach would be quite unwise for a country as large and diverse as ours. This is particularly true at this juncture when on one hand, high focus states such as Assam and Uttar Pradesh struggle with an MMR of more than 280/lakh live births and on the other hand, states such as Kerala, Maharashtra, Tamil Nadu and Andhra Pradesh have achieved the MMR level of below 100.

Considering this, it is important for us to learn from a large multi-country survey on Maternal and Newborn Health, conducted by the World Health Organization and its partners, which reflects a phenomenon called '*Obstetric Transition*'. As per the survey, "there is a change in the causes of maternal deaths as countries gradually shift from high maternal mortality to low maternal mortality. There is transition from predominance of direct obstetric causes of maternal mortality to an increasing proportion of indirect causes, non-communicable causes.

Overall five stages of obstetric transition have been defined as follows:
- Stage I (MMR>1000 maternal deaths per 100 000 live births)
- Stage II (MMR 999–300 maternal deaths per 100 000 live births)
- Stage III (MMR 299–50 maternal deaths per 100 000 live births)
- Stage IV (MMR <50 maternal deaths per 100 000 live births)
- Stage V (MMR lower than five maternal deaths per 100 000 live births)
India falls in stage III of the transition.

States with High MMR
- Ensure quality antenatal care (ANC), timely detection, basic management and timely referral of complicated cases, assured transport with wide awareness to the people on toll free number.
- Identify areas with high home deliveries and focus on increasing institutional deliveries and skilled attendance at birth in these areas. Introduce home-based distribution of misoprostol in these areas and simultaneously focus on strengthening health facilities in the nearby areas for provision of basic obstetric care.
- Focus on quality 'care at birth' including skilled attendance at birth. Plan for training/handhold the health workers for improving intrapartum care at health facilities.
- Labour room protocols have to be in place, adherence to infection prevention measures and protocols must be a priority. Labour room staff must be trained and not rotated.
- Focus on ensuring availability of comprehensive emergency obstetric care (CEmOC) services. States must monitor the functionality of identified first referral units (FRUs) to ensure that there is at least one FRU/5 lakh population. States may, however, need additional FRUs in hand to reach areas and hilly areas with sparse population based on time to care approach.
- Good quality PNC both at facility and at home ensured.
- Focus on availability of PPIUCD services in these areas.
- Focus on action on social determinants such as age at marriage in collaboration with concerned departments of the government.

Committees and Nodal Persons for MDSR (Flowchart 10.1)
1. National level Maternal Death Surveillance and Response Committee (NMDSRC)
2. State Level Taskforce (SLT)
3. State Level Monitoring and Review Committee for MDSR (SMRC-MDSR)

Nodal Persons for Implementing MDSR at Various Levels
Training is a key step for building the capacity of the human resources involved in implementation, good quality monitoring and review for taking corrective actions with ultimate objective of reducing the burden of maternal death in the states and UTs.

MDSR Guidelines as per State Level Workshop Held in Pune on 29/6/2019
- Every maternal death to be informed to State authorities within 24 hours in Form 1
- PPH box and eclampsia kit to be available at all centres

Flowchart 10.1

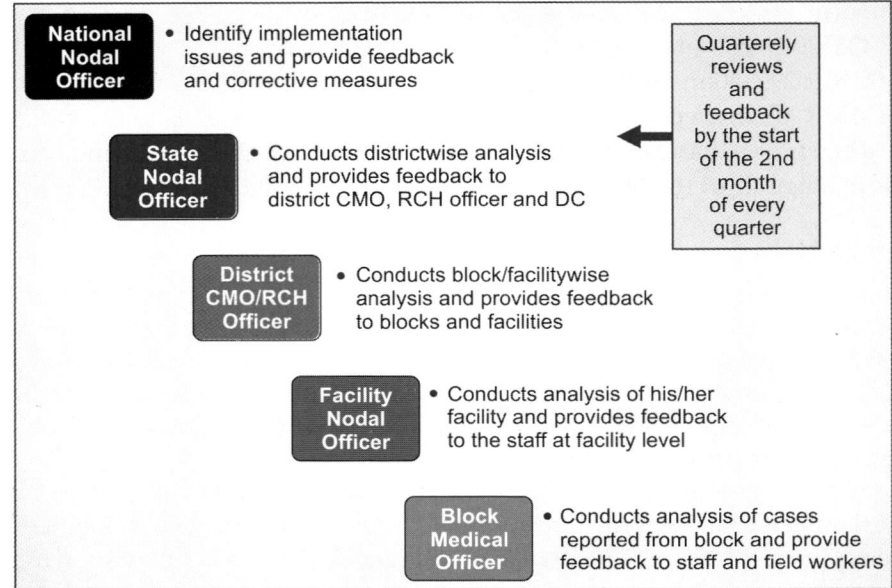

Maternal Death Notification Form

Sr. No.	Activity	Details/Remark
1.	Name of District/ Corporation	
2.	Name of Block/Facility	
3.	Name of the deceased Woman	
4.	Name of Husband	
5.	Address	
6.	Date and Time of Death	
7.	Place of Death 1. Home 2. Health Facility 3. Others	
8.	When did Death occur 1. During Pregnancy 2. During Delivery 3. Within 42 days after delivery 4. Others	
9.	Name of reporting Person	
10.	Brief history	

Signature of reporting persons

Designation:

Date: To be submitted to district nodal officer within 24 hours of maternal death. All other MDR Reporting Formats can be obtained from the MDSR Guidelines 2017 by National Health Mission.

- Delayed cord clamping and AMTSL
- District Quality Assurance Committee to meet monthly for analysis and review of maternal deaths
- Referral protocol for high risk cases
- One ICU bed to be reserved for obstetric cases. This ICU should be fully equipped.
- While sending the patient in 108 Ambulance, carry Inj. Pitocin in a vaccine carrier.
- Gynaecologist from Government Medical College to be called for DQAC.
- 24-Column Line list of each maternal mortality case to be filled correctly and completely.
- Summary of cases and observations and suggestions of DQAC to be sent to state authorities.
- All districts and corporations to complete MDSR training.

BIBLIOGRAPHY

1. Arora P. Maternal Mortality - Indian Scenario. Med J Armed Forces India. 2005 Jul;61(3):214-5. doi: 10.1016/S0377-1237(05)80155-8. Epub 2011 May 30. PMID: 27407761; PMCID: PMC4925460.
2. Chawla Sushil, T. Jose, Paul Manish – Critical Care in Obstetrics – Where are we. Official Journal of FOGSI 2018 May-June; 68(3).
3. Guidelines for MDSR by National Health Mission 2017.
4. Implementing maternal death surveillance and response: a review of lessons from country case studies. Helen Smith, Charles Ameh, Natalie Roos, Matthews Mathai and Nynke van den Broek; BMC Pregnancy and Childbirth volume 17, Article number: 233 (2017).
5. Moving from maternal death review to surveillance and response: A paradigm shift. Kansal A, Garg S, Sharma M. Indian J Public Health. 2018 Oct-Dec;62(4):299-301.Doi:10.4103/ijph.IJPH_37_18.
6. State Family Welfare Bureau Pune Circular dated 19-09-2019/58152-253.
7. State Family Welfare Bureau Pune Circular dated 05-08-2019 47205-309 containing Minutes of the MDSR Meeting held on 29-06-2019.

Chapter 11

Maternal Death Review: Facility-Based MDR

○ Deepika Nandanwar Sadawarte   ○ Mandar K Sadawarte   ○ YS Nandanwar

WHO commends India for its groundbreaking progress in recent years in reducing the maternal mortality ratio (MMR) by 77%, from 556 per 100 000 live births in 1990 to 130 per 100 000 live births in 2016. India's present MMR is below the Millennium Development Goal (MDG) target and puts the country on track to achieve the Sustainable Development Goal (SDG) target of an MMR below 70 by 2030. This achievement is possible due to combined efforts of every healthcare professional in proper and timely reporting to respective authorities.

Four key actions are responsible for India's remarkable achievement:
1. India has made a concerted push to increase access to quality maternal health services. Since 2005, coverage of essential maternal health services has doubled, while the proportion of institutional deliveries in public facilities has almost tripled, from 18% in 2005 to 52% in 2016 (if private facilities are included, institutional deliveries now stand at 79%).
2. State-subsidized demand-side financing like the Janani Shishu Suraksha Karyakram, which allows all pregnant women delivering in public health institutions to free transport and no-expense delivery, including caesarean section, has largely closed the urban–rural divide traditionally seen in institutional births. Overall, 75% of rural births are now supervised, as compared to 89% of urban deliveries.
3. India has put significant emphasis on mitigating the social determinants of maternal health. Women in India are more literate than ever, with 68% now able to read and write. They are also entering marriage at an older age, with just 27% now wedded before the age of 18.
4. Government of India, Ministry of Health and Family Welfare, has decided to investigate maternal deaths at various levels like community based and facility based.

Facility-Based Maternal Death Review

Facility-based maternal deaths reviews (FDMDR) will be taken up for all teaching hospitals, referral hospitals and other hospitals (district, subdistrict, CHCs) where more than 500 deliveries are conducted in a year.

Steps

1. All maternal deaths occurring in the hospital, including abortions and ectopic gestation related deaths, in pregnant women or within 42 days after termination of pregnancy irrespective of duration or site of pregnancy should be reported immediately by the medical officer who has treated the mother and was on duty at the time of occurrence of death to the Facility Nodal officer (FNO). In medical colleges, the Professor and Head, Department of Obstetrics and Gynaecology, should do the reporting.
2. The FNO of the hospital should report maternal death to the District Nodal Officer (DNO) and State Nodal Officer by telephone/fax within 24 hours of the occurrence of death. The nodal officer of the hospital should complete the Primary Informant Format (Form 1) and send it to the DNO within 24 hours of the occurrence of maternal death.
3. Any maternal death which occurred in the hospital should be immediately investigated within 24 hours by the medical officer/teacher who had treated the mother and was on duty at the time of occurrence of death using the Facility Based Maternal Death Review (FBMDR) Format (Form 4).
4. The form would be submitted under the guidance and approval of the FNO. The FBMDR format should be filled in triplicate, one copy would be retained by the FNO, one would be sent by the FNO to the DNO within 24 hours and the other to the Facility Maternal Death Review (MDR) committee of the hospital.
5. All medical officers, teachers, postgraduate students and administration of the college in the facility must be aware about the MDR program and oriented on the use of the FBR form. All pregnant and postpartum women that were treated, and died, in other departments, e.g. medicine, intensive care areas like ICCU, IRCU, MICU, neurology, trauma, etc., and OB/GYN department, must also be reported and investigated.
6. All pregnant and postpartum women that were treated, and died, in other departments than the OB/GYN department, must also be reported and investigated.
7. MO has to prepare a case summary and send it to the facility based maternal death review committee along with a copy of the case sheet. The case sheet should be numbered and have the patient name and registration number on each page.
8. Each health facility reporting maternal death will keep a register of all maternal deaths in the facility (Form 3: Line listing of maternal deaths). Even if there is no death in a month, the facility should report that there was no death in that month (nil death report).
9. FNO will be the nodal person for organizing the FBMDR Committee at the hospital. He/she will attend the FBMDR Committee meeting at the district level and also the review conducted by the District Magistrate (DM). Another senior officer may be nominated in his/her absence. In Mumbai, this is being done at F South Parel and Mantralaya.

10. The FDMDR Committee is constituted by Government of Maharashtra, Ministry of Health and Family Welfare. The members nominated for 3 years are: Gynaecologist, anaesthesiologist, pathologist, physician, nurse, layman, member of obstetrics society or IMA. EHO is chairperson and special officer secretary. AMC (medical education and major peripheral hospitals), all Deans and EHO are in steering committee for proper functioning.

Office of DNO will receive the notification form (Form 1) from FNO within 24 hours of maternal death
↓
Office of DNO will receive the investigation form (Form 4) from FNO within 48 hours of maternal death
↓
FNO will also send the line list of maternal deaths (Form 3) electronically to DNO every month. In case there is no death in a month, the facility should report that there was no death in that month (nil death report)
↓
DNO will prepare the line list of all the maternal deaths (Form 3) received from all the facilities conducting MDSR including facilities in urban area
↓
By the 7th of every month, line list of maternal deaths (Form 3) will be updated and submitted to SNO
↓
All the data will be entered in the MDSR software.

Cause of Death: Classification

Direct Obstetric Deaths

Maternal deaths resulting from obstetric complications of the pregnant state (pregnancy, labour and the purperium), from interventions, omissions or incorrect treatment, or from a chain of events resulting from any of the above.

A classification of dual causes of maternal death is more useful. It allows for two levels of causes: An essential level and a specific level. The essential level identifies a minimum list of causes that can be identified in all settings, whatever the level of sophistication of the cause of death.

The list of specific causes improves the degree of detail achieved. Examples: Antepartum haemorrhage following placenta previa, postpartum haemorrhage following prolonged labour, PPH following cervical tear, ecclampsia, sepsis following prior foetal death.

DEFINITIONS

Maternal Death

The death of a woman while pregnant or within 42 days of termination of pregnancy, irrespective of the duration and site of the pregnancy, from any cause related to or aggravated by the pregnancy or its management but not from accidental or incidental causes (WHO).

Maternal Mortality Ratio (MMR)

The maternal mortality ratio is the number of maternal deaths per 100,000 live births per year (WHO).

Indirect Obstetric Deaths

Maternal deaths resulting from previous existing disease or disease that developed during pregnancy and that was not due to direct obstetric causes but was aggravated by the physiological effects of pregnancy. Indirect maternal deaths are relatively few in number. The classification should list the causes of importance according to the local epidemiology of diseases. The diseases representing relatively large proportions should be listed as such rather than hidden in a broader category. Examples: Heart diseases, Hepatitis, malaria, TB, AIDS, tetanus (WHO).

Non-obstetric Causes

Death of pregnant woman resulting from accidental or incidental causes. (Examples: Accident, assault, suicide, snakebite, burns.)

MODULES

1. Module I
Should be used for collection of general information for all maternal deaths irrespective of whether deaths occurred during antenatal or intranatal or postnatal period or due to abortion.

2. Module II
Should be used for the deaths occurring during the antenatal period including abortion.

3. Module III
Should be used for the deaths occurring during delivery or postnatal period.

MDR Case Summary

To be filled by the medical officer and the investigation team for each maternal death.

1. *Delay in Seeking Care*
Unawareness of danger signs, illiteracy and ignorance, delay in decision making, nil birth preparedness, beliefs and customs, non-availability of healthcare professional, any other/specify _____ Fill in appropriate cause of Delay 1.

2. *Delay in Reaching First Level Health Facility*
Delay in getting transport, delay in mobilizing funds, not reaching appropriate facility in time, difficulty in, any other/specify _____ Fill in appropriate cause of Delay 2.

3. Delay in Receiving Adequate Care in Facility

Delay in initiating treatment, substandard care in hospital, lack of blood, equipment and drugs, lack of adequate funds, any other/specify ——Fill in appropriate cause of Delay 3.

Maternal death after the sterilization operation also has to follow the same procedures and as per the guidelines given in the "Standards for Female and Male Sterilization Services"published by Division of Research Studies and Standards: Ministry of Health and Family Welfare, Govt. of India, Oct 2012. It is essential to have a surgeon/gynaecologist on panel for compensation to client as per government programme, by ICICI Lombard Insurance Company.

A study of Near Miss cases as per NIRRH project reflects more details of causes with a proof of prevention of death will be the best guideline to be implemented to prevent the maternal death. For example, golden hour treatment, prevention of antenatal preventable conditions, institutional deliveries, identification of high-risk cases and early reference, blood and blood products availability, prostaglandins availability, qualified trained obstetricians with good infrastructure. These all prevent approximately 70% of the deaths (unpublished data).

Maternal Deaths Reporting: Practical Aspects

There are not many Acts for the maternal deaths directly but be aware that the cases of maternal deaths can be fitted in Acts/legislation in many ways as desired by lawyers. In the absence of any act, the guidelines and rules made by the Government are treated as the law. The cases are investigated by designated members of committee.

BIBLIOGRAPHY

1. A study of Near Miss cases as per NIRRH project.
2. http://www.censusindia.gov.in/vital_statistics/SRS_Bulletins/MMR%20Bulletin-2014-16.pdf
   Forms: Available online from www.nhm.gov.in: maternal health: guidelines: guideline for MDSR
3. http://www.gujhealth.gov.in.
4. Maternal Death Review GuideBook (WHO)
5. Maternal Health Division Guidebook, Ministry of Health and Family Welfare, Government of India, Nirman Bhawan, New Delhi.
6. Standards for Female and male sterilization Services published by Division of Research Studies and Standards: Ministry of Health and Family Welfare, Govt. of India Oct 2012.
7. Textbook of Preventive and Social Medicine- AFMC.

Maternal Death Review: Facility-Based MDR

Form 1
Notification Form

Format to be filled by Primary informant for all Women's Death (15-49) years

S. No.		Place of Current Residence	Native Place
1	Name of State		
2	Name of District		
3	Name of Block		
4	Name of village/ Description of location		
5	Name of the deceased woman		
6	Name of Husband		
7	Name of Father		
8	Age of the woman		
9	MCTS ID		
10	Mobile No		
11	Date and time of death	Date ....DD/ MM/ YYYY Time _____ : _____ am/pm	
12	Place of death	Yes	No (tick)
	I. Home		
	II. Health Facility		
	III. Transit		
	IV. Others		
13	When did death occur	Yes	No (tick)
	a. During pregnancy		
	b. During delivery		
	c. Within 42 days after delivery		
	d. During abortion or within 6 weeks after abortion		

| If either a, b, c, d, =yes in Q 13: **Suspected maternal death** |
| If all- a, b, c, d, =no in Q13 ; **Non- maternal death** |

Name of reporting Person: _____

Designation: _____

Signature of reporting person:

Date:

Verification by ANM of the respective Sub-center that death of women occurred during pregnancy or within 42 days of delivery/abortion:

Name of the sub center:

                                      Signature: _____

                                      Name: _____

                                      Date: _____

Form 2
Block Level MDR Register for All Women's Death (15-49 years)

(Fill in one form for every month)

Name of Block _____

District _____ State _____

Month _____ Year _____

S. No.	Name of deceased	Age	Date of death	Address	Husband's name	Cause of death (tick √)		Name/ designation of Primary informant (Annex 6)	Date of field investigation	If died due to maternal causes, specify reasons	Action Taken
						Maternal	Non-maternal				
1.											
2.											
3.											
4.											
5.											

Signature of MO I/C of the block with date:

Form 3
MDR Line Listing Form for All Cases of Maternal Deaths

Line listing for use by ANM, BMO, FNO and DNO

District _____ State _____

FB MDR: Name of facility: _____ or CB MDR: _____

SHC/Block _____

S. No.	Date of death	Name of deceased	Place of death			When did the death occur				Probable cause of death	Status of newborn (Delivery outcome)	Name of investigator/ date of interview
			Home	Health facility	In transit	During pregnancy	During delivery	During abortion or within 6 weeks after the abortion	Within 42 days after delivery			

Name of reporting person: _____ Signature: _____

Designation: _____ Date of reporting: _____

Form 4
Confidential

Facility Based Maternal Death Review Form

Name and Type of Health Facility (specify)_____

Address_____

Name of Nodal Person _____ Contact No_____

FOR OFFICE USE ONLY

FBMDR No. (Specific to the Place)   MCTS No   Month   Year

Please fill up the Performa given below

NOTE:
- MDR Number must be put serially 0001 & so on.
- This form must be filled for all Maternal Deaths.
- Mark with √ wherever applicable.
- For Date use Day/Month/Year format. For time use 24 hours clock format.
- Complete within 24 hrs.
- Make 2 photocopies & send original to MRD, a copy to DNO, and one retained with Nodal Officer for further action.

Background information of deceased Mother

Full Name_____ Age _____ Inpatient No_____

Medico-legal admission: Yes ☐ No ☐

Complete Address _____

Contact/ Mobile No_____

Education: Illiterate ☐   Upto 5th class ☐   6th to 12th class ☐   Beyond 12th class ☐

Below Poverty Line: BPL Certified ☐   Self certified BPL ☐   Not BPL ☐

1. a. Date and Time of admission: Day☐☐ Month☐☐ Yr.☐☐ at Hours☐☐ Min.☐☐
   b. Date and time of Death: Day☐☐ Month☐☐ Yr.☐☐ at Hours☐☐ Min.☐☐
   c. Duration of Hospital stay: ☐☐ Days ☐☐ Hours
   d. Duration of ICU stay: Days ☐☐   Hours ☐☐ if any

Maternal Death Review: Facility-Based MDR

	Days	Hrs.	N.A.	DNK
e. Admission- delivery interval:	☐☐	☐☐	☐☐	☐
f. Admission – death interval	☐☐	☐☐	☐☐	☐

g. Outcome of pregnancy:

1) Abortion ☐	2) Ectopic ☐	3) Live birth ☐
4) Still birth ☐	5) Undelivered ☐	

2. On Admission
a. Complaints at time of admission: _____
b. Obstetric formula on admission   **M F**
1. Gravida ☐☐   2. Para ☐☐   3. Abortions ☐☐   4. No. of Living children ☐☐
c. Period of gestation:

1) Before 22 weeks ☐	2) Antenatal 22-34 weeks ☐	3) Antenatal ≥34 weeks ☐	4) Intrapartum ☐
5) Post- Partum up to 24hrs ☐	6) Post-natal 24hrs- 1 week ☐	7) Post-natal- More than 1 week to 42 days ☐	

3. Condition on Admission: 1) Stable ☐   2) Semi conscious responds to verbal commands ☐   3) Semi conscious responds to painful stimuli ☐   4) Unconscious ☐
5) Brought dead ☐

a. **Referral:** If referred from outside: i. No. of places visited prior ☐

b. Please fill the table below for the details on transport, referral and type of care given			
Place	**Home/ Village**	**Facility 1**	**Facility 2**	**Facility 3**
Date (DD/MM/YY)				
Time of onset of complication or onset of labour				
Time of calling/ arrival of transport				
Transport used/type				
Time to reach				
Money spent on transport (Rs.)				
Name of Facility/ Level of referral				
Attended by Doctor/ nurse/ other staff/none				

Place	**Home/ Village**	**Facility 1**	**Facility 2**	**Facility 3**
Reason for referral				
Referral slip (given or not, if yes, attach)				
Treatment given				
Money spent on treatment/ medicine/ Diagnostics				
Time spent in facility				

4. Diagnosis at time of admission:
(Please make sure to fill the table with underlying cause given for each condition)

S. No.	Diagnosis	Underlying Cause		
1.	Hemorrhage ☐	I. Abortion ☐		
		II. Ectopic Pregnancy ☐		
		III. Gestational Trophoblastic Disease ☐		
		IV. Antepartum Bleeding	a) Placental causes- Placenta Previa ☐	
			- Placental abruption ☐	
			b) Late pregnancy Bleeding other than placental causes-	
			- Scar dehiscence ☐	
			- Rupture uterus ☐	
			- Others, ☐ Specify_____	
		V. Intrapartum Bleeding		
		VI. Postpartum bleeding- Atonic ☐ Traumatic ☐ Mixed ☐		
2.	Hypertensive disorders of pregnancy ☐	i. Gestational Hypertension ☐	ii. Pre-eclampsia ☐	
		iii. Eclampsia ☐	iv. Others ☐	
3.	Labour related Disorders ☐	i. Normal labour ☐	ii Prolonged / Obstructed labour ☐	
		iii. Inversion of Uterus ☐	iv. Retained placenta ☐	
		v. Any other ☐		
4.	Medical Disorders ☐	i. Anaemia ☐	ii. Heart disease ☐	iii. TB ☐
		iv. Diabetes ☐	v. Others ☐	

S. No.	Diagnosis	Underlying Cause	
5.	Infection ☐	I. Post abortal ☐	a) Viral such as Hepatitis/HIV AIDS/ Others, ☐
		II. Antepartum ☐	b) Malaria, ☐
		III. Intrapartum ☐	c) Dengue, ☐
		IV. Post-partum ☐	d) Lower Respiratory Tract Infection, ☐
			e) Other infections, ☐ Specify_____
6.	Incidental/ Accidental Disorders E.g. Surgical including Iatrogenic, Trauma, Violence, Anaesthetic complications, ☐	Specify	
7.	Any other, ☐	Specify	

2. Abortion (to be filled if applicable)

a. Spontaneous ☐ Induced ☐
i. If spontaneous, - Complete ☐ Incomplete ☐
ii. If induced   -Legal ☐   Illegal ☐
b. What was the procedure adopted? Medical methods ☐   MVA ☐   D&E/ S&E ☐
                                              Extra Amniotic Installation ☐ Hysterotomy ☐   Others ☐
c. Post Abortal Period   Uneventful ☐   Sepsis ☐   Hemorrhage ☐   Others ☐
d. Was the termination procedure done in more than one center   Yes ☐   No ☐
(If yes, specify the centres visited before coming to this facility)..
....

Maternal Death Review: Facility-Based MDR

3. Antenatal Care

a. Did she receive ANC? Yes ☐ No ☐ Don't know ☐
b. If Yes, Type of Facility: SC ☐ PHC ☐ CHC ☐ SDH ☐ DH ☐ Medical College ☐ Private hospital ☐ Others ☐ specify_____
c. Services provided by: ANM ☐ MO ☐ Obstetrician ☐ AYUSH ☐ Nurse ☐ Other specialists, ☐ specify_____
d. If yes, was she told about any disorder/complication? Yes ☐ No ☐ Don't know ☐
e. If yes, what was the risk factor identified?

1. Abortion ☐	2. Ectopic pregnancy ☐	3. Vesicular Mole ☐	4. APH ☐
5. Hydramnios / Oligohydramnios ☐	6. Short stature ☐	7. PIH/PE ☐	8. Previous C section ☐
9. Multiple pregnancy ☐	10. Grand multi ☐	11. Abnormal presentation/position ☐	12. Big baby ☐
13. Anemia ☐	14. Diabetes/GDM ☐	15. Medical conditions (Specify____) ☐	16. Others (Specify____) ☐

4. DELIVERY, PUERPERIUM AND NEONATAL INFORMATION   **If applicable**

a. Did she have labour pains? Yes ☐ No ☐
b. If yes, was a partograph used to monitor labour?
i.) Past facility: Yes ☐ No ☐ Don't know ☐
ii.) Current facility: Yes ☐ No ☐

c. Complications during labour:

1. Eclampsia/pre-ecclampsia ☐	2. Prolonged labour ☐	3. Obstructed labour /Rupture Uterus ☐	4. Intra partum Hemorrhage ☐
5. Inversion of Uterus ☐	6. IP sepsis ☐	7. Others ☐ Specify_____	

d. Mode of Delivery

1. Undelivered		☐
2. Vaginal	a. Normal - With episiotomy b. Assisted - Forceps - Vacuum c. Breech d. Multiple Pregnancy	☐ ☐ ☐ ☐ ☐ ☐ ☐
3. Caesarean Section	Elective	☐
	Emergency	☐
4. Laparotomy	Rupture uterus	☐
	*Ectopic Pregnancy	☐
5. Indication (CS/Instrumental)		☐

* Although in Ectopic pregnancy woman does not deliver but fetus may be removed during Laparotomy

e. Anaesthesia (any adverse reaction):

a) General Anaesthesia ☐	b) Regional Epidural / Spinal ☐	c) Local ☐

f. In which phase of labor did she develop complications?

a) First stage ☐	b) Second stage ☐	c) Third stage ☐	d) Post Birth ☐		
			a. Within ≤ 6 hrs. of birth ☐	b. > 6 - ≤ 24 hrs. of birth ☐	c. > 24 hrs. after birth ☐

g. Neonatal Outcome: Alive ☐   Fresh Still birth ☐
                        Macerated still birth   Neonatal death ☐

h. If baby died, probable cause of death:

1. Birth Asphxia ☐	2. Respiratory distress ☐	3. Aspiration including MAS ☐	4. Sepsis ☐
5. Cong Anomalies ☐	6. Preterm ☐	7. Others ☐ Specify_____	

i. Postnatal period: - Uneventful Eventful ☐
                   - If Eventful, specify probable cause of death: ☐

1. PPH ☐	2. PE / Eclampsia ☐	3. CVA/Pulmonary Embolism ☐	4. Sepsis/ ARDS ☐
5. Anemia ☐	6. Post op complication ☐	7. Medical conditions Specify_____ ☐	8. Others Specify_____ ☐

5. INTERVENTIONS (Tick appropriate box), Specify other in the last row

Early pregnancy	Antenatal	Intrapartum	Postpartum	Anaesthesia/ICU
1. Evacuation ☐ 2. Trans-fusion ☐ 3. Laparotomy/laparoscopy ☐ 4. Hyster-ectomy ☐	1. Trans-fusion ☐ 2. Version ☐ 3. Other surgeries ☐	1. Instrumental del. ☐ 2. Caesarean section ☐ 3. Hyster-ectomy ☐ 4. Manual removal of placenta ☐ 5. Conservative surgery ☐ 6. Trans-fusion ☐	1. Removal of retained POC ☐ 2. Laparo-tomy ☐ 3. Hyster-ectomy ☐ 4. Trans-fusion ☐	1. Anaesthesia -GA ☐ 2. Spinal ☐ 3. Local ☐ 4. Epidural ☐ 5. ICU monitoring ☐

a. Blood transfusion given? Yes ☐   No ☐
b. If yes, No of units ☐☐☐☐   Whole Blood ☐ /PRBC ☐ /FFP ☐ /Platelets ☐ /Cryo ☐
c. Specify if any transfusion reaction occurred?: Yes ☐   No ☐

6. Primary diagnosis/condition leading to death_____

7. **CAUSE OF DEATH:**_____

Part 1: Antecedent causes (Please mention the cause of death from Box below)
     a. Due to or as a consequence of _____
     b. Due to or as a consequence of _____
     c. Due to or as a consequence of _____

8. **IN YOUR OPINION WERE ANY OF THESE FACTORS PRESENT?**

System	Example	Y	N	Not known
Personal/Family	Delay in woman seeking help			
	Refusal of treatment or admission			
Logistical Problems	Lack of transport from home to health care facility			
	Lack of transport between health care facilities			
	Lack of assured referral system			
Facilities	Lack of facilities, equipment or consumable			
	Lack of blood/ blood products			
	Lack of OT availability			
Health personnel problems	Lack of human resources			
	Lack of Anesthetist			
	Lack of Obstetricians			
	Lack of expertise, training or education			

9. **AUTOPSY:** Performed ☐ Not performed ☐
- **If performed please report the final diagnosis and send the detailed report later**

_____

_____

10. **CASE SUMMARY** (please supply a short summary of the events surrounding hospital stay and the death of the patient)

[   ]

Form filled by the MO on duty   **Nodal Officer of the Hospital:**

Name & Signature   **Name & Signature**

Form 6
MDR Case Summary

Name of the Block/PHC/District OR/Name of facility				
Particulars of the Deceased Woman	MCTS ID	Name _____ Age:	Religion:	Caste:
Address (when death occurred)	Place of Residence:		Native Place:	
Place of Death				
Date and Time of death	D D M M Y Y Y Y	At	H H : M M .AM/PM	
Timing of Death	Pregnancy	During or within 6 weeks of abortion	In labour or during Delivery	Within 1 week after delivery	7 - 42 days after Delivery
Obstetric History	Gravida	Para	Previous Abortions	Infant outcome	Number of alive children
			Spontaneous	Induced		
Investigation	Date of interview	Date of Interview-2 (if second visit made)	Name and contact details of main respondents:		

Maternal Death Review: Facility-Based MDR

1. **Delay in seeking care**
   - Unawareness of danger signs
   - Illiteracy & Ignorance
   - Delay in decision making
   - No birth preparedness
   - Beliefs and customs
   - Lack of assured services
   - Unawareness about services available in nearby facility
   - Any other, specify_____

2. **Delay in reaching health facility**
   - Delay in getting transport for first facility
   - Delay in mobilizing funds
   - Not reaching appropriate/referral facility in time
   - Difficult terrain
   - Any other, specify_____

3. **Delay in receiving adequate care in facility**
   - Delay in initiating treatment
   - Substandard treatment in hospital
   - Lack of blood, equipments and drugs
   - Lack of adequate funds
   - Any other, specify_____

_____

Probable direct obstetric cause of death: _____

_____

_____

Indirect obstetric cause of death: _____

_____

_____

Contributory causes of death: _____

_____

_____

Initiatives suggested: _____

_____

Name and designation of investigation team:

1. Name:_____ Designation: _____

2. Name:_____ Designation: _____

3. Name:_____ Designation: _____

Signatures and Name of Block Medical Officer/Facility Nodal Officer (with stamp)

Chapter 12

Guidelines for Postmortem in Obstetric Deaths

○ Kusum Jashnanai

Autopsy is called

The House of Wisdom, because
Death does not lie, where
Pride is laid low,
Humility triumphs
Obscure is brought to light'
Truth is made simple, and the
Most arrogant diagnosticians strike their breasts and
Bite the cement floor

—Anonymous

Even in an era of declining autopsy rates, the autopsy continues to play a prominent role in medical quality improvement, particularly in healthcare facilities that support educational or academic programs. Despite advances in imaging techniques and laboratory diagnosis, an autopsy is still the most accurate way to identify the cause of death.

The autopsy in maternal death is in no way different from any other adult autopsy. However, maternal death autopsies assume greater significance than most other deaths since all the maternal autopsy reports are scrutinized closely in preparation for reports for the MCGM (Municipal Corporation of Greater Mumbai) Confidential Enquiry into the Maternal Death. Since these reports make recommendations for improving the obstetric practice, optimum quality of reports, clearly determining what actually happened to cause the death, are critical.

The first step in performing an autopsy is the review of the medical record. The pathologist must obtain a clear understanding of the patient's present and past medical history, therapeutic interventions, and the terminal events leading to the patient's death. Whether the delivery took place at home or in hospital, and whether patient transfer was involved. When drafting the final report, care needs to be taken over sensitive issues such as previous terminations and pregnancies if they may not be known to relatives.

Information on the delivery process, e.g. vaginal, caesarean, forceps, any blood transfusions given; Clinical and drug information on pre-existing medical conditions, including pre-eclampsia, renal disease, cardiac disease and hematological conditions such as sickle cell disease. Past or family history of thrombosis and thromboembolism.

The fetal/neonatal information is also relevant, e.g. infection peri-partum, small-for-dates, etc. It would be preferable if the pathologist can get in touch with the obstetrician/physician to discuss the case before beginning the prosection. The clinical team should be invited to visit the autopsy room during or after the autopsy.

External examination: Look for signs of pallor, icterus, edema feet, anasarca, any injuries, etc. External signs of disease should be sought, for example, vaginal discharge (genital tract infection and possible systemic sepsis), generalized bleeding from multiple sites (DIC) and examination of external genitalia for signs of injury which may be related to medical intervention, e.g. use of forceps and episiotomy.

Evisceration and organ dissection: After external assessment and before evisceration proceeds, any samples required for microbiological, biochemical or other analysis should be taken. In septic cases, blood sample for culture should be collected. Swabs from localized septic sites to be sampled for microbiological investigation. In cases of acute febrile illness, blood sample should be processed for MP, RMAT, dengue, etc. if not already done antemortem.

In situ examination: Amniotic fluid embolism (AFE), air embolism, pneumothorax and pulmonary thromboembolism (PTE) need to be tested on *in situ* examination. The buffy coat of blood sample from the pulmonary artery may reveal evidence of tell-tale fetal squames in patients suspected of death from AFE. Close inspection of the uterus, cervix, vagina and adjacent soft tissue for tears or rupture is mandatory to identify macroscopic evidence of AFE. The final diagnosis of AFE requires histopathologic examination of lung vasculature for presence of squames, fat, bile, etc. Particular attention should be paid to identifying the presence or absence of air embolism, pneumothorax, and pulmonary thromboembolism. The skin over the neck and anterior chest should initially be palpated for evidence of crepitus and soft tissue emphysema which may give a clue to an associated pneumothorax. The skin and subcutaneous tissue is then reflected from the midline to about the mid-axillary line and traction is then applied to produce an angle between chest wall and subcutaneous tissue. This area is then filled with water, and the intercostal muscles incised watching closely for air bubbles indicating an underlying pneumothorax. Air emboli usually occur during labor or surgical intervention in delivery of the baby or products after miscarriage. Air gains access to the venous circulation and travels to the right side of the heart where it interferes with blood flow and results in rapid collapse of the cardiovascular system. The sternum is then removed being careful not to puncture the pericardial sac. The anterior pericardium is now opened and water is introduced to fill the pericardial space. The right atrium and ventricle are incised and see for escape of any air bubbles. The great vessels of the heart especially pulmonary artery should be opened before removal of the heart from the body. A pulmonary artery saddle embolus may be identified or the presence of frothy blood within may be an indicator of air embolism.

Internal systemic examination: Examination of all the systems does not differ from any other autopsy. Particular attention must be paid in view of maternal death in all the following systems:

Central nervous system: Look for intracranial hemorrhage consequent upon eclampsia. Histologic examination is mandatory, since these hemorrhagic lesions can be a manifestation of metastatic choriocarcinoma. Infarction and sagittal sinus/cerebral venous thrombosis are other lesions to be looked for.

Cardiovascular system: The heart should be weighed and examined for irregularities in shape, which may indicate cardiomyopathy. In this condition, the heart becomes enlarged with left ventricular dysfunction and may be viral in etiology. There are no characteristic histologic features, but focal fibrosis, variability in myocyte caliber and scattered chronic inflammatory cells may be noted. Dilated cardiomyopathy is also recognized increasingly in association with HIV infection as this pandemic increasingly affects women. The valves should be examined for possible infective endocarditis and appropriate swabs taken for microbiological studies. Chronic rheumatic heart disease with mitral stenosis is often a surprise finding.

Respiratory system: The upper air passages and laryngeal inlet should be examined for trauma consequent upon intubation. Stomach contents may be present in the upper air passages; this finding needs to be interpreted with caution since regurgitation can occur during resuscitation measures and even after death by movement of the body. A more reliable guide to assess aspiration is a thorough histological examination of the lungs. Look for varying morphologic lesions of tuberculosis and angry red boggy lungs of acute respiratory distress syndrome (ARDS).

Gastrointestinal system: In situ, the stomach and intestines should be examined for gaseous distention which may indicate misplacement of the endotracheal tube. Perforative peritonitis can be a common finding in the intestines. The liver can be involved in a number of disease processes during pregnancy, including intrahepatic cholestasis, acute fatty liver of pregnancy (AFLP) and submassive to massive hepatic necrosis, especially in hepatitis E infection. It can be seriously affected in eclampsia. Frozen section of the liver with Oil Red O staining for fat is essential, as is 'routine' histological examination. Figure 12.1 shows a slice of liver with wrinkled capsule, and soft foldable hepatic parenchyma suggestive of massive necrosis, a common finding in viral hepatic necrosis. Hepatitis E infection is a common cause of hepatic necrosis with hepatic encephalopathy in pregnancy apart from HBV and HCV infections. Figure 12.2 shows a slice of liver which is enlarged and yellow suggestive of AFLP, commonly seen in third trimester of pregnancy and can be fatal.

Urinary system: The kidneys can be affected by several disease processes in pregnancy. The kidneys may show signs of acute pyelonephritis, eclampsia and renal cortical necrosis due to a number of causes. Appropriate histological examination is essential in all cases including diabetic mothers. Fibrin thrombi in the glomerular capillaries are an important histopathological

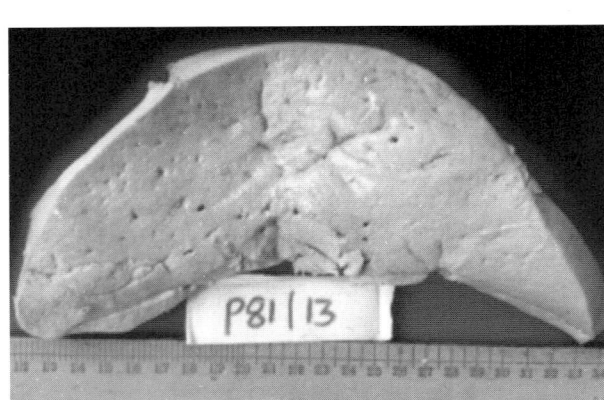

Fig. 12.1: A slice of liver with wrinkled capsule, and soft foldable hepatic parenchyma suggestive of massive necrosis, a common finding in viral hepatic necrosis. Hepatitis E infection is a common cause of hepatic necrosis with hepatic encephalopathy in pregnancy apart from HBV and HCV infections

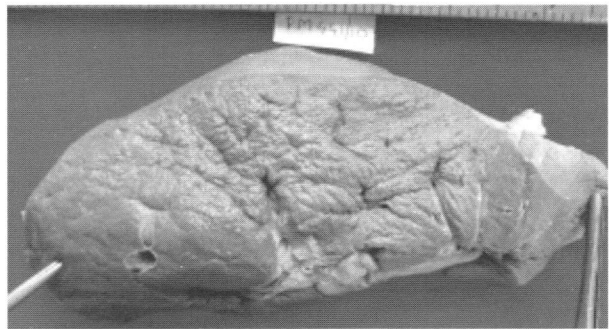

Fig. 12.2: A slice of liver which is enlarged and yellow suggestive of AFLP, commonly seen in third trimester of pregnancy and can be fatal

finding in DIC. Special stain Martius scarlet blue (MSB) for fibrin can be used to highlight these thrombi.

Genital tract: In any event, the cervix, vagina, uterus and placental site should be examined. Evidence should be sought for retained products of conception, abnormal placental adherence (accreta), placenta previa, rupture of uterine scar, retroplacental blood clot, etc. In cases of uterine rupture, the extent, size and weight/volume of blood clot/hemorrhage should be documented. The size and site of rupture; whether LSCS scar, previous myomectomy scar etc. should be noted. If placenta previa is suspected, ante-mortem ultrasound data should be sought in the notes before autopsy, and the uterus opened away from the site of placental attachment.

Figure 12.3 shows rupture of uterus along the anterolateral border. Histopathologic examination showed adherent placenta (placenta accreta) at the site of previous LSCS scar. The dead fetus was lying partly outside the uterus.

External examination should be followed by internal examination. On cut surface of uterus, the endometrial surface should be examined for any greenish yellow purulent exudate suggestive of puerperal sepsis. The myometrium and the serosal aspect should be examined for any yellow white areas of abscesses. Figure 12.4 shows presence of yellowish exudate over the endometrial surface. This was a case of home delivery followed by complaints of fever and abdominal pain few days postpartum for which she was admitted. The causes of death in such cases may vary from septic shock to DIC. Fallopian tube and ovary need to be examined properly in cases of ectopic pregnancy

Examination of products of conception: These include the placenta, membranes, fetal material and occasionally, molar tissue and other products of gestational trophoblastic disease.

Placenta, if available, should be subjected to standard examination, with measurements and weight, and histopathology for inflammation, infection, and placental bed arterial lesions.

Fetus: There may be a fetus retained within the mother; autopsy of the fetus is usually unnecessary as this will contribute little or nothing to the understanding of the mother's cause of death. Gender of the fetus along with the weight to be documented and any external anomalies to be looked for.

Review of the pathology of any previous surgical resection specimens of relevance to the pregnancy, e.g. obstetric hysterectomy specimen, products of conception may help. This may require liaison with other laboratories.

A provisional cause of death is given on completion of the autopsy after gross examination of various organs and clinicopathologic correlation. Sections are taken from each and every

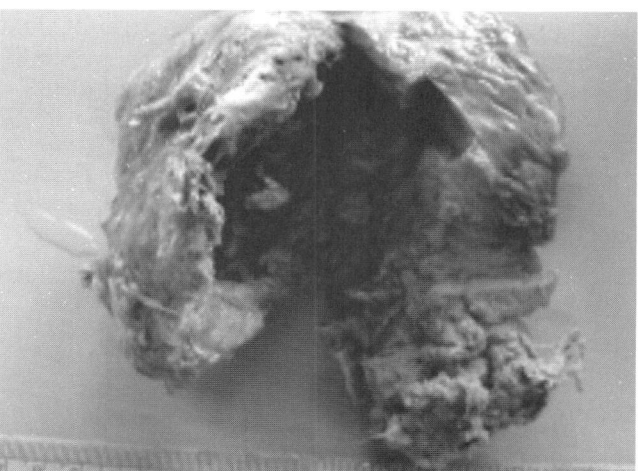

Fig. 12.3: Rupture of uterus along the anterolateral border. Histopathologic examination showed adherent placenta (placenta accreta) at the site of previous LSCS scar. The dead fetus was lying partly outside the uterus

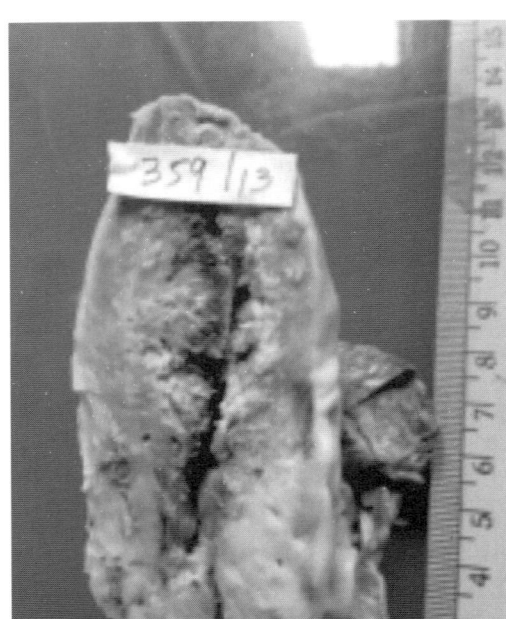

Fig. 12.4: Presence of yellowish exudate over the endometrial surface. This was a case of home delivery followed by complaints of fever and abdominal pain few days postpartum for which she was admitted. The causes of death in such cases may vary from septic shock to DIC. Fallopian tube and ovary need to be examined properly in cases of ectopic pregnancy

organ for histopathologic examination followed by final cause of death. The final autopsy report should be completed in 30 calendar days or less. Clinicians should receive their autopsy report while the clinical issues of the case are still fresh in their minds.

Anaesthetic deaths: These include those related to biochemical, toxicological or oxygenation problems which may not give rise to specific gross or microscopic findings even after thorough examination. Anaphylaxis and hyperthermia are other anaesthetic complications leading to death.

Criminal (unsafe) abortion is one of the important causes of maternal death. Medical or surgical termination of pregnancy should receive attention for
  i. Uterus rupture from prostaglandin induction
  ii. Trauma to genital tract and perforation of uterus
  iii. Infection and air embolism

The negative autopsy: Occasionally, after a thorough gross and histopathologic examination has been performed, no satisfactory cause of death can be found. In fact, if no specific gross findings are found, the provisional cause of death is given as "after histopathologic examination" (HP). We may find a cause after a thorough HP examination. Sometimes no cause of death is found even after HP examination. This does not imply that the pathologist has failed in the autopsy investigation: Negative findings are just as valid as positive ones. The terminology of the cause of death in such cases can be given as 'Unascertained'. A full and frank summary set in understandable terms will assist the deceased's relatives' enquiries, and may provide some small comfort to relatives at a time when certainly one and possibly two lives have been lost. The other option is to discuss this case in detail during a multidisciplinary meeting with the treating obstetrician, physician, intensivist, anaesthetist, etc. who then may give a consensus opinion on cause of death based on clinical circumstances.

I would like to share some of our institute findings of maternal death. In a three-year period from end of year 2008 to 2011, there were a total of 118 maternal deaths. Autopsy was carried out in 58 cases. Maternal deaths in these autopsy cases were divided into direct and indirect causes after histopathologic examination. Fulminant hepatic failure (FHF) due to submassive to massive hepatic necrosis was the predominant cause of death in 16 cases with positive serology for Hepatitis E (HEV) infection in 6 cases. All these 16 patients had presented with jaundice and variable levels of consciousness, ranging from mental confusion state to hepatic coma. Liver function tests like SGOT and SGPT were elevated with values ranging from 450 units/dl to 1600 units/dl. Acute fulminant hepatic necrosis was also the predominant cause of death in 41.5% cases where autopsy had been performed in our previous study. On auditing the maternal autopsies, that is, when we compared the current practices with the standard criteria laid down, it was noticed that in most of the referral cases, complete clinical details including the antenatal details were not available. The high incidence of viral hepatitis in the autopsy group is probably due to the fact that this hospital manages pregnant patients of the nearby municipal public hospital for infectious diseases. Table 12.1 gives the causes of maternal deaths in the period from January 2014 to December 2015.

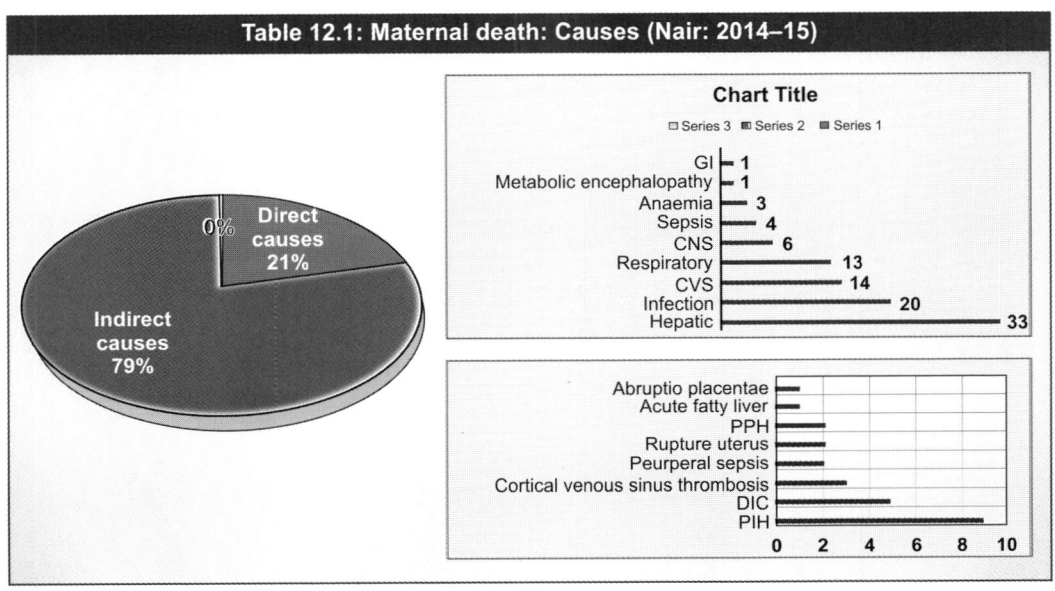

Table 12.1: Maternal death: Causes (Nair: 2014–15)

Sections from the uterus are important to study physiological and pathological changes during pregnancy and have to be specifically taken from the placental bed, especially for conditions like PIH and puerperal sepsis. Trophoblastic invasion of the myometrium as well as vessel wall, thinning of myometrial vessels with evidence of fibrinoid necrosis are the normal physiological changes noted in the placental bed which are not seen in cases of PIH. Similarly, in puerperal sepsis, endometritis usually begins from the placental bed. The pituitary gland also commonly shows physiological and pathological changes in pregnancy. Pituitary gland necrosis/Sheehan's syndrome is one of the most common causes of hypopituitarism in under-developed or developing countries in the postpartum period. Pituitary gland infarction is also known in HIV-positive individuals. Sections should be taken from the pituitary gland routinely. The medicolegal aspects of autopsies in maternal death will not be dealt here.

BIBLIOGRAPHY

1. Christiansen LR, Collins KA. Pregnancy-associated deaths: A 15-year retrospective study and overall review of maternal pathophysiology. Am J Forensic Med Path2006; 27:11–9.
2. Essentials of Autopsy Practice: Recent Advances, Topics and Developments edited by Guy N. Rutty. Springer-Verlag London Limited 2004.
3. Guidelines on Autopsy Practice Maternal death May 2010, http://www.rcpath.org/index.asp
4. Gwyneth Lewis (ed). Saving Mothers Lives: Reviewing maternal deaths to make motherhood safer-2003-2005. The Seventh Report of the Confidential Enquiries into Maternal Deaths in the United Kingdom. Available at:http://www.cemach.org.uk/getattachment/8f5c 1 ed
5. Jashnani KD, Rupani AB, Wani RJ. Maternal mortality: an autopsy audit. J Postgrad Med. 2009; 55(1):12–6.
6. Lucas S. Maternal death, autopsy studies, and lessons from pathology. PLos Med 2008;5:e48.
7. Shamshad, Saadia Shamsher, Bushara Rauf: Puerperal sepsis -still a major threat for parturient. J Ayub Med Coll Abbottabad 2010;22(3), 18–22.
8. The Hospital Autopsy, 2nd ed, J L Burton, G N Rutty. http://www.arnoldpublishers.com
9. The Royal College of Pathologists. Guidelines on Autopsy Practice; Scenario 5: Maternal Death, Jan 2005. Available from: http://www.rcpath.org.

Chapter 13

Maternal Deaths: Global Scenario and Practitioner's Perspective

○ Preeti Deshpande

The **UNICEF** Report 2019 states that 800 women still die in child birth everyday globally. As far as institutional delivery is concerned, the UNICEF analysis says that though improved in last decade variations between different countries were glaring. The obstetricians role comes into play where institutional deliveries are involved. "For far too many families, the sheer costs of child birth can be catastrophic. If a family cannot afford these costs, the consequences can be fatal," said UNICEF Executive Director, Henrietta Core. "When families cut corners to reduce material healthcare costs, both mothers and their babies suffer."[1] This assumes significance because according to WHO 216 mothers still die per 1 lakh live births while the sustainable development goals aim to reduce this to less than 70 by 2030.[1]

Between 2016 and 2030, a part of sustainable development goals of **WHO** targets, is to reduce the global maternal morality ratio to less than 70 per 1 lakh live births and with no country having a maternal mortality rate of more than twice the global average.[2]

The maternal mortality ratio in developing countries in 2015 was 239 per 1 lakh live birth versus 12 per 1 lakh live birth in developed countries.[2] Maternal mortality is unacceptably high in developing countries. Maternal mortality is high in rural areas and poorer communities. There are still a large number of patients delivering at home.

Table 13.1: MMR in developed and developing countries (as per WHO)

MMR	Developing countries	Developed countries	World over average
Current scenario 2015	239/lakh	12/lakh	216/lakh
Goal 2030	Less than 140/lakh for all	-	70/lakh

Women die due to complications during pregnancy and following childbirth. Most of these complications develop during pregnancy. However, some complications may be pre-existing,

but may worsen during pregnancy. The major complications that account for nearly 75% of all maternal deaths as per WHO are:[2]
1. Severe bleeding (mostly bleeding after childbirth)
2. Infections (usually after child birth)
3. High blood pressure during pregnancy (pre-eclampsia and eclampsia)
4. Complications from delivery
5. Unsafe abortions

The remainders are causes associated with diseases such as malaria and AIDS during pregnancy.

All women need access to antenatal care in pregnancy, skilled care during childbirth along with care and support in the weeks after childbirth Most maternal deaths are preventable, as healthcare solutions to prevent and manage complications are well known. Maternal and newborn health are closely linked.[2] Improving maternal health is one of WHO's key priorities

Severe bleeding after childbirth can kill a healthy woman within hours if she is unattended.

Infection after childbirth can be eliminated if good hygiene is practiced and if early signs of infection are recognized and treated in a timely manner.

Pre-eclampsia should be detected and appropriately managed before the onset of convulsions or other life-threatening complications.

It is also vital to prevent unwanted and too young age pregnancies. All women, including adolescents, need access to contraception, safe abortion services to the full extent of the law and quality abortion care.

During **United Nations** General Assembly 2015 in New York, United Nations Secretary General Ban Ki Moon launched the global strategy for women's, children's and adolescents' health, 2016–2030.

The strategy is a **roadmap for post 2015 agenda as described by the sustainable development goals** and seeks to end all preventable deaths of women, children and adolescents.

As a part of the global strategy and goal of ending preventable maternal mortality, **WHO** is working with partners towards:
1. Addressing inequalities in access to and quality of reproductive, maternal and newborn health services.
2. Ensuring universal health coverage for comprehensive reproductive, maternal and newborn healthcare
3. Addressing all causes of maternal mortality, reproductive and maternal morbidities and related disabilities
4. Strengthening health system to collect high quality data in order to respond to needs and priorities of women
5. Ensuring accountability in order to improve quality of care equity[2]

So as we do acknowledge, access to healthcare can be a major barrier during pregnancy and childbirth. Poverty, distance, lack of information, inadequate services and cultural practices play a role.

Each country has to layout its own path to tackle these issues. India also witnesses such barriers preventing women from accessing healthcare. In India, various programmes such as

Janani Suraksha Yojna have been implemented by the government with ASHA workers to serve at the grass roots level to help women access healthcare facilities (as mentioned in the concerned chapter in our book).

While the government has to ensure access to healthcare, our role as obstetricians, is important in giving clinical care to prevent mortality and morbidity, collecting data and ensuring accountability.

As per **WHO and Pan American Health Organisation (PAHO)** more than 1 out of 5 maternal deaths are from haemorrhage (bleeding).

Almost all maternal deaths by haemorrhage are preventable.[3]

Zero Maternal Death by Haemorrhage is an initiative taken up by **PAHO**. This programme involves and encourages:

- *Families and communities:* To take steps to make sure women are able to reach a health centre in case of emergency and should support them in getting to their prenatal appointments. Everyone should donate blood to make sure it is available for transfusion.
- *Mothers:* To visit their healthcare providers and avoid unnecessary C-sections.
- *Health professionals and service workers:* To offer pregnant women proper treatment that respects their culture and ensures no woman is turned away from health services
- *Health workers:* To provide pregnant women and their families with information on the risks and warning signs of obstetric haemorrhage
- *Decision makers:* To ensure support for health systems including staff training and equipment and means to employ them.[3]

The **Zero Maternal Death by Haemorrhage** is one of the projects taken up by **FIGO** President Carlos Fuchtner.[4] Dr Carlos Fuchtner is a Bolivian by origin. He intends to integrate associations of Gynaecology and Obstetrics of the region. Zero Maternal Death by Haemorrhage is also taken up by FLASOG (Federacion Latinamerica na de Sociedades de Obstetricia Y Ginecologia) and FEBRASGO (Federacao Brasileria das Associacoes de Ginecologia e Obstetricia).

Patients safety is most important for doctors. However, the approach to this has changed in the last few years. In **UK**, the current approach to patients safety has been defined by the *principles of risk management* similar to those used in psychology, aviation and high reliability organisations.[7]

The basic questions addressed in risk management principles include:
1. Risk identification as to what could go wrong
2. Risk analysis as to what is the chance it could go wrong
3. Risk treatment to minimize the chance of it happening or mitigate damage
4. Risk control as to what we can learn from things that go wrong

Risk management may be reactive or proactive.

Incident reporting is on the reactive side of the risk management strategies. Incident reporting and documentation will definitely be a step forward for these projects for staff training and to ensure support for health system.

Emphasis needs to be placed on the proactive side as risk management is more effective when resources are used to minimize the occurrence of patient safety incidents instead of "fire fighting" after things have gone wrong. Scenario training drills is one method of proactive risk management. Risk management is the business of all stakeholders in the organization, clinicians and non-clinicians. The critical element for all specialists is *primum non-nocere* "firstly, do no harm".

The term 'clinical risk management' is sometimes used to refer to the application of risk management in clinical setting.

As a practitioner what does this mean to us and how do we apply it. It is a sort of 'triage system' we need to follow in antenatal care and obstetric management. Let us discuss in perspective with some common situations and examples.

Risk Identification

Risk identification is like being prewarned about a disaster. "Forewarned is forearmed."

We could either use prospective systems to flag up possible sources of patient safety incidents before the event has actually happened or we could look back at things that actually go wrong. (Incident Reporting).

Incident reporting may use the 'London Protocol' which includes steps like identifying the incident, investigating, gathering data in chronology, identifying unsafe actions and contributing factors and devising future action.

One prospective method of identifying what could potentially go wrong is failure mode and effect analysis (FMEA). This method has been used extensively in aviation, aerospace and automobile industries also. But it is also applicable to healthcare. It identifies risks, contributory factors, its likelihood and effects. It also identifies controls to mitigate risks, to prioritize and devise action plans.

Let us see some examples as to how we can apply this **prospective method in our obstetric practice.**

The first step to a successful management is to identify the high risk factors. Patients with medical risk factors such as anaemia and thrombocytopenia are at a high risk of haemorrhage. Also obstetric risk factors such as twins, polyhydramnios and placenta previa make the patient prone to bleeding.

What action do we take once the risk is identified?

Such patients need adequate reservation of blood. Ideally such patients should be delivered in a tertiary set up with blood and blood products available in-house to minimize the time loss. This would be a primary precaution to ensure patients safety.

Other medical risk factors like gestational diabetes and hypertension in pregnancy increase fetal risks and also maternal risks. Having a physician on board and close monitoring by tests for fetal well-being such as Doppler and non-stress test would help.

Although mild hypertension may be manageable in a smaller set up, we need to be aware that hypertension in pregnancy can aggravate suddenly. If we are well-prepared, half the battle is won. Moderate to severe hypertension should ideally be managed in a tertiary set up.

Risk Analysis

Risk analysis would ensure adequate utilization of resources and prevent wastage of human and economic resources. We must assign a 'risk score' based on severity and likelihood.

A twin pregnancy is a high risk for PPH. So also a grand multipara is at a high risk for PPH. We must be well equipped when we take on such high risk cases.

Just as the phrase goes a gynaecologist must be "ectopic minded", an obstetrician should be "PPH minded".

Though a primigravida is unlikely to suffer from postpartum haemorrhage (PPH), an awareness of the small risk even in such cases must always be present at the back of our mind. Basic precautions must be taken even in low risk situations like "universal precautions".

As relevant to the condition in cases with oligohydramnios, IUGR, hypertension in pregnancy or diabetes in pregnancy we must analyze the fetal risk and maternal risk. All decisions must be calculated based on a risk versus benefit ratio.

Risk Treatment

The management must be instantly assessed and tailored to fit the patients condition.

For example, let us take a most catastrophic obstetric complication which gives us only a few minutes to think: **Postpartum haemorrhage.**

In case of postpartum haemorrhage, the amount of bleeding should be assessed and charted. This should include the blood collected in the suction drains, soaked mops and sheets as well. A fully soaked mop accounts for about 50 ml of blood loss, whereas a partially soaked mop is equivalent to about 30 ml of blood loss. The decision for the the number of pints of blood or blood products to be transfused must be based on this assessment. The anaesthesia chart must include intraoperative vitals and SpO_2 readings. Also intraoperative fluids given crystalloids and colloids need to be charted.

A pre-operative crossmatch reservation slip for blood reserved is a good evidence of precautions taken (risk identification and risk analysis).

Intraoperatively blood lost and blood transfused must be charted. In case of acute haemorrhage whole blood is more beneficial than packed cells for volume replacement (risk treatment).

In case of antepartum haemorrhage, a record of the time of detection of the condition like scar rupture or abruption should be charted. Thereafter steps taken like blood transfusion and interval to delivery or surgery should be documented.

We cannot play God, we can play the best role to save lives in "the golden hour" of action.

Risk Control

This defines what we have learnt from the situations that have gone wrong.

The key objective is to transform the prevailing culture of blame into a culture of safety and openness. Its remit is to look at systems rather than individuals. It aims at disseminating safety alerts and facilitates development of solutions to identified risks.

Patient safety incidents and near miss incidents can be reported to an anonymous data base. The aim is not a punitive action but accountability. Additionally it is important to report changes implemented and demonstrable benefits. Women who survive life-threatening conditions arising from complications related to pregnancy and childbirth have many common aspect with these who die of such complications. This similarly led to the development of the near miss concept in maternal health. Comparison between women who died and those who survived life-threatening conditions provide a more complete assessment of quality in maternal healthcare.

Knowledge about situations that go wrong will help comprehensive dialogues with government professionals, civil societies and health facilities for promoting best practices.[6]

For example, the system of **confidential enquiry** into maternal deaths in **UK** has been very successful in improving outcomes and reducing deaths by highlighting deficiencies in care.

Similarly in India, *maternal death review* was started in **Maharashtra State** as per Government resolution of 2010. As per guidelines it was expected that every maternal death whether institutional or at community level, be reported and reviewed.[5] This move has promoted the need for proper record-keeping and has motivated many institutes to streamline the reporting and recording systems. Notes and records are not a chore. They are actually checklists to ensure safety of our patients and in today's times even for the safety of doctors in medicolegal matters.

The maternal mortality ratio in Maharashtra declined from 68 in 2011–2013 to 61 in 2014–2016. India's national average for maternal mortality is 130.

Over the last five years, maternal deaths have declined by around 30% in Mumbai. Though this is good news, Mumbai still remains worse than most parts of India when it comes to maternal mortality. Mumbai's maternal mortality rate is 144 which is really high as compared to the state and national average. This may be associated with referrals from outside the city and those admitted in critical condition. Also the role of infections and antibiotic resistance cannot be ruled out. Earlier pre-partum haemorrhage and postpartum haemorrhage were the main causes of maternal mortality. These seen to have declined relatively after introduction of Maternal Death Review.[8]

Autopsies assume a great significance in maternal deaths since all maternal autopsy reports are scrutinized closely in preparation of reports for MCGM (Municipal Corporation of Greater Mumbai) Confidential Enquiry in Maternal Death. Since these reports make recommendations for improving obstetric practice, optimum quality of reports, clearly determining what actually happened to cause the death are critical.[9]

As an **obstetrician in private practice** one may sometimes be faced with a most trying situation when a **maternal death occurs in your hospital/ nursing home or on table! What is one meant to do in such a situation**?

Firstly, the doctor has to declare the death.[10]

Having done that, he or she must inform the local police station by a letter written in triplicate about the occurrence of the death for further action. He or she must mention the details of the patient's history.

The doctor cannot issue a death certificate.[10]

This automatically ensures that the body cannot be cremated or buried.

After taking over the body, the investigating police officer proceeds with the inquest and cause of death will be decided by medicolegal postmortem at the local government or Municipal Hospital. The Death Certificate will be filled by the Medical Officer who does the autopsy or hospital administration. This Death Certificate will be forwarded to the investigating Police

Officer/Magistrate or Coroner as the case may be. The required part of the death certificate will then be handed over to the relative for cremation or burial.[10]

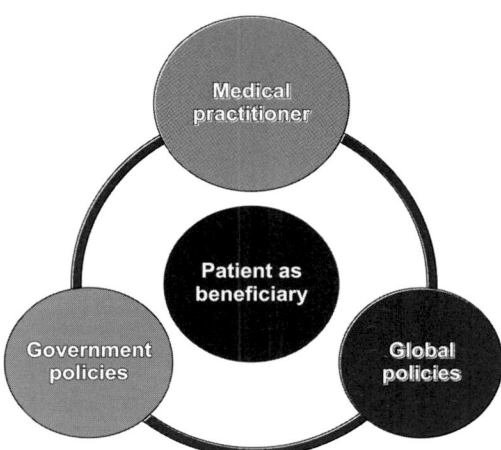

Fig. 13.1: The patient is the ultimate beneficiary of all medical services, government health policies and global policies

In conclusion, we as practitioners are 'microunits' in the world scenario. Each practitioner plays a part in improving the world statistics by giving the best quality of care to his/her patients. It goes without say that in his/her biosphere, things cannot improve unless the recipient also tries to imbibe the best quality of care. The patients who are informed, educated and empowered are most likely to benefit.

Next comes the role of the governments in improving the status of women, empowering women and ensuring access to quality healthcare. This may involve strengthening peripheral hospitals, rural healthcare facilities and door to door services. Also statistical reviews, analysis and audits like the Confidential Enquiries (UK) and Maternal Death Reviews (India) help assessing the scenario from time to time.

Global organisations are playing their part by increasing awareness, laying down strategies, analyzing the healthcare scenarios as a whole. This will help focus the energies of the practitioners in areas of need and serve as a guide to improve the healthcare sector as a whole.

REFERENCES

1. www.downtoearth.org.in/news/health /800-women-still-die-in-childbirth-every-day-globally-unicef report.
2. www.who.int/news-room/facts-sheets/detail/maternal-mortality
3. www.paho.org/cero-muertes-maternas-hemorragia
4. What the new president of FIGO, Carlos Fuchtner thinks/FIGO 2018/World Congress of gynecology and obstetrics http://figo2018.org/what-the-new-president-of-figo-carlos-fuchtner-thinks/

5. Addl Director, State Family Welfare Bureau, Pune, No. SFWB/RCH/CBMDR/report/file24B/D-10B/41177-220/2012
6. The WHO Near-miss approach www.who.int/reproductivehealth/topics/maternal_perinatal/nmconcept/en/
7. Improving Patient Safety: Risk Management for Maternity and Gynaecology. RCOG Clinical Governance Advice No. 2, Sept 2009
8. http://timesofindia.indiatimes.com/city/mumbai/maternal-death-in-mumbai-fall-30-in-five-years/articleshow/69381613.cm
9. Guidelines for Postmortem in Obstetric Deaths: Dr Kusum Jashnani, Playing By the Rules, An Update on Government Policies, Regulations and Acts for Practicing Obstetricians and Gynaecologists, First Edition, 2015, FOGSI Publications
10. Medical Certification of Death: Lt Col RB Kotabagi, Col RK Chaturvedi, Lt Col A Banerjee;MJAFI 2004; 60: 261–272.

Chapter 14

Human Milk Banking in a Developing Country

○ Jayashree Mondkar ○ Swati Manerkar

The benefits of mother's own milk (MOM) for her baby are universally acknowledged. The Lancet Child Survival Series has identified exclusive breastfeeding for the first six months as one of the most effective low-cost strategy for reducing infant and child mortality and together with appropriate institution of complementary feeding accounting for a 19% reduction in the under 5 mortality.[1]

Mother's milk is of particular importance for tiny preterm babies. Paradoxically, it is mothers of these babies who are more likely to have lactation problems due to tremendous stress of having a newborn in an intensive care unit, prolonged hospital stay of babies and may find it difficult to keep up their breast milk supply. For the survival of these babies, it is important that we guarantee a constant and adequate supply of human milk. This is possible with the presence of a human milk bank.

A human milk bank can be defined as an institution, established for the purpose of collecting, screening, processing, storing and distributing donated milk to recipients who are not the biological offspring of the donor mother. It is the technological alternative to the age old concept of wet nursing, ensuring that the milk fed to these needy babies is safe in all respects. The objectives of the milk bank are to ensure that every high risk baby born or admitted to the hospital who for some reason does not have access to her/his own mother's milk, gets the next best alternative, i.e. pasteurized donor human milk (PDHM), till mother's own milk is available or till discharge. It also ensures avoidance of use of animal and formula milk, to heighten breastfeeding awareness. Thus, the human milk bank acts as an ancillary support service to promote baby-friendly practices in the NICU and post-natal care wards.

The first human milk bank was set up in our country at the Lokmanya Tilak Municipal Medical College in 1989. It is only in the past decade that the importance of pasteurized donor milk (PDHM) to improve outcomes for the vulnerable very low birth weight (VLBW) and extremely low birth weight babies (ELBW) resulting in increase in the number of milk banks. Currently, there are over sixty human milk banks in the country and numbers are on the rise.

The first guidelines in our country were published by IAP in 2014.[2] In 1917, the Government of India brought out the guidelines for milk banking, thereby providing a basis for setting up milk banks in the country.[3] These guidelines are entitled "National Guidelines on Lactation Management Centres in Public Health Facilities" rather than Milk Banking Guidelines. Thus, the focus is on the importance of breastfeeding and need for breastfeeding support of which donor milk banking is a form of ancillary support. The national guidelines envisage a three tier system: Donor Milk Banks called "Comprehensive Lactation Management Centres" (CLMC) are to be established at Medical College NICUs or large District SNCUs; Lactation Management Units (LMUs) at Level II hospitals and SNCUs for safe management of expressed mother's own milk (MOM) for feeding her own baby at the SNCUs; Lactation Support Units (LSUs) have been recommended at every delivery centre.[3]

ORGANISATION OF A COMPREHENSIVE LACTATION MANAGEMENT CENTRE (CLMC)/ HUMAN MILK BANK

Prerequisites, Space and Location of The Milk Bank

An institution desirous of starting a CLMC or human milk bank should fulfil some basic requirements.
- The hospital should be certified as baby friendly and must practice early exclusive breastfeeding for normal and Caesarean section deliveries.
- It must be compliant with IMS Act 2003 and must not indulge in promotion of infant formula feed.
- The milk bank should be associated with an NICU facility.
- It should have an adequate delivery load from where donor mothers can be recruited.

It is recommended to have a milk bank in association with a 20 bedded NICU or more with a good case load of sick newborns.[3]

Location and Size of A Milk Bank/Comprehensive Lactation Management Centre

The CLMC should be ideally located as close to the postnatal care wards and NICU as possible. Proximity to the post-natal wards ensures convenience for the potential donor mothers and proximity to the NICU facilitates collection and disbursal. The National Guidelines recommend an average of 350 sq meters for setting up the CLMC. It should have a reception cum administrative area, a counselling area, milk expression area with facility for 4–6 expression stations with adequate provision for the donor mother's privacy, a milk processing area and a cleaning and autoclaving room.

The cost incurred for setting up a basic milk bank is equivalent to the cost of one neonatal ventilator, i.e. approximately Rs. 10–15 lakhs. The equipment required for setting up a bank is listed below:[4–6]

Equipment

At Site of Milk Collection

- Hospital grade, electric breast milk pumps—for milk collection.
- Sterilized containers—for milk storage.

In the Milk Bank

- **Deep freezer: (–20°C)** for storing milk. Ideally separate freezers for raw donor human milk (DHM), post-pasteurization milk storage awaiting culture reports and one for safe culture negative milk ready for distribution, should be available. Both vertical and horizontal models are available.
- **Refrigerator:** For storage of milk as soon as DHM containers arrive at the CLMC till its pasteurization within 24 hours of arrival. It is also used for thawing the frozen milk.
- **Laminar air flow/biosafety cabinet** for aseptic pooling of milk is preferable to have but not mandatory.
- **Pasteurizer/shaker water bath** for heat treatment: Holder pasteurization of milk. Local, microprocessor controlled, shaker water bath can be used for pasteurization. Imported, fully automatic pasteurizers may also be used but are expensive.
- Generator/UIPS: In case of power failure.
- Hot air oven for sterilization of the milk containers, glassware, etc.

Staff

The head of the Neonatal services serves as the Milk Bank Director who assisted by the faculty is responsible for overall supervision and for planning, developing, implementing and evaluating milk bank services.

Lactation management nurses form the backbone of lactation services. Their job is to help mothers with lactation problems, to motivate mothers to donate milk, to organize the milk collection, to dispatch the donated milk to the bank and to ensure sterilization of pumps.

A milk bank technician, who is responsible for pasteurization of milk, microbiological surveillance, maintenance of records and disbursement of milk.

A **microbiologist** who carries out the cultures from the milk samples from each container.

A **milk bank assistant/hygiene helper** who transports milk to bank from the collection sites, washes and sterilizes the containers and the lacta sets, assists in OPD milk donation activities.

MILK BANKING PROCESSES

Donor Population

Unlike milk banks in the West, where donors express and collect milk at home and periodically deposit the milk in the bank over an extended period of time, in our milk bank, donor population is cross sectional.[3-6] The system of milk donation includes supervised collection of milk from donor mothers in hospital and in the outpatient department. Mothers in the postnatal wards and those following up in the post-natal well baby follow-up clinics are motivated to donate milk. A second group of donors are those mothers whose babies are admitted in the NICU and are not in a position to be fed or are on minimal enteral feeds. Mothers are encouraged to express milk frequently through the day to maintain their milk output and the excess of milk is then banked. Another emerging group of donor mothers are educated mothers who are willing to express surplus milk at home, store in the deep freezer and have the milk periodically picked up by the milk bank van. All donor mothers are screened before registration as per criteria mentioned below.

Donor Selection Criteria

The following donor selection criteria is used in our milk bank:[3]
- Healthy and well-nourished mothers
- No evidence of tuberculosis or other infectious diseases
- Not consuming medication that are contraindicated during breastfeeding
- Screened and documented to be non-reactive for HIV, VDRL, hepatitis B.
- No history of blood transfusions/hepatitis in the recent past.
- Willing to donate.

Milk Expression and Collection Procedure

Donor mothers are recruited after appropriate screening and written informed consent is taken.
All mothers are given specific instructions regarding washing their hands with soap and water and cleaning their breast. Milk is expressed manually to feed their own babies. For the purpose of milk banking, hospital grade electric pumps are preferred as they result in better volumes of expressed milks and are relatively painless and comfortable to use.

Collection and Storage Containers

Containers include milk storage bags, plastic containers, glass and pyrex containers and stainless steel containers. In developing countries, cylindrical, wide mouthed stainless steel containers with tight fitting caps are used, as they are easily available, durable, easy to clean and autoclave. There is no significant decrease in nutrient composition on storage, however, cellular components are reduced. The imported pasteurizers require polypropylene or glass containers.

TRANSPORT OF MILK TO THE BANK

Freshly expressed milk should be stored in the refrigerator at the site of collection and should be transported to the milk bank in an ice box with gel packs to maintain the cold chain. Transport should be at the earliest, not later than 24 hours of collection.

POOLING OF MILK

Milk from 3–5 donors can be pooled as soon as it reaches the bank. Prior to freezing, the milk is pooled separately as colostrum and mature milk. Pooling should be done with all aseptic precautions preferably under the laminar air flow system.

HEAT TREATMENT OF BANKED MILK (PASTEURIZATION)

Pasteurization not only increases the shelf-life of the milk but also preserves the unique composition of human milk while preventing transmission of disease. It is carried out by the Holder method by heating the milk containers at 62.5°C for 30 minutes followed by rapid cooling to 4°C. Heat treatment is carried out using a shaker water bath with a thermostatic control and is found to be equally effective and economical. Imported, fully automatic pasteurizers are also available. The benefit is that both the heating and cooling cycles are carried out in the same machine with continuous recording of temperature throughout the process. The heating process is done in the shaker water bath however cooling is achieved by keeping the containers in a slurry of ice, till cooling is achieved.

Pasteurization is found to preserve more than 80% of total IgA, lactoferrin and 100% of lysozyme, destroying 99% of pathogens including HIV virus.

POSTPASTEURIZATION CULTURE OF MILK

After heat treatment, an aliquot of processed milk from each container is immediately sent for bacteriological testing and the containers are placed in the freezer at –20°C. Containers showing any culture positivity are discarded. Once a negative culture report is available, the milk is considered ready for distribution.

It is important to store raw donor human milk, pasteurized milk awaiting culture report and safe, culture negative PDHM in separate deep freezers. In case of cost constraints, they may be stored on different shelves of the freezer and only safe, culture negative milk should be dispensed for use.

Pasteurized milk can be kept up to 6 months at –20°C without much change in the composition. Milk frozen for several months may have a soapy odor and taste due to change in the molecular structure of milk lipids, but this does not harm the baby. Unpasteurized milk, pending pasteurization should not be stored for more than three months.

DISTRIBUTION OF BANKED MILK

Milk from the bank is distributed on a "first in first out" basis, the oldest milk being used first. Milk is shifted out to the fridge in the neonatal unit as per the day's requirements. Stored heat processed milk can be kept at 4°C for 72 hours only. Prior to use, the milk is thawed by standing the container at room temperature or in lukewarm water. Gently shaking the container distributes the heat more evenly. Once the milk is warmed to room temperature, it is used within 2–4 hours in our institution although studies have shown that it may be utilized within 6–8 hours.

Microwave or heating the breast milk destroys anti-infective properties of breast milk.

As we can see the supply–demand ratio is just met. Hence banked milk is only used for babies in the hospital and is not supplied on an outpatient basis or to babies in other hospitals.

RECIPIENTS

The largest group of recipients of banked milk in our unit is preterm (VLBW and ELBW) and term SGA babies especially in the first few days, till their mothers are able to secrete adequate milk. Babies of mothers with problems like eclampsia, PPH, acute illnesses, LSCS deliveries, are also supplemented with banked milk whenever needed. Extra mural babies admitted to the unit till their mothers are available and babies whose mothers have lactation failure also receive banked milk.

RECORDKEEPING

CLMCs must ensure that records regarding donor health status, informed consent forms for donors and recipients, pasteurization procedure logs, culture records, disbursement logs, tracking logs, stocks, inventory, etc. are meticulously maintained.

MEASURES TO ENSURE SAFETY OF BANKED MILK

In order to ensure bacteriological safety of milk in the developing countries, the following guideline must be adhered to.
1. Selection criteria for donor should be strictly followed.
2. Donor mothers should wash hands and clean breasts before milk collection.
3. All pumps and milk containers should be sterile. Random cultures from pumps and containers should be sent to ensure sterility.
4. All milk samples should be subjected to heat treatment or pasteurization.
5. Post-pasteurization samples of milk should be sent for microbiological culture of milk. Containers showing any growth should be discarded immediately.
6. Each milk bank should follow "Hazard analysis and Critical Control Points" guidelines and should have its own written, standard operating procedures for maintenance of asepsis and cleanliness.

REFERENCES

1. Jones G, Steketee R, Robert E Black, Bhutta Z, Morris S, and the Bellagio Child Survival Study Group. Lancet 2003; 362: 65–71.
2. Bharadva K, Tiwari S, Mishra S, Mukhopadhyay K, Agarwal R, Kumar V; for the Infant and Young Child Feeding Chapter, Indian Academy Of Pediatrics. Human Milk Banking Guidelines. Indian PediatricsVolume 51, 2014: 469–474.
3. National Guidelines on Lactation Management Centres in Public Health Facilities. Child Health Division, Ministry of Health and Family Welfare, Government of India 2017.
4. Guidelines for the establishment and operation of a donor human milk bank. Italian Association of Human Milk Banks Associazione Italiana Banche del Latte Umano Donato (AIBLUD: www.aiblud.org). The Journal of Maternal-Fetal and Neonatal Medicine, September 2010; 23(S2): 1–20.
5. Human Milk Banking Association of North America (HMBANA) Guidelines for the establishment and operation of a donor human milk bank. Sandwich, MA: HMBANA; 2009.
6. Donor breastmilk banks: The operation of donor breastmilk bank services.NICE clinical guidelines. Issue dated February 2010. www.nice.org.uk/guidance/CG93.

Chapter 15

Role of Paramedical Staff

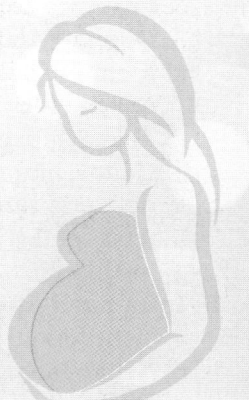

○ Pushpa Thorat

Maternal mortality ratio is a very sensitive index of health status of the country.

Statistics on maternal mortality ratio (MMR) are of great value to the planners, administrators, decision makers and medical professionals.

The Family Planning Programme and Maternal Child Health (MCH) Programme was introduced in 1952 and subsequently changed to Family Welfare Programme, then to the Child Survival and Safe Motherhood (CSSM) in 1992 and later into Reproductive Child Health (RCH) phase I in 1997 and then phase II in 2005 for Comprehensive Health in National Rural health mission (NRHM). The objective was to provide services with equality especially to the underprivileged group, i.e. mothers and children, people below poverty line and those from remote areas from backward community.

Accelerated achievement of goal for health is due to combined efforts of health staff, paramedical staff and voluntary organizations along with community participation. The role of paramedical staff is of great importance in improving the quality of services from the actual to the desired services with a view to reduce Maternal Mortality Rate (MMR)<100 per lac live births, infant mortality rate (IMR) <15 per thousand and TFR <1.8% and to achieve comprehensive health services in rural and urban areas.

Role of Female Multipurpose Health Worker (MPW) in Field

In RCH and NRHM Programme

1. To prepare an action plan at subcentre level on need base of the community
2. **A. Antenatal care:**
   a. At least four visits in ANC
   b. Registration (within 1st trimester)

c. Physical examination, weight, height, blood pressure, abdominal examination.
d. Essential laboratory investigations (Hb, urine for albumin/ sugar, pregnancy test)
e. Ensuring consumption of at least 100 iron and folic acid tablets (IFA) (for all pregnant women), 200 tablets (for anemic women); referral for severe anemia
f. Identification of danger signs for prompt treatment and early referral. Assured referral linkage for complicated cases.
g. Tetanus toxoid immunization (two doses at one-month interval)
h. Counseling on nutrition, birth preparedness and complication readiness, institutional delivery, safe abortion and exclusive breastfeeding, family planning measures.
i. At level II (PHC), linkages with ICTC/ PPTCT centre for voluntary counseling and HIV testing.

B. Intra-natal care
a. Institutional normal delivery with use of partograph (training of skilled birth attendant)
b. Active management of third stage of labour (use of misoprostol tablets)
c. Infection prevention, use of 5 cleans formula, use of DDT, antibiotics—ampicillin, metronidazole, gentamicin, etc.
d. Identification and referral of danger signs.
e. Pre-referral management for obstetric emergencies, e.g. eclampsia, PPH, shock, obstructed labor, severe anemia, etc.
f. Assured referral linkages to higher centres with transport facility.

Newborn care: Integrated management of neonatal and childhood illness (IMNCI).
a. Neonatal resuscitation
b. Keep baby clean and warm, maintain humidity
c. Infection prevention
d. Initiation of breastfeeding within an hour of birth and exclusive breastfeeding till six months.
e. Screening for congenital anomalies.
f. Weighing of newborn and management of premature babies.
g. Referral to higher center for pediatric care.

C. Postnatal and newborn care
a. Minimum 6 hours stay post delivery
b. Counseling for feeding, nutrition, family planning, hygiene, postnatal examination, immunization, infection prevention.
c. Home visits on 3rd, 7th and 42nd day. Additional visit for the newborn on 14th, 21st and 28th days.
d. Timely identification of danger signs and complications and referral to higher centre.

Newborn care
a. Hygiene and cord care.
b. Identification, management and referral of low birth weight (LBW), preterm and sick babies.
c. Immunization: Zero-day OPV, BCG, hepatitis B and routine immunization and vitamin A.

Role in Adolescent Reproductive and Sexual Health (ARSH) Programme

Counseling regarding healthy diet, cleanliness, hygiene, sanitation, pure drinking water, communicable disease, sexually transmitted diseases (STIs), reproductive tract infections (RTI) and AIDS, menstrual cycle, MTP law, and reproductive health physiological, mental and emotional changes.

Role of Health Assistant

One health assistant is posted for 15,000 people in rural population and for 10,000 people in tribal area to look after the implementation of programme in 3 subcentres.

1. A. To supervise and guide the work of female MPW and to help her in planning, implementation and development of skill and knowledge.
   B. Weekly preplanned visits to subcentre and sending the report to PHC.
2. Team-work:
   A. To work in coordination with male and female health workers and dais at Committee and Surpanch level
   B. To attend meetings with Block Development Officers (BDO), Child Development Programme Officer (CDPO) and Medical Officers and to review the work.
   C. To help as a team leader in camps and Mother and Child Protection Clinic
3. A. To maintain the supply of medicines and materials at the subcentre and to check the kits (delivery and medicine kit)
   B. In Mother and Child Protection (MCP) session, to maintain the cold chain of vaccine.
4. A. To check and correct the reports and registers of subordinates.
   B. To review the work, compile it and submit the report regularly.
5. A. Training of dais, ASHA workers, Anganwadi workers.
   B. To help the medical officer in planning the training programme.
6. Reproductive and Child Health (RCH) programme:
   A. To motivate and counsel the resistant cases to adopt family planning measures.
   B. Refer the needy client for MTP to an authorized center.
   C. To help subordinates promote spacing methods.
7. Nutrition:
   A. To detect malnourished children below 5 years of age, arrange supplementary diet from Anganwadi and to refer children with disease to the PHC or nearest RH with free transport.
   B. To ensure regular and free supply of IFA tablets and vitamin A solution in prescribed doses.
   C. To educate mothers for breastfeeding (exclusive up to 6 months)
   D. Health education for weaning feeds (complimentary food)
8. Medical treatment
   A. Management of minor ailments and provision of first aid treatment in accidental cases.
9. Health education, communication skills and counseling in RCH and immunization
10. Discuss the health problems with local leaders, village health committee staff, Integrated Child Development Services (ICDS) staff, social workers, Mahila Mandals, etc.

11. Propaganda of implementation of newer obstetric care schemes like Janani Suraksha Yojana, Savitribai Phule Yojana and special schemes in Melghat.

Aim is to reduce maternal mortality. To ensure skilled attendance at every birth and access to quality emergency obstetric care for timely management of complications, a skill-based training programme is arranged. A residential training program of 2 to 3 weeks for staff nurses and 3 to 6 weeks for Auxiliary Nursing Midwife (ANMs)/Lady Health Visitors (LHVs) is designed. This training involves imparting skills like ANC care to identify high risk pregnancy, pelvic assessment, managing all stages of labor involving antepartum, intrapartum and postpartum care, newborn resuscitation and timely identification and management of complications. The Government of India has taken policy initiatives to empower the ANMs/LHVs/staff nurses to make them competent to undertake certain life saving measures. These measures are:

1. Permission to use uterotonic drugs for prevention of postpartum hemorrhage, e.g. misoprostol tablets and oxytocin.
2. Permission to use drugs in emergency situations prior to referral for stabilizing patients: Use of injection magnesium sulphate in eclampsia.
3. Permission to perform basic procedures at community level, e.g. assistance to Medical Officer in evacuation, manual removal of the products of conception in incomplete abortions.
4. Partograph training for every skilled birth attendant.
5. Treatment of infection with use of drugs like broad spectrum antibiotics, e.g. ampicillin, gentamycin, metronidazole, etc.
6. Permission to establish intravenous line and infusion of fluids.
7. To prepare the checklist of drugs and materials for basic skills.
8. Awareness programmes in the community for blood donation and national programs.

Paramedical staff at the subcentre level are responsible for implementation of activities under national programme, local health programme and health development programme for rural people. They are trained for quality services and to bring medical and minimum essential health services within easy reach to the rural population. They are responsible for providing promotive, preventive, curative and rehabilitative services with the help of community health workers, teachers, health guides, trained dais, private practitioners, and voluntary organizations. It will help in achieving the health goals of the country.

"Empower Women, Empower India"

BIBLIOGRAPHY

1. NRHM RCH-II 8th joint review mission 2011.
2. Guidelines for operationalizing SBA training in RCH-II.
3. BEMOC, SBA module public health institute.

Chapter 16

Training of Medical and Paramedical Staff in Obstetric Care

○ Reena J Wani ○ Rashmi Jalvee

INTRODUCTION

Maternal mortality in India continues to remain unacceptably high. Majority of births in India takes place at home and a large proportion are assisted by unskilled persons. It is estimated that nearly 15 percent mothers will develop one or other life-threatening obstetric complications during intrapartum and immediate postpartum period but which mother will develop complications cannot be predicted. Keeping this in view, it is essential that all mothers have access to a birth attendant, who has requisite midwifery skills to recognize complications, manage as per scope of practice and refer if needed. Government of India is committed to ensure universal coverage of all births with skilled attendance both in the institution and at community level and to provide access to emergency obstetric care services for women experiencing serious complications.[1]

AIMS

To reduce maternal mortality.

Maternal mortality reduction remains a priority under "Goal 3: Ensure healthy lives and promote well-being for all at all ages" in the new Sustainable Development Goals (SDGs)[2] agenda through 2030 which aims to reduce the global Maternal Mortality Ratio (MMR) to fewer than 70 maternal deaths per 100,000 live births. In India, reduction in maternal mortality ratio is one of the goals of the National Population Policy and the Reproductive and Child Health Programme (RCH-II). Ensuring skilled attendance at every birth and access to quality emergency obstetric care for timely management of complications are critical interventions to achieve programmed goals. Keeping this in view, a skill-based training programme of 2–3 weeks' duration for Staff Nurses (SNs) and 3–6 weeks' duration for Auxiliary Nurse

Midwife (ANMs)/Lady Health Visitors (LHVs) has been designed. This training involves acquisition of skills like abdominal examination, pelvic assessment, managing all the stages of labour involving intrapartum care, newborn resuscitation, timely identification and management of complications, etc.[1]

RCH II goal indicator	All India status (year and source)	RMCH + A (2017) goal[3]
MMR	301 (SRS 2001-03) 254 (SRS 2004-06) 212 (SRS 07-09) 178 (SRS 2010-12)	<100

Role of Skilled Birth Attendant (SBA) in Reducing MMR

A skilled birth attendant is defined as "an accredited health professional—such as midwife, doctor or nurse—who has been educated and trained to achieve proficiency in the skills needed to manage normal (uncomplicated) pregnancies, childbirth and immediate postnatal period and in the identification, management and referral of complications in women and newborns." Government of India considers the "Skilled Birth Attendant" as a person who can handle common obstetric and neonatal emergencies, recognize when the situation reaches a point beyond his/her capability and refers the woman or the newborn to a First Referral Unit (FRU)/appropriate facility without delay (Ref: Government of India Guidelines for ANC and Skilled Attendance at Birth by ANMs and LHVs). Government of India has taken policy initiatives to empower the ANMs/LHVs/SNs to make them competent for undertaking certain lifesaving measures. These measures are as follows:

- Permission to use Uterotonic drugs for prevention of PPH.
- Permission to use drugs in emergency situations prior to referral for stabilizing the patient.
- Permission to perform basic procedures at community level in emergency situations.[1]

Checklist for Training Site Readiness[1]

Emergency Drug Tray

- Injection oxytocin
- Injection diazepam
- Tablet nifedipine
- Injection magnesium sulphate
- Injection lignocaine hydrochloride
- Tablet misoprostol
- Sterilized cotton and gauze
- At least 2 pairs of gloves
- Sterile syringes and needles (different sizes)
- Sterile I/V sets (at least 2)
- Equipment, supplies and other drugs
- Delivery kits including those for normal deliveries and assisted deliveries (forceps and Ventouse extraction)—at least two each

- Cheattle forceps in a dry bottle
- Foetal stethoscope
- Baby weighing scale
- Radiant warmer
- Table lamp with 200 watt bulb
- Phototherapy unit
- Self-inflating bag and mask (neonatal size)
- Oxygen hood (neonatal)
- Laryngoscope and endotracheal tubes
- Mucus extractor with suction tube and foot operated suction machine
- Feeding tubes
- Blankets
- Clean towels
- Baby feeding cup
- BP apparatus and stethoscope
- Sterile/clean pads
- Bleaching powder
- Povidone iodine solution
- Spirit
- Micropore tape
- Antenatal card
- Partograph
- Inj. Gentamycin
- Inj. Ampicillin
- Oral Metronidazole

Checklist for Basic Skills
- Antenatal history taking
- Antenatal physical examination:
  - Measure height
  - Measure weight
  - Measuring BP
  - Pallor
- Abdominal examination:
  - Measuring symphiso-fundal height
  - Measuring fundal height in weeks
  - Measuring abdominal girth
  - Identifying foetal lie and presentation other than normal
  - Hearing foetal heart sound
- Hemoglobin estimation

- Urine examination
- Ante-natal counselling and interventions
- Identification of danger signs during pregnancy, labour, delivery and postpartum period.
- Health education and counselling

Additional Skills (Desirable)

- Conducting normal delivery and newborn care
- Providing postpartum care to normal delivery mothers and newborns
- Giving deep intramuscular injections
- Establishing IV line and giving fluids
- Trainer's remarks and signatures

REFERENCES

1. Guidelines for Operationalizing SBA Training in RCH II
2. https://www.undp.org/content/undp/en/home/sustainable-development-goals.html
3. https://www.nhp.gov.in/reproductive-maternal-newborn-child-and-adolescent-health_pg

Section III

Surgical Procedures and TL

17. National Guidelines for Female Sterilization and Male Sterilization
18. National Guidelines for Mini-Lap Tubal Sterilization
19. National Guidelines for Laparoscopic Tubal Ligation and Managing Its Complications
20. Criteria for Selection of Patients for Tubal Ligation
21. MTP and Tubal Ligations—Problems at Rural Areas of India
22. Medicolegal Issues and Informed Consent Format in Sterilization Operation

Chapter 17

National Guidelines for Female Sterilization and Male Sterilization

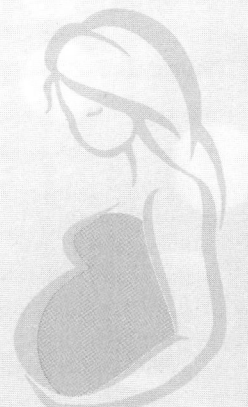

○ Asha Advani

INTRODUCTION

Under National Welfare Programme, it is an important step to develop standardized national guidelines for female and male sterilization in India. Guidelines for male and female sterilization have been prepared with an objective to develop the skills of medical officers to perform tubectomies and vasectomies in a standardized manner across the country, minimizing complications.

AIMS

1. To adopt a strategy, which would provide assured, accessible and quality sterilization services, throughout the year, nearest to the doorsteps of the couples desiring permanent contraception.
2. To ensure uniformity of sterilization policies throughout the country.
3. To provide medicolegal security to medical practitioners performing sterilization operations, and
4. To lay down clear guidelines as to the indications, contraindications and prerequisites for sterilization operations in India.

A. Eligibility Criteria for Service Providers for Performing Female/Male Sterilization

Female sterilization	*Male sterilization*
Basic qualification requirement of service provider	Basic qualification requirement of service provider
Minilaparotomy services—trained MBBS doctor	Conventional vasectomy—trained MBBS doctor
Laparoscopic sterilization—DGO, MD (obstetrics and gynaecology), MS (surgery) (trained in laparoscopic sterilization)	No scalpel vasectomy—trained MBBS doctor

Only those qualified and trained doctors who are eligible and whose name appears on the panel will be entitled to carry out sterilization operations (male and female) in government or accredited institutions.

Physical Eligibility Criteria of Female/Male Sterilization for Clients

Case selection: Female	*Case selection: Male*
1. Age: 22 to 49 years	1. Age: 21 to 60 years
2. Married	2. Married
3. Couple should have at least one child, above the age of 1 year. Unless the sterilization is medically indicated, the child should be fully immunized and healthy	3. Couple should have at least one child, above the age of 1 year. Unless the sterilization is medically indicated, the child should be fully immunized and healthy
4. Clients or spouse should not have undergone sterilization operation earlier (except failure of sterilization)	4. Clients or spouse should not have undergone sterilization operation earlier (except failure of sterilization)
5. Client must be in sound state of mind and not under the influence of drugs/alcohol so that she understands the implications of the sterilization procedure	5. Client must be in sound state of mind and not under the influence of drugs/alcohol so that he understands the implications of the sterilization procedure
6. Mentally ill clients must be certified so by a psychiatrist and a statement should be given by the legal guardian/spouse regarding the soundness of the clients state of mind	6. Mentally ill clients must be certified so by a psychiatrist and a statement should be given by the legal guardian/spouse regarding the soundness of the clients state of mind.
7. Spouse consent not required	7. Spouse consent not required

Clinical Process

1. *Preliminary Steps*
- Counseling of patient by healthcare providers for sterilization operations.
- Motivation
- Written informed consent before surgery by the client as under Annexure 4. It should not be obtained under coercion (force) or when the client is under sedation.
- Checklist to be filled in and signed by MO in Annexure 3
- Preoperative assessment can also provide an opportunity for overall health screening and treatment of RTIs/STIs.
- Preoperative instructions, review of the surgical procedure.

2. *Operation*

3. *Postoperative Care*

Counselling

This is the process of helping clients make informed and voluntary decision about sterilization procedure.

The following steps must be taken before clients sign the consent form:

Female client	Male client
1. Clients must be informed of all the available methods of family planning and should be made aware that for all practical purposes, this operation is a permanent one	1. Client must be informed of all the available methods of family planning and should be made aware that for all practical purposes, this operation is a permanent one
2. Clients must make an informed decision for sterilization voluntarily	2. Clients must make an informed decision for sterilization voluntarily
3. Clients must be counseled in the language that they best understand	3. Clients must be counseled in the language that they best understand.
4. Clients should be made to understand what will happen before, during and after the surgery, its side effects and potential complications.	4. Clients should be made to understand what will happen before, during and after the surgery, its side effects and potential complications
5. The following features of the sterilization procedure must be explained to the client • It is a permanent procedure for preventing future pregnancies • It is a surgical procedure that has a possibility of complications, including failure, requiring further management • It does not affect sexual pleasure, ability or performance • It will not affect the clients strength or her ability to perform normal day-to-day functions • Sterilization does not protect against RTIs, STIs or HIV/AIDS • Clients must be told that a reversal of this surgery is possible, but that the reversal involves major surgery and its success cannot be guaranteed	5. The following features of the sterilization procedure must be explained to the client • It is a permanent procedure for preventing future pregnancies • It is a surgical procedure that has a possibility of complications, including failure, requiring further management • It does not affect sexual pleasure, ability or performance • It will not affect the clients strength or his ability to perform normal day-to-day functions • After vasectomy, it is necessary to use a back-up contraceptive method until azoospermia is achieved (usually this takes three months) • Sterilization does not protect against RTIs, STIs or HIV/AIDS • A reversal of this surgery is possible but the reversal involves major surgery and its success cannot be guaranteed
6. Clients must be encouraged to ask questions to clarify their doubts, if any	6. Clients must be encouraged to ask questions to clarify their doubts, if any
7. Clients must be told that they have the option of deciding against the procedure at anytime without being denied their rights to other reproductive health services	7. Clients must be told that they have the option of deciding against the procedure at anytime without being denied their rights to other reproductive health services

Clinical Assessment and Screening of Clients

Prior to the surgery, compilation of the clients medical history, physical examination and laboratory investigations as specified below need to be done in order to ensure the eligibility of the client for surgery.

Demographic information: As per the checklist and the consent form (Annexures 3 and 4)

Medical history: History of any illness as per medical eligibility criteria, must rule out present pregnancy by menstrual history/UPT.

Physical examination: General, systemic and obstetric (P/A, P/V) examination.

Laboratory examinations: Hb should be above 7 gm%, and urine albumin and sugar is must, other laboratory tests must be carried out if indicated.

Timing of the Surgical Procedure

Female client	Male client
a. Interval sterilization should be performed within 7 days of the menstrual period (in the follicular phase of the menstrual cycle) b. Postpartum sterilization should be done after 24 hours up to 7 days of delivery c. Sterilization with medical termination of pregnancy (MTP) can be performed concurrently d. Sterilization following spontaneous abortion can be performed provided the client fulfils the medical eligibility criteria e. Laparoscopic tubal ligation should not be done concurrently with second trimester abortion and in the postpartum period up to 6 weeks	It can be done at any convenient time on healthy clients as per the checklist

Preoperative Instructions

Female client	Male client
1. Bath and clean, loose clothing is a must for client. 2. Nil by mouth (even water) for minimum 4 hours prior to surgery and no solids, milk or tea for 6 hours prior to surgery 3. Empty bowels (laxative or enema) and trimming of hair, no shaving 4. Empty bladder 5. The health worker or a responsible relative to accompany the patient 6. Clean the parts with antiseptic solution such as betadine (povidone iodine) or cetavlon (savlon). It should be applied liberally twice in a circular motion beginning at the site of incision and working out. To prevent the recontamination of the site with local skin bacteria. 7. Spirit or alcohol preparation should not be applied to the genitalia.	1. Bath and clean, loose clothing is a must for client 2. No NBM. Light breakfast before surgery 3. Trim the hairs from the scrotum and pubic region—no shaving 4. Empty bladder 5. The health worker or a responsible relative to accompany the patient 6. Clean the parts with antiseptic solution such as betadine (povidone iodine) or cetavalon (savlon) 7. Spirit or alcohol preparation should not be applied to the genitalia.

Preoperative Medication

Female client	Male client
Reassurance	Reassurance
Antianxiety/sedation/tab. alprazolam (0.25 to 0.50 mg)/ tab. diazepam (5 to 10 mg) just before the operation	Sedation not required except very anxious client tab. diazepam 10 mg
Local anaesthesia—lignocaine without adrenaline— doses 3 mg per kg body weight	Local anesthesia—lignocaine 1–2% without adrenaline—doses 10 ml of 2% and 20 ml of 1%
IV line before the procedure	
Drugs for the intraoperative sedation and analgesia	
Inj. pethidine 25 to 50 mg + Inj. promethazine (pherargan) 12.5 to 25 mg or Inj. pentazocin (fortwin) (15 to 30 mg) + Inj. promethazine (phenargan) 12.5 to 25 mg IM 30–45 min before surgery. Repeat pethidine 10 mg or fortwin 5 mg IV if required 5 min prior to surgery if required.	
Dosage by body weight: Pethidine 0.5 to 1 mg/kg; promethazine 0.3–0.5 mg/kg. Only once to be given after 45 minutes of the initial dose	
General anaesthesia rarely necessary only if patient is non-cooperative, excessive obesity or history of allergy to LA	No anaesthetist required
Monitoring: Constant communication with the client throughout the operation	Monitoring: Constant communication with the client throughout the operation
SOP for preoperative monitoring TPR, BP chart	SOP for preoperative monitoring TPR, BP chart
Resuscitation kit to be kept ready	Resuscitation kit to be kept ready

Medical Eligibility Criteria of Female/Male Sterilization for Clients

There are no medical contraindications for performing male or female sterilization. However, certain criteria to apply as follows:

Case selection: Female	Case selection: Male
1. A—Accept	A—Accept
• Nulliparous • Parous • Breastfeeding • Postpartum after 24 hrs< 7 days, after 42 days • Mild PIH • Post-abortion • Post-ectopic pregnancy • Patient with history of smoking	• High risk of HIV • HIV infected • Anaemias—sickle cell disease

Case selection: Female

- History of high BP but current BP is normal
- History of superficial venous thrombosis/DVT and pulmonary embolism
- Hyperlipidaemias
- Non-migrain headache/migraine
- Menorrhagia (DUB) or heavy/regular menses
- Benign ovarian tumours (including cysts)
- Severe dysmenorrhoea
- Benign gestational trophoblastic disease
- Cervical ectropion
- Cervical intraepithelial neoplasia (CIN)
- Benign breast disease
- Family history of cancer
- Past and no evidence of current disease for 5 years
- Past PID with subsequent pregnancy
- Other STIs (excluding HIV and hepatitis)
- Vaginitis (including *Trichomonas vaginalis* and bacterial vaginosis)
- Increased risk of STIs
- High risk of HIV
- HIV infected
- Tuberculosis—non-pelvic
- Malaria
- Diabetes-controlled—non-vascular disease and non-insulin dependent
- Thyroid disorders—simple goiter
- Gall bladder disease—symptomatic—treated by cholecystectomy
- Asymptomatic gall bladder disease
- History of cholestasis—pregnancy related
- Viral hepatitis—carrier
- Sterilization concurrent with caesarean section

Case selection: Male

2. C—Caution	C—Caution
Procedure is conducted but with extra preparations and precautions	
• Young age	• Young age
• Obesity with >30 kg/m² body mass index (BMI)	• Depressive disorders
• Hypertension adequately controlled	• Diabetes
• Elevated BP levels with systolic values 140–159 or diastolic 90–99 mm Hg	• Previous scrotal injury
• Current ischaemic heart disease	• Large varicocele
• Stroke—history of cerebrovascular accident	• Large hydrocele
• Valvular heart disease—uncomplicated	• Cryptorchidism
• Epilepsy	
• Depressive disorders	
• Breast cancer—current	
• Uterine fibroids without distortion of the uterine cavity	

- Uterine fibroids with distortion of the uterine cavity
- Pelvic inflammatory disease without subsequent pregnancy
- Diabetes—non-vascular disease—non-insulin dependent
- Insulin dependent
- Hypothyroid
- Cirrhosis mild (compensated)
- Benign (adenoma)
- Malignant (hepatoma)
- Thalassaemia
- Sickle-cell disease
- Iron deficiency anaemia: Hb 7 to 10 gm%
- Diaphragmatic hernia
- Kidney disease
- Severe nutritional deficiencies
- Previous abdominal or pelvic surgery
- Elective sterilization along with abdominal surgery

3. D—Delay	D—Delay
The procedure is to be delayed until the condition is evaluated or corrected	
• Pregnancy	• Local infections—scrotal skin infection, active STI, balanitis, epididymitis or orchitis
• Postpartum—from days 7 to 42	• Systemic infections or gastroenteritis
• Severe PIH	• Filariasis, elephantiasis
• Prolonged rupture of membranes (PROM) more than 24 hours	• Intrascrotal mass
• Puerperal sepsis/fever	
• Severe APH/PPH	
• Severe trauma to the genital tract	
• Acute haematometra	
• Current DVT/PE	
• Major surgery with prolonged immobilization	
• Current ischaemic heart disease	
• Unexplained vaginal bleeding before evaluation	
• Trophoblastic disease—malignant/gestational/trophoblastic disease	
• Cervical cancer (awaiting treatment)	
• Endometrial cancer	
• Ovarian cancer	
• Current PID	
• Current purulent cervicitis, chlamydial infection or gonorrhea	
• Current gall bladder disease	
• Viral hepatitis—active	
• Iron deficiency anaemia with Hb< 7 gm%	
• Local infection abdominal skin infection	

- Respiratory diseases—acute bronchitis or pneumonia
- Systemic infections or gastroenteritis
- Sterilization concurrent with abdominal surgery—emergency (without previous counseling)
- Infectious conditions

4. S—Special	S—Special
Procedure done in a setting where experienced surgeon, anaesthetist, equipment for GA and backup medical support are available with special precautions	
• Uterine rupture and perforation (postpartum or postabortal). If the patient is stable during the exploratory surgery or laparoscopy, tubal ligation may be performed if there is no additional risk involved.	• AIDS
• Systolic BP > 160 or diastolic > 100 mm of Hg	• Coagulation disorders
• Vascular disease	• Inguinal hernia
• Valvular heart disease—complicated (pulmonary hypertension, atrial fibrillation, history of sub-acute bacterial endocarditis)	
• Endometriosis	
• AIDS	
• Known case of genital tuberculosis	
• Diabetes—diabetic nephropathy/retinopathy/neuropathy	
• Other vascular disease or diabetes lasting > 20 years	
• Hyperthyroidism	
• Cirrhosis—severe (decompensated)	
• Coagulation disorders	
• Respiratory diseases—chronic asthma, bronchitis, emphysema, lung infection	
• Fixed uterus due to previous surgery or infection	
• Abdominal wall or umbilical hernia	

Postoperative Monitoring

Female vasectomy case

1. TPR, BP, bleeding, abdominal girth monitoring and input–output charting is done 1 hourly for 4 hours
2. Follow-up instructions given with discharge card
3. Postoperative medication and advice—oral and liquids started after bowel sounds appear. Normal diet resumed as soon as possible. Rest for 24–48 hours Resume the light work after 48 hours and normal activity after two weeks
4. Keep the wound and stitches dry till stitches are removed. Bath after 24 hours

Male vasectomy case

1. Client observed for vital signs for half an hour after surgery
2. Follow-up instructions given with discharge card
3. Postoperative normal diet on NBM, rest for 24 hours. No cycling for 48 hours, normal activity after 48 hours to 1 week
4. Keep the wound and stitches dry till stitches removed. Bath after 24 hours

National Guidelines for Female Sterilization and Male Sterilization

Female vasectomy case	Male vasectomy case
5. Client can have sexual intercourse after 1 week or when comfortable	5. Client can have sexual intercourse whenever he feels comfortable. Use condoms for 3 months if wife is not using any contraception. Do a semen analysis after 3 months
6. Return if missed periods or suspected pregnancy	6. Return if excessive pain or increase in the scrotal size or fever
7. Medications—painkillers, antibiotics for a week	7. Medications—painkillers, antibiotics for a week
8. Keep the contact number of the client for verbal follow-up	8. Keep the contact number of the client for verbal follow-up

Denial of the Operation

In case if the operation is denied intraoperatively, or it is difficult to get the second tube or the vas, take the consent of the client or the relative that the client is not sterilized and the client should then use alternative methods of contraception. Signature of the counselor or doctor should also be taken in Annexure 4 (informed consent form).

The family planning indemnity scheme by GOI for giving the compensation to the clients getting complications, failure or death following sterilization operation.

Prerequisites for Patient to be Eligible for Compensation

a. As per the GR the facility for doing the sterilization should be accredited
b. Surgeon should be qualified and trained as a service provider and surgeon should be impanel. Available benefits under the family planning indemnity scheme are as under:

Section	Coverage	Limits
I A	Death following sterilization (inclusive of death during process of sterilization operation) in hospital or within 7 days from the date of discharge from the hospital.	2 Lakhs
I B	Death following sterilization within 8–30 days from the date of discharge from the hospital.	50,000/-
I C	Failure of sterilization	30,000/-
I D	Cost of treatment **in hospital and up to 60 days** arising out of complication following sterilization operation (inclusive of complication during process of sterilization operation) from the date of discharge.	(actual not exceeding) 25,000/-
Sec. II	Indemnity per doctor/health facilities but not more than 4 times in a year	Up to 2 lakh per claim

This updated manual is available on the Ministry's website: www.mohfw.nic.in, click www.nrhm.gov.in and then click http://nrhm.gov.in/nrhm-components/rmnch-a/family-planning/schemes.html

DQAC will investigate the above cases and the claims are to be paid within 60 days of the incident by the local committee after the approval of the DQAC and executive health officer.

Documents Required for the Indemnity Scheme

Death	Complication	Failure
Claim form sign by the spouse	Claim form signed by the client	Claim form signed by the client
Original consent form and checklist	Original consent form and checklist	Original consent form and checklist
Sterilization certificate	Sterilization certificate	Sterilization certificate
Death certificate	Bills original	Sonography/UPT/medical examination report
Case papers	Case papers	Case papers and old discharge card for the previous TL operation or sterilization certificate/papers, if any

Submit all the above documents along with the institution covering letter to the office of the Special Officer—Family Welfare within 1 week of incident so that claims can be processed in time.

BIBLIOGRAPHY

1. Manual for Family Planning Indemnity Scheme Family Planning Division. Ministry of Health and Family Welfare, Government of India, October 2013.
2. Manual for Minilap Tubectomy Family Planning Division. Ministry of Health and Family Welfare, Government of India, November 2009.
3. Standards for Female and Male Sterilization Services Division of Research Studies and Standards, Ministry of Health and Family Welfare, Government of India, October 2006.

National Guidelines for Mini-Lap Tubal Sterilization

○ Rashmi Jalvee ○ Reena J Wani

Provision of quality contraception services is vital to stabilise population and to improve maternal and child health. Surgical methods of sterilization are the most commonly used form of contraception worldwide, with the prevalence in developing countries ranging from 20 to 35%.

Tubal ligation offers a highly effective protection against pregnancy; it carries a very low risk of complications when done according to accepted medical standards; and as a once only procedure, it eliminates the need for long-term contraceptive supplies. Under National Welfare Program, it is important to develop standardized national guidelines for female sterilization in India. Guidelines for female sterilization have been prepared with an objective to develop the skills of medical officers to perform tubal sterilization in a standardized manner across the country, minimizing complications.

Aims

1. To adopt a strategy, which would provide assured, accessible and quality sterilization services, throughout the year, nearest to the doorsteps of the couples desiring permanent contraception.
2. To ensure uniformity of sterilization policies throughout the country.
3. To provide medicolegal security to medical practitioners performing sterilization operations and
4. To lay down clear guidelines as to the indications, contraindications and prerequisites for sterilization operations in India.

A. Eligibility Criteria for Service Providers for Performing Female Sterilization

- Mini-laparotomy sterilization—trained MBBS doctor
- Laparoscopic sterilization—DGO, MD (OBGY), DNB (OBGY), MS (Surgery) (trained in laparoscopic sterilization)

Additional certification for a doctor holding a postgraduate diploma/degree in OBGY is NOT required for laparoscopic sterilization.

The Government of India with Oriental Insurance Company has taken a National Insurance Scheme for all the doctors across the country for tubal ligation (TL). The National Insurance Scheme benefits all empanelled doctors to avail of compensation in case of any major complication or death due to TL procedure. As per the rules of the National Insurance Scheme, only doctors empanelled with state government will be eligible for the benefits under the National Insurance Scheme.

B. Physical Eligibility Criteria of Female Sterilization for Clients

1	Age	22–49 years
2	Marital status	Married (including ever married)
3	Parity	Couple should have at least one child more than 1 year age. Unless the sterilization is medically indicated, the child should be fully immunized and healthy
4	Sterilization status	Clients or spouse should not have undergone sterilization operation earlier (except failure of sterilization)
5	Consent	• Client must be in sound state of mind and not under the influence of drugs/alcohol so that she understands the implications of the procedure. • Mentally ill clients must be certified so by a psychiatrist and a statement should be given by the legal guardian/spouse regarding the soundness of the client's state of mind. • **Consent of the spouse is not required** (but desirable)

Spousal consent for tubal ligation is not required legally, but because tubectomy is a permanent procedure, a joint decision usually will mean more satisfied clients and fewer complaints to health workers following surgery. It may be advisable to find out how the spouse feels about adopting the method. If the spouse is not in favour of it, the provider should caution the client about going ahead with the procedure.

Clinical Process

Preparation for surgery includes counselling, pre-operative assessment, pre-operative instructions, review of the surgical procedure and postoperative care.

Counselling

Counselling enables clients to make an informed and voluntary decision about sterilization procedure. The following points should be included:

All available methods of family planning should be informed

An informed decision for sterilization must be made voluntarily

Clients must be counselled in the language that they best understand

Clients should be made to understand what will happen before, during and after the surgery, its side effects and potential complications.

The following features of the sterilization procedure must be explained to the client:
- It is a permanent procedure for preventing future pregnancies.
- It is a surgical procedure that has a possibility of complications, including failure, requiring further management.
- It does not affect sexual pleasure, ability or performance.
- It will not affect the client's strength or her ability to perform normal day-to-day functions.
- Sterilization does not protect against RTIs, STIs or HIV/AIDS.
- Clients must be told that a reversal of this surgery is possible, but that the reversal involves major surgery and its success cannot be guaranteed.

Clients must be encouraged to ask questions to clarify their doubts, if any.

Clients must be told that they have the option of deciding against the procedure at any time without being denied their rights to other reproductive health services

Clinical Assessment and Screening of Clients

Prior to the surgery, compilation of the client's medical history, physical examination and laboratory investigations as specified below need to be done in order to ensure the eligibility of the client for surgery.

a. *Demographic information*—age, marital status, occupation, religion, educational status, number of living children, and age of the youngest child.
b. *Medical history*—history of any illness as per medical eligibility criteria, must rule out present pregnancy by menstrual history/UPT.
c. *Physical examination*—general, systemic and pelvic (P/A, P/V) examination.
d. *Laboratory examinations*—Hb should be above 7 gm%; urine albumin and sugar; other laboratory tests to be carried out if indicated.

Timing of the Surgical Procedure

Interval sterilization	Should be performed within 7 days of the menses (in the follicular phase of menstrual cycle)
Postpartum sterilization	Should be done after 24 hours up to 7 days of delivery.
Sterilization with medical termination of pregnancy (MTP)	Can be performed concurrently. Sterilization following spontaneous abortion can be performed provided the client fulfils the medical eligibility criteria.
Laparoscopic tubal ligation	Should not be done concurrently with 2nd trimester abortion and in the postpartum period up to 6 weeks.

Preoperative Instructions
- Bath and wear clean, loose clothing.
- Nil by mouth (even water) for minimum 4 hours prior to surgery and no solids, milk or tea for 6 hours prior to surgery
- Empty bowels (laxative or enema) and trimming of hair, no shaving
- Empty bladder
- Health worker or a responsible relative to accompany the patient
- Clean the parts with antiseptic solution such as Betadine (Povidone iodine) or Cetavalon (Savlon). It should be applied liberally twice in a circular motion beginning at the site of incision and working out to prevent the recontamination of the site with local skin bacteria.
- Spirit or alcohol preparation should not be applied to the genitalia.

Pre-medication Anaesthesia Analgesia
1. Reassurance
2. Tab. Alprazolam (0.25 to 0.5 mg) or Tab Diazepam (5 to 10 mg) on the night before surgery if required
3. Inj. Atropine 0.6 mg, given intramuscularly before the surgery, reduces oral secretions and the possibility of vasovagal syncope or cardiac arrest
4. IV line before the procedure
5. Drugs for the intraoperative sedation and analgesia:
   - Inj. Pethidine 25 to 50 mg + Inj. Promethazine (Phenargan) 12.5 to 25 mg OR
   - Inj. Pentazocin (Fortwin) 15 to 30 mg + Inj. Promethazine (Phenargan) 12.5 to 25 mg IM 30–45 min before surgery.
   - A repeat dose (if required) is given slow IV as Pethidine 10 mg or Pentazocine 30 mg, 45 minutes after the first dose.
   - Dosage by body weight: Pethidine 0.5 to 1 mg/kg; Promethazine 0.3–0.5 mg/kg; Pentozocine 0.5 mg/kg.
6. General anaesthesia is rarely necessary only if patient is non-cooperative, excess obesity or with history of allergy to LA. Spinal anaesthesia is preferred in cases where surgery is likely to be prolonged.
7. Monitoring: Constant communication with the client throughout the operation
8. SOP for monitoring:
   - Preoperative: TPR and BP should be taken prior to pre-medication and every 10 minutes thereafter.
   - Intraoperative: TPR and BP every 5 minutes.
   - Postoperative: TPR and BP every 15 minutes for at least one hour after surgery or longer if the patient is unstable or not awake.
9. Resuscitation kit to be kept ready

Medical Eligibility Criteria of Female Sterilization

There are no medical contraindications for performing female sterilization. However, certain criteria to apply are as follows:

A	Accept	No medical reason to deny sterilization to a person with this condition.
C	Caution	Procedure is normally conducted in a routine setting, but with extra preparation and precautions.
D	Delay	Procedure is delayed until the condition is evaluated and/or corrected. Alternative temporary methods of contraception should be provided.
S	Special	Procedure to be undertaken in a setting with an experienced surgeon and staff, equipment needed for providing GA and other back-up medical support. Alternative temporary methods of contraception to be provided if referral is required or if there is otherwise any delay.

Accept
- Nulliparous women
- Parous women
- Breastfeeding
- Postpartum after 24 hours <7 days, after 42 days
- Mild PIH
- Postabortion
- Postectopic pregnancy
- Patient with h/o smoking
- H/o High BP but current BP is normal
- H/o superficial venous thrombosis/DVT and pulmonary embolism
- Hyperlipidaemia
- Headache/migraine with or without aura
- Menorrhagia (DUB) or heavy/regular menses
- Benign ovarian tumours (including cysts)
- Severe dysmenorrhoea
- Benign gestational trophoblastic disease
- Cervical ectropion
- Cervical intraepithelial meoplasia (CIN)
- Benign breast disease
- Family h/o cancer
- Past h/o breast cancer and no e/o current disease for 5 years
- Past PID with subsequent pregnancy
- Other STIs (excluding HIV and hepatitis)
- Vaginitis (including *Trichomonas vaginalis* and bacterial vaginosis)
- Increased risk of STIs
- High risk of HIV
- HIV infected
- Tuberculosis: Non-pelvic
- Malaria
- Diabetes: Controlled—non-vascular disease and NIDDM
- Thyroid disorders: Simple goiter
- Gall bladder disease: symptomatic—treated by cholecystectomy

Caution	• Asymptomatic gall bladder disease • History of cholestasis—pregnancy related • Viral hepatitis carrier • Sterilization concurrent with caesarean section • Young age • Obesity with >30 kg/m² body mass index (BMI) • Hypertension adequately controlled • Elevated BP levels with systolic values 140–159/diastolic 90–99 mm Hg • H/o ischaemic heart disease • Stroke—history of cerebrovascular accident • Valvular heart disease – Uncomplicated • Epilepsy • Depressive disorders • Breast cancer: Current • Uterine fibroids without distortion of the uterine cavity • Uterine fibroids with distortion of the uterine cavity • Pelvic inflammatory disease without subsequent pregnancy • Diabetes: Non-vascular disease–NIDDM • Insulin dependent DM • Hypothyroid • Cirrhosis mild (compensated) • Benign (adenoma) • Malignant (hepatoma) • Thalassaemia • Sickle-cell disease • Iron deficiency anaemia Hb 7 to 10 gm% • Diaphragmatic hernia • Kidney disease • Severe nutritional deficiencies • Previous abdominal or pelvic surgery • Elective sterilization alongwith abdominal surgery
Delay	• Pregnancy • Postpartum: From days 7 to 42 • Severe PIH • Prolonged rupture of membranes (PROM) more than 24 hours • Peurperal sepsis/fever • Severe APH/PPH • Severe trauma to the genital tract • Acute hematometra • Current DVT/PE • Major surgery with prolonged immobilization • Current ischaemic heart disease • Unexplained vaginal bleeding before evaluation • Trophoblastic disease: Malignant gestational trophoblastic disease

	• Cervical cancer (awaiting treatment) • Endometrial cancer • Ovarian cancer • Current PID • Current purulent cervicitis, chlamydial infection or gonorrhea • Current gall bladder disease • Viral hepatitis: Active • Iron deficiency anaemia with Hb <7 gm% • Local infection abdominal skin infection • Respiratory diseases: Acute bronchitis or pneumonia • Systemic infections or gastroenteritis • Sterilization concurrent with abdominal surgery: Emergency (without previous counselling) • Infectious conditions
Special	• Uterine rupture or perforation (postpartum or postabortal). If the patient is stable during the exploratory surgery or laparoscopy, tubal ligation may be performed if there is no additional risk involved. • Systolic BP > 160 or diastolic >100 mm of Hg. • Vascular disease • Valvular heart disease—complicated (pulmonary hypertension, atrial fibrillation, history of subacute bacterial endocarditis) • Endometriosis • AIDS • Known case of genital tuberculosis • Diabetes—diabetic nephropathy/retinopathy/neuropathy • Other vascular disease or diabetes lasting >20 years • Hyperthyroidism • Cirrhosis—severe (decompensated) • Coagulation disorders • Respiratory diseases—chronic asthma, bronchitis, emphysema, lung infection • Fixed uterus due to previous surgery or infection • Abdominal wall or umbilical hernia

Steps of Surgery

- Once the patient is under suitable anaesthesia, parts are painted and draped.
- In **postpartum tubal ligation**, a skin incision 2–3 cm long is made beneath the umbilicus, just below the upper border of the palpable uterus.
- Using forceps or retractors, subcutaneous fat is gently dissected by blunt dissection until the rectus fascia is visualized and exposed with retractors.
- The rectus sheath is grasped with Allis forceps in the midline at the inferior and superior portions and using scissors, the fascia is incised transversely and extended slightly beyond the skin incision on both sides.
- Peritoneum is elevated with artery forceps to protect the underlying viscera from injury during incision and a small opening is made in the peritoneum with a scissors.

- Once entry into the abdominal cavity is confirmed and with gentle retraction, the fallopian tube is visualized and grasped atraumatically with Babcock forceps.
- The fallopian tube is identified and confirmed by tracing it to the fimbriated end.
- Modified Pomeroy technique is most commonly used. The basic principle is to tie a knot onto a loop of an avascular area of the fallopian tube (in the area of the isthmus, 2 to 3 cm from the cornual end), excise a portion of the tube and use absorbable suture.
- Rapidly absorbable suture (chromic or plain catgut) No 0 is recommended, to allow the two cut ends of the tube to withdraw quickly from each other. This reduces the risk of failure as a result of spontaneous recanalization.
- Procedure involves placing an anchor tie around the proximal side of the loop of fallopian tube using a square knot. Tie the same suture on the other side of the looped tube using a square knot.
- 1 cm of the loop of fallopian tube above the knot is cut off using the scissors, leaving at least a 0.5 cm tubal stump above the knot. Check the stump for bleeding.
- Procedure is repeated on the other side.
- The abdomen is closed in two layers—the fascia and the skin. Peritoneal closure is not necessary. The fascia using a continuous suture with absorbable suture number 0 and the skin with interrupted stitches 1 cm apart using either absorbable or non-absorbable suture number 0.
- For **interval tubal ligation**, a transverse skin incision is made 2–3 cm above the pubic symphysis. The abdominal entry is similar to the procedure described above. Access to fallopian tube requires manipulation of the uterus and tubes to position the fallopian tubes near the incision area. The index finger is inserted inside the incision to feel the uterine fundus, slide laterally to feel the fallopian tube which is hooked and brought out through the incision. The rest of the procedure is similar to as described above.

Postoperative Monitoring

1. TPR, BP, bleeding, abdominal girth monitoring and input output charting is done 1 hourly for 4 hours.
2. The client can be discharged after at least 4 hours of procedure when she has been seen and evaluated by a healthcare provider to check that the vital signs are stable, she is fully awake, has passed urine and can talk, drink and walk and is accompanied by a responsible adult while returning home. Whenever necessary the client should be kept overnight at the facility.
3. Follow-up details along with a detailed discharge summary mentioning all relevant details should be given. Both written and verbal postoperative instructions must be provided in the local language.
4. Postoperative medication and advice—liquids and orals started after bowel sounds appear. Normal diet resumed as soon as possible. Rest for 24–48 hours. Resume light work after 48 hours and normal activity after one week.
5. Keep the wound and stitches dry till stitches are removed. Bath after 24 hours.
6. Establish contact with health worker within 48 hours, return for a follow-up visit on the 7th day of surgery or as early as possible after 7 days and a 2nd follow-up after 1 month or if menses do not return.

7. Client can have sexual intercourse after 1 week of interval sterilisation or 2 weeks of postpartum sterilisation or when comfortable.
8. Return if missed periods or suspected pregnancy.

Certificate of Sterilization

Certificate of sterilization should be issued after the second follow-up after ruling out any pregnancy.

Complications of Female Sterilization

Intraoperative complications:
- Nausea and vomiting
- Vasovagal attack
- Respiratory depression or arrest
- Cardiac arrest
- Uterine perforation
- Bleeding from the mesosalpinx
- Injury to the urinary bladder
- Injury to intra-abdominal viscera: Small or large bowel and blood vessels
- Convulsions and toxic reactions to local anaesthesia

Postoperative complications:
- Wound sepsis
- Haematoma in the abdominal wall
- Intestinal obstruction, paralytic ileus and peritonitis
- Tetanus
- Incisional hernia

All complications arising intraoperative or even postoperative, should be evaluating and managed as per the standard surgical guidelines. Any complication arising during surgery or after surgery must be reported to the District Quality Assurance Committee.

Failure of Operation, Leading to Pregnancy

This may be due to either technical deficiency in the surgical procedure or spontaneous recanalization. The patient should be offered MTP or be medically supported throughout the pregnancy. She should be offered repeat surgery. Ectopic pregnancy must be ruled out as tubectomy predisposes this condition.

Denial of the Operation

In case the operation is denied intraoperatively, or there is difficulty to reach the second tube, take the consent of the client or the relative that the client is not sterilised and the client should then use alternative methods of contraception. Signature of the counsellor or doctor should also be taken in Annexure 4 (informed consent form). The family planning indemnity scheme by GOI gives compensation to clients for complications, failure or death following sterilization operation.

Prerequisites for Patient to be Eligible for Compensation
- As per the GR, the facility for doing the sterilization should be accredited,
- Surgeon should be qualified and trained as a service provider and surgeon should be empanelled.

Available benefits under the family planning indemnity scheme are as under:

Section	Coverage	Limits (₹)
I A	Death following sterilization (including death during sterilization operation) in hospital or within 7 days from the date of discharge from the hospital.	2 Lakh
I B	Death following sterilization within 8–30 days from the date of discharge from the hospital.	₹50,000
I C	Failure of sterilization	₹30,000
I D	Cost of treatment in hospital and up to 60 days arising out of complication following sterilization operation (inclusive of complication during process of sterilization operation) from date of discharge.	Not exceeding ₹25000
II	Indemnity per doctor/health facilities but not more than 4 times in a year	Up to 2 Lakh per claim

This updated manual is available on the Ministry's website: www.mohfw.nic.in, click www.nrhm.gov.in and then click http://nrhm.gov.in/nrhm-components/rmnch-a/familyplanning/schemes.html. DQAC will investigate the above cases and the claims are to be paid within 60 days of the incident by the local committee after the approval of the DQAC and executive health officer.

Documents Required for the Indemnity Scheme

Death	Complication	Failure
• Claim form signed by the spouse	• Claim form signed by the spouse	• Claim form signed by the spouse
• Original consent form and checklist	• Original consent form and checklist	• Original consent form and checklist
• Sterilization certificate	• Sterilization certificate	• Sterilization certificate
• Death certificate	• Death certificate	• USG/UPT/medical examination report
• Case papers	• Case papers	• Case papers and old discharge card for previous TL operation or sterilization certificate

All documents along with the institution covering letter must be submitted to the office of the Special Officer—Family Welfare within 1 week of incident so that claims can be processed in time

BIBLIOGRAPHY

1. Guidelines for Training in Female Sterilization for Program Officers, Training Co-ordinators and Trainers. Family Planning Division, Ministry of Health and Family Welfare. 2010.
2. ICOG FOGSI Recommendations for Good Clinical Practice: Female Sterilization. March 2009.
3. Manual for Family Planning Indemnity Scheme, Family Planning, Division Ministry of Health and Family Welfare Government of India October 2013.
4. Manual for Minilap Tubectomy, Family Planning Division, Ministry of Health and Family Welfare Government of India November 2009.
5. Reference Manual for Minilap Tubectomy. Family Planning Division, Ministry of Health and Family Welfare. 2014.
6. Standards for Female and Male Sterilization: Services Division of Research Studies and Standards, Ministry of Health and Family Welfare, Government of India. October 2006.
7. World Contraceptive Use 2012 [Internet] Department of Economic and Social Affairs, United Nations Population Division; [cited 2015 Jun 23]. Available from: http://www.un.org/en/development/desa/population/publications/family/contraceptive-wallchart-2013.shtml

Chapter 19

National Guidelines for Laparoscopic Tubal Ligation and Managing Its Complications

○ Madhuri Patel ○ Amol P Pawar

Family planning in India is based on efforts largely driven by the government. All efforts are nearly concentrated around the initiatives and guidelines regularly put in place by the Government of India. However, the initiative of the government has now rightly focused from family limitation to family welfare. As a result, the focus of the guidelines has shifted from rules and regulations to standards and quality control to effectively implement the National Guidelines.

From 1965–2009, contraceptive usage has more than tripled (from 13% of married women in 1970 to 48% in 2009) and the fertility rate has more than halved (from 5.7 in 1966 to 2.4 in 2012), but the national fertility rate remains high, causing concern for long-term population growth. India adds up to 1,000,000 people to its population every 20 days.[1–5] Extensive family planning has become a priority in an effort to curb the projected population of two billion by the end of the twenty-first century.

In 2015, 15.6 million abortions were performed, with an abortion rate of 47.0 abortions per 1000 women aged between 15 and 49 years.[6] With high abortion rate follows a high number of unintended pregnancies, with a rate of 70.1 unintended pregnancies per 1000 women aged 15–49 years.[6] Overall, the abortions occurring in India make up for one-third of pregnancies and out of all pregnancies occurring, almost half were not planned.[7]

Laparoscopic Tubal Ligation Guidelines

The National Technical Resources Group on family planning, a part of the family planning division of the National Rural Health Mission, has introduced the **Reference manual for Female Sterilization** in 2014. These guidelines are set to standardize the female sterilization services in the country and to enable the provider to recognize and manage potential problems as well as provide appropriate follow-up. It has also set up uniform standards of training across the country and can be used for monitoring and ensuring quality in provision of sterilization services.

This manual supersedes the previous guidelines of 2009 and 2010 developed by Ministry of Health and Family Welfare of Government of India.

Some of the salient features in the reference manual are given below.

Guiding Principles of Sterilization

- Clients must be provided informed choice.
- Written consent should be taken prior to surgery.
- Doctors and staff should be trained and skilled in the female sterilization techniques, use of appropriate anesthesia and managing emergencies.
- All instruments and equipment must be in optimum working condition.
- The facility must be equipped with drugs and equipment to handle emergencies as appropriate.
- Standard infection prevention practices must be adhered to.
- Clients must be screened for medical eligibility for female sterilization.

Eligibility of Provider

For laparoscopic sterilization:

DGO, MD/MS in OBGY, specialists in other surgical fields, MBBS performing Minilap sterilization (trained in laparoscopic sterilization).

- The state government has been directed to maintain a district-wise list of doctors empaneled for performing sterilization operations in public and accredited private/NGO facilities based on the above criteria.
- The state maintains a separate list for minilap, laparoscopic tubectomy, conventional and no scalpel vasectomy providers.
- Only those doctors whose names appear on the panel are entitled to carry out sterilization operations in public and accredited private/NGO facilities. The panel should preferably be updated every three months or sooner if warranted. A doctor empaneled with one state/district of India is eligible to perform sterilization operation in other states/districts of India).
- States can empanel doctors who are already performing sterilization operation in the public facilities for the last 3 years.

When to Perform Female Sterilization

Laparoscopic tubal occlusion is usually performed in the 'interval' period (6 weeks after delivery or any time when the woman is not pregnant) or following first trimester abortion.

For interval procedures, laparoscopy may be performed at any time in the menstrual cycle although it is preferable to do it at the end of the menstrual period or shortly thereafter to ensure that the client is not pregnant.

It is not recommended in the immediate (up to 6 weeks) postpartum period or after 2nd trimester postabortion because of the possibility of injury to the larger, more vascular postpartum uterus. It is also not recommended to do sterilization procedure till the next menstrual period after medical abortion.

Informed Choice and Informed Consent

- Clients have been counseled wherever required in the language they understand.
- Clients have been informed of all the available methods of family planning and procedures.
- Clients have been made to understand what may happen before, during and after the surgery, its side effects and potential complications.
- Clients have made an informed decision for sterilization voluntarily.
- Client needs to understand that it is a permanent method of sterilization, and though reversal is possible, its success rate and outcomes are unpredictable.
- In the unlikely event of any complication/failure/death, there is a redressal mechanism available in the form of indemnity coverage.
- The consent of the partner is not required for sterilization. However, the partner should be encouraged to come for counseling.
- Advise client to return to the facility if there is any missed period/suspected pregnancy, within two weeks to rule out pregnancy.

Eligibility Criteria for Female Client undergoing Sterilization Procedure

(Self-declaration by the client will be the basis for compiling this information. No eligible client should be denied female sterilization service)

- Clients should be ever-married.
- Clients should be >22 years and <49 years.
- The couple should have at least one child, whose age is above one year, unless sterilization is medically indicated.
- Clients or their spouses/partners must not have undergone sterilization in the past (not applicable in cases of failure of previous sterilization).
- Clients must be in a sound state of mind as to understand the full implications of sterilization.
- Mentally ill clients must be certified by a psychiatrist and a statement should be given by the legal guardian/spouse regarding the soundness of the client's state of mind.
- A relevant medical history, physical examination and laboratory investigations need to be completed to ascertain eligibility for surgery.

Client assessment for eligibility to undergo female sterilization is a key factor in minimizing risk of complications and ensuring quality of service delivery (Annexure I).

For medical eligibility criteria for sterilization, refer previous Chapter 18.

Pre-procedure Steps

The client should:
  i. Preferably trim pubic and perineal hair. Shaving of pubic hair, if warranted, should be done just prior to surgery.
 ii. Bathe and wear clean and loose clothes to the OT.

iii. Not have a meal on the morning of the surgery (nothing orally, not even water, at least 4 hours prior to surgery and any solids, milk or tea, at least 6 hours prior to surgery).
iv. Empty bowels on the morning of surgery and empty bladder before entering OT.
v. Should remove her glasses, contact lens, dentures, jewellery and lipstick.
vi. Have a responsible adult accompanying her to take her home after surgery.

Analgesia and Anesthesia

Local anesthesia, when properly administered and managed, meets both these goals and is recommended both for minilap tubectomy and laparoscopic tubal occlusion. Although general and regional anesthesia can be used safely and effectively for abdominal tubectomy and laparoscopic tubal occlusion, the number of unexpected and life-threatening complications related to general or regional anesthesia is higher than the number associated with local anesthesia (WHO, 1992). Thus, general and regional anesthesia should be used only in settings that are properly equipped and staffed to provide such anesthesia and to handle emergencies.

The anxiolytic, sedative, light muscle relaxant and amnesic effect produced in the client following administration of sedation allow sterilization procedure to be performed smoothly under local anesthesia.

- Lignocaine is the recommended local anesthetic (LA) and the recommended concentration is 1% lignocaine without adrenaline.
- The usual dose for local infiltration is 3 mg/kg body weight and onset of action is typically within three to five minutes, with anesthetic effect lasting up to 45 minutes.

Approximate weight/ build of client	Name of the drugs (Dose)	Route and time of administration	Repeat dose if required on the table**	Route and time of administration**
Thin (<40 kg)	Pethidine 25 mg + Promethazine 12.5 mg	IM: 30–45 min prior to surgery OR	Pethidine 10 mg	IV: 5 min prior to surgery
	Pethidine 15 mg + Promethazine 12.5 mg	IM: 30–45 min prior to surgery	Pentazocine 15 mg	IV: 5 min prior to surgery
Average (40–50 kg)	Pethidine 37.5 mg + Promethazine 12.5 mg	IM: 30–45 min prior to surgery OR	Pethidine 10 mg	IV: 5 min prior to surgery
	Pethidine 22.5 mg + Promethazine 12.5 mg	IM: 30–45 min prior to surgery	Pentazocine 15 mg	IV: 5 min prior to surgery
Well built (<40 kg)	Pethidine 50 mg + Promethazine 25 mg	IM: 30–45 min prior to surgery OR	Penthidine 10 mg	IV: 5 min prior to surgery
	Pethidine 30 mg + Promethazine 25 mg	IM: 30–45 min prior to surgery	Pentazocine 15 mg	IV: 5 min prior to surgery

**Dosage according to body weight is: Pethidine 0.5 to 1 mg/kg, Pentazocine 0.5 mg/kg and Promethazine 0.3 to 0.5 mg/kg. Repeat dose (if required) is given slowly intravenously as Pethidine 10 mg or Pentazocine 15 mg, 45 minutes after the first dose. The drugs should be diluted with equal quantity of normal saline or distilled water.

- 2% lignocaine solution must be diluted to 1% using normal saline or sterile water.
- Confirm effect of anesthesia before surgery.
- Client must be continuously monitored during and after parenteral administration.
- Oral communication must be maintained with the client throughout the procedure.
- If required, an IV line is to be secured before the start of the procedure.

Skin sensitivity test for lignocaine has no established predictive value for anaphylactic reaction. Therefore, it is not mandatory to perform a skin sensitivity test prior to infiltration of lignocaine.

Complications of LA

Major complications from LA are extremely rare. Rarely, convulsions and deaths have been reported in cases where excessive doses were used or inadvertent injections into a vein occurred.

In most cases, 10 ml of 1% lignocaine is adequate. In no case should the total dose exceed 3 mg per kg body weight of the client (i.e. about 15 ml). The key to safe use of a LA is to ensure that it is not injected directly into a vein and to use the lowest effective dose.

The following sequence indicates increasingly toxic levels of LA:

Mild effects:
- Numbness of lips and tongue
- Metallic taste in mouth
- Dizziness and light-headedness
- Ringing in ears
- Difficulty in focusing eyes

Severe effects:
- Lack of verbal response
- Sleepiness
- Disorientation
- Muscle twitching and shivering
- Slurred speech
- Generalized tonic-clonic convulsions
- Respiratory depression or arrest

For mild effects, wait a few minutes to see if symptoms subside, talk to the client and then continue the procedure.

Immediate treatment is needed for severe effects: Keep airway clear and give oxygen by mask or ventilation by Ambu bag. Should convulsions occur or persist despite respiratory support, small dose of injection Midazolam 1 to 2 mg may be given intravenously slowly or 5 to 10 mg of injection Diazepam intravenously slowly.

In all cases of sterilization, monitoring is an important aspect for patient safety.

    i. Medical records are to be maintained on monitoring of vital signs (pulse, respiration and blood pressure), level of consciousness, vomiting and other relevant information. The name of the drug(s), dosage, route and time of all administered drugs must be recorded.

ii. Pre-operatively: Pulse, respiration and blood pressure should be taken prior to pre-medication and every 10 minutes thereafter.
iii. Intraoperatively: (a) Maintain Verbal communication with client; and (b) check pulse, respiration and blood pressure every 5 minutes, especially during time of gas insufflation and at the time of tubal ligation.
iv. Postoperatively: Pulse, respiration and blood pressure are to be monitored and recorded every 15 minutes for at least one hour after surgery or even longer if the patient is unstable or not awake.

Procedure of Laparoscopic Sterilization

i. Position the client flat on her back on the operating table and ensure that bladder is empty.
ii. Determine that sterile or high-level disinfected laparoscopic instruments, fiber-optic cable and insufflator tubing are present and working.
iii. Ensure that emergency tray is available and all emergency equipment are in working order. Check that insufflator apparatus and light source units are working.
iv. Ensure that vital signs of the client are observed and recorded.
v. Give IV/ IM pre-medication (repeat if needed).
vi. Wash hands thoroughly with soap and water and air dry or dry with a clean cloth.
vii. Put new sterile gloves on both hands.
viii. Ensure that client is in a lithotomy position.
ix. Perform a gentle bimanual pelvic examination to assess uterine size, determine position, mobility and shape of the uterus and whether there is any pelvic abnormality.
x. Perform surgical scrub and put on sterile surgical gown and sterile disposable gloves on both hands.
xi. Apply antiseptic solution two times to the incision area (sub-umbilical). Use a sterile or high-level disinfected sponge forceps to hold a cotton or gauze swab soaked with antiseptic.
xii. Begin by wiping at incision site and move outward in a circular motion for 15 to 20 cm (6 to 8 inches or as for any abdominal procedure) and allow to air dry (about 2 minutes) before proceeding.
xiii. Drape the client with a sterile surgical drape.
xiv. Check functioning of laparoscope (both lens and ring applicator), trocar assembly unit and Veress needle.

Local Anesthesia

i. Raise a small skin wheal at the center of incision site using 1% lignocaine in a 10 or 20 ml sterile syringe (Fig. 19.1)
ii. Starting at the center of incision line, insert needle into skin and infiltrate 1 cc LA solution, then proceed into fascia at 45 degrees angle with the needle slightly caudal to the incision line. Aspirate to be sure the needle is not in a blood vessel. Then, withdraw the needle slowly while injecting 3–5 ml of lignocaine.
iii. Massage the skin to spread the anesthetic within the tissues. Wait for 2–3 minutes and then test the incision site with tissue forceps for adequacy of anesthesia. If the client feels

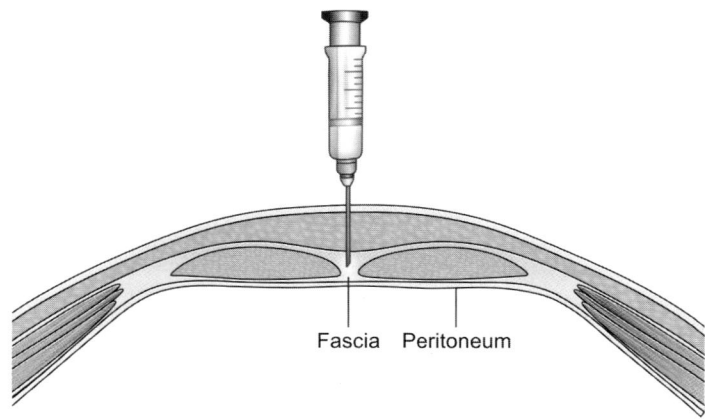

Fig. 19.1: Infiltration of LA at 90° angulation

pain, wait 2–3 minutes more and retest the incision site and inject 2 ml of 1% lignocaine, if necessary.

Creating Pneumoperitoneum

i. Place client in a head down (Trendelenburg) position of not more than 20 degrees.
ii. Make a small incision at the inferior umbilical margin (Fig. 19.2). Size of skin incision should not be more than the diameter of the trocar.
iii. Gently lift the infra-umbilical part of abdominal wall using the thumb and the forefingers to lift the abdominal wall away from the intestines.
iv. Grasp the shaft of the Veress needle (Fig. 19.3) and insert it at a 45 degree caudal angle to the abdominal wall. Two distinct 'gives' (feeling of release from a slight resistance) will be felt as the fascia is penetrated and the peritoneum is entered.
v. Check for correct abdominal entry by placing a drop of the anesthetic on the Veress needle Luer Lock opening and observing its ingress when the abdominal wall is lifted manually.

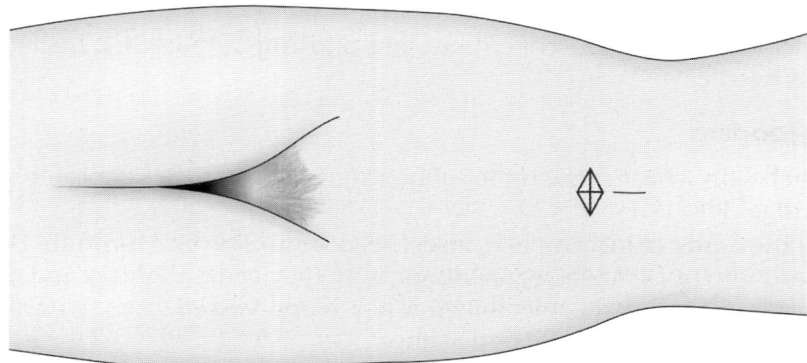

Fig. 19.2: Infra-umbilical incision

National Guidelines for Laparoscopic Tubal Ligation and Managing Its Complications

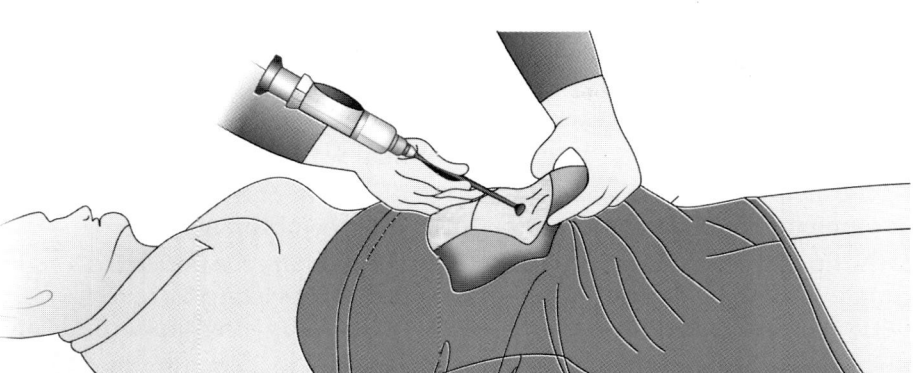

Fig. 19.3: Insertion of Veress needle for creating pneumoperitoneum

(Alternatively, use the pressure gauge of the insufflator apparatus to check for negative intra-abdominal pressure).

vi. Connect the sterile or high-level disinfected insufflator tubing to the Veress needle stop cock. Ask the assistant to connect the other end to the insufflator unit.

vii. Insufflation of abdomen should be done preferably with carbon dioxide (CO_2). Slow insufflation with graded insufflator and gradual de-sufflation should be done. Use the high flow switch to introduce CO_2 at the rate of 1 litre per minute. Intra-abdominal pressure should not exceed 15 mm of mercury (in field situations where availability of carbon dioxide is an issue, air may be used).

viii. Percuss the hypogastric area and listen for a drum-like sound, which will indicate pneumoperitoneum.

ix. Remove the Veress needle after insufflating 1.5 to 2.0 litres of CO_2.

x. Tell assistant to load Falope rings on the ring applicator of the laparoscope.

Alternatively, pneumoperitoneum can be created by directly introducing the trocar, if the surgeon is experienced and confident.

Falope Ring Loading

i. Lubricate Falope ring with sterile water or remaining LA but they should never be dipped in spirit or alcohol. Place the Falope ring dilator onto the inner tube of the laparoscope.

ii. Firmly hold the laparoscope at the middle area. Shift the two ring switch to position no.1 when applying the first ring (position no. 2 when loading the second ring). Place the end of the Falope ring guide against the tip of the dilator and in a steady motion, slowly push the band along the dilator until it rests on the inner tube. Remove guide and dilator. Repeat the first two steps to load the second ring. Remember to move the switch to the No. 2 position. Do not leave the Falope rings into the ring dilator for more than 5 minutes.

Abdominal Entry

i. Recheck the trumpet valve and rubber seal of the trocar sleeve to ensure air tightness. Assemble the trocar unit by inserting the obturator into the trocar sleeve.
ii. Manually grasp and raise the anterior abdominal wall directly beneath the umbilicus.
iii. Hold the fully assembled trocar (Fig. 19.4) on the palm of the hand, making sure that the thenar eminence is resting on the superior end of the obturator.
iv. Direct the tip of the obturator to an imaginary point where the pouch of Douglas is located at an angle of 60 to 70 degree. Apply downward and twisting force to traverse the fascia and peritoneum directed towards the pelvic cavity. Stop after the second "give" is felt.
v. Slightly retract obturator and advance trocar sleeve 1 to 2 cm into the abdominal cavity. Completely remove obturator.
vi. Connect insufflator tubing to the trocar stopcock and open. Insufflate air as needed.
vii. Connect the fiber-optic light cable to the laparoscope and ask the assistant to switch on the light source.
viii. Hold trocar trumpet valve mechanism between middle finger and thenar eminence of the hand in palms down position.
ix. Hold the hand grip assembly of the laparoscope using the thumb, middle and ring fingers of the hand. Allow the index finger to remain free.
x. Insert the tip of the laparoscope into the trocar sleeve before opening the trumpet valve.
xi. Insert laparoscope slowly under direct vision. Maneuver the laparoscope-trocar unit toward the pelvic cavity.
xii. Inspect and identify pelvic cavity structures.
xiii. In case of difficulty in viewing of pelvic structures, elevate the uterus per vagina preferably using the uterine elevator and by depressing handle of the uterine elevator/manipulator in a downward direction.

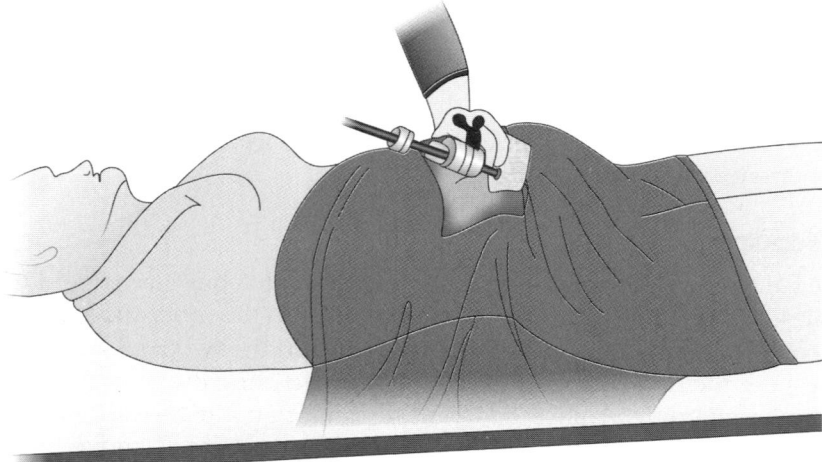

Fig. 19.4: Insertion of trocar with cannula followed with laparoscope

Laparoscope Guided Tubal Occlusion (Fig. 19.5)

i. Locate and verify the fallopian tube by visually identifying anatomical landmarks such as the cornu and fimbrial end.
ii. Extend forceps tongs fully by pushing the trigger operating slide away from the hand grip.
iii. Rotate the prong in order to position it at right angle to the axis of fallopian tube, ensuring that the slightly longer limb of the prong is below the tube. Also reconfirm that correct structure has been picked up.
iv. Place the posterior limb of the prong under the inferior aspect of the tube about 4 cm away from the cornu. Slightly lift it toward the anterior abdominal wall to allow excess mesosalpinx to fall off. Slowly retract the tongs by pulling the trigger operating slide toward the hand grip. Move the laparoscope forward during tong retraction to reduce risk of lacerating or injuring the tube. Continue retracting until spring tension is felt.
v. Using the index finger, check that the ring adaptor is in position no.1 without taking eyes off from the laparoscope eyepiece. Apply additional pressure to the operating slide to overcome the spring tension and to release the Falope ring. Slowly push away the operating slide to extend the forceps tongs and release the occluded fallopian tube.
vi. Inspect for adequacy of occlusion, i.e. a 2 cm loop of tube above the Falope ring showing the acute angle in mesosalpinx and for any active bleeding. Completely retract forceps

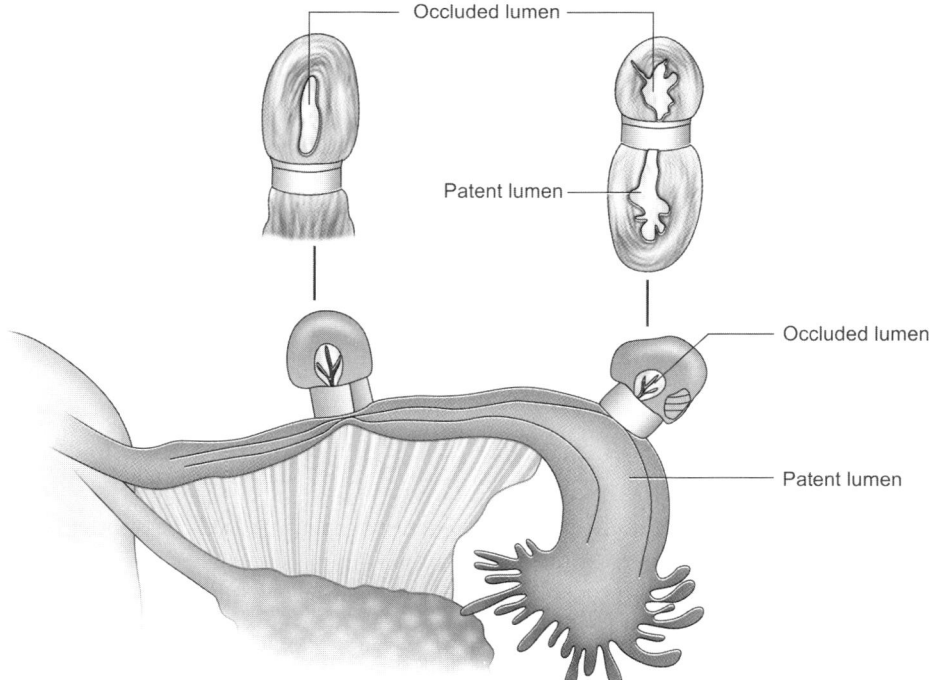

Fig. 19.5: Complete/correct occlusion on left side while incorrect/incomplete occlusion on right side

tongs prior to inspection. Always retract the tongs of the Ring Applicator into its sleeve after releasing the tubal loop.
vii. Locate and verify the other tube.
viii. Place two ring adaptors in no. 2 position. Repeat steps vi to ix to occlude the other tube.
ix. Inspect pelvic cavity for bleeding and other organ injuries. Keep tongs retracted after occlusion of the tubes.
x. Bring the operating table from Trendelenburg position to horizontal position.
xi. Remove laparoscope from the abdominal cavity under direct vision and disconnect external light source. Keep open the trocar trumpet valve to enable intra-abdominal gas escape slowly.
xii. Replace the obturator inside the trocar halfway and remove both of them together from the abdominal cavity.
xiii. Close incision with a single, simple stitch using absorbable or non-absorbable suture material.
xiv. Clean the wound and surrounding area and apply a small dressing.

Postoperative Care

- Remove uterine elevator/manipulator and vulsellum (if not done earlier) and place in 0.5% chlorine solution for decontamination.
- Dispose needle and syringe in a puncture-proof container.
- Place instruments in 0.5% chlorine solution for decontamination and soak for 10 minutes.
- Dispose materials according to infection prevention guidelines.
- Briefly immerse gloved hands in chlorine solution. If disposing off gloves, place in leak proof container or plastic bag. If reusing gloves, soak gloves in chlorine solution for 10 minutes.
- Wash hands thoroughly with soap and water and dry with a clean cloth or air dry.
- Ensure that the client is monitored at regular intervals and that vital signs are taken before wheeling the client out of OT.
- Ensure that the client is safely transferred to the postoperative (recovery) area.
- Determine that the client is ready for discharge after 4–6 hours.

Determining Discharge

- After at least 4 hours of procedure, when the vital signs are stable and the client is fully awake, has passed urine and can talk, drink and walk.
- The client has been seen and evaluated by the healthcare provider. Whenever necessary the client should be kept overnight at the facility.
- The client is accompanied by a responsible adult, while returning home.
- Analgesics, antibiotics and other medicines may be provided and/or prescribed as required.
- After sedation has worn off and before discharge, a trained staff member should repeat the postoperative instructions to the client or designated accompanying person. A written copy of the postoperative instructions should also be provided.

Advise and Follow-up (See Annexure II)

- Rest for the remainder of the day and resume light work after 48 hours.
- Should avoid lifting heavyweight or putting tension on the incision for 1 week.
- Be able to return to full activities within 1 week after surgery.
- Bathe after 24 hours but if the dressing becomes wet, it should be changed so that the incision area is kept dry until the stitches are removed.
- Report to the doctor or clinic if there is excessive pain, fainting, fever, bleeding or pus discharge from the incision, not passed urine, not passed flatus and feels bloating of abdomen.
- Return to the clinic, if there is any missed period/suspected pregnancy within two weeks of missed period for confirmation of pregnancy.
- Be instructed to go for routine and emergency follow-up.
- Establish contact with health worker within 48 hours.
- Return for a follow-up visit on the 7th day of surgery or as early as possible after 7 days.
- Have 2nd follow-up after 1 month or if menses do not return.
- In case of interval sterilization (minilap and laparoscopic), client may have sex one week after sterilization or whenever she feels comfortable thereafter.
- Certificate of sterilization should be issued one month after the surgery or, after the next menstrual period by the medical officer of the facility.
- If the client does not have her periods even after one month of surgery, rule out pregnancy before issuing sterilization certificate.

Complications of Laparoscopic Tubal Ligation and Its Management

Relatively, female sterilization has very few complications. The rate of complications is less than 2% for both minilap sterilization and laparoscopic sterilization. Identification of complication with prompt management decreases the probable morbidity associated with it.

Intraoperative Complications

1.	Vaso-vagal attack	• Make the OT table horizontal and raise the leg end and lower the head end • Give oxygen • Administer atropine (0.6 mg) IV if there is bradycardia (pulse below 60 per min). Repeat, if the baseline pulse rate is not achieved within 1 to 2 minutes
2.	Respiratory depression or cardiac arrest	Keep the airway open; assist breathing using manual resuscitation equipment with oxygen; assess the circulation by monitoring pulse, blood pressure and respiration; and other supportive therapy to be given as indicated.
3.	Cardiac arrest	On confirming cardiac arrest, give an immediate chest thump and begin external cardiac massage; assist breathing of the patient as described in Annexure 8; cannulate a vein and given appropriate resuscitative drugs; apply external counter-shock if an electrical defibrillator is available.

4.	Convulsions and toxic reactions to local anaesthesia	Maintain airway and administer 100% oxygen. If convulsions still persist, administer injection Midazolam 1–2 mg IV slowly. If Midazolam is not available, injection diazepam 5–10 mg IV can be given. Administration of IV fluid is not generally requird but may be given, if necessary. Surgery should be stopped and the patient is allowed to recover. Futher surgery should be performed at a centre with full range of services.
5.	Gas embolism	(When gas gets introduced into vascular system during insufflation of abdomen or needle inserted into vessel. Promptly turn client on her left side to keep gas on right side of heart; aspirate gas from the right atrium and ventricle with a central venous catheter or a direct intracardiac needle.
6.	Uterine perforation	(May occur due to introduction of uterine elevator from below). Repair immediately if there is bleeding; otherwise, these patients need to have further hospital observation to ensure they are stable.
7.	Bleeding from the mesosalpinx	If during minilap procedure—tie the bleeder with 2-0 chromic catgut. If during laparoscopic procedure—treat through the laparoscope with cautery or ring/clip application. If the bleeder cannot be controlled immediately, perform laparotomy.
8.	Injury to urinary bladder	Close in two layers and put self-retaining catheter in the bladder for 7 days or as long as necessary. If surgeon is available, ask for help.
9.	Injury to intra-abdominal viscera (i.e. small or large bowel) and blood vessels	Repair immediately and maintain IV line. If the operating surgeon is not confident of repairing, he/she must ask for help from a competent surgeon.
10.	Subcutaneous emphysema	(May occur when gas gets introduced into abdominal subcutaneous tissue during insufflation when trocar/veress needle tip is above the peritoneum). Stop insufflation and remove veress needle/trocar. Allow air to escape from the incision by gently pressing the surrounding skin.

Postoperative Complications

1.	Wound sepsis	Small stitch abscess is to be treated with drainage and dressings. However, severe sepsis needs opening of the incision and drainage of pus. Further treatment will be with dressing, antibiotics and analgesics.
2.	Hematoma in the abdominal wall	A small non-expanding, non-infected hematoma will resolve with no therapy, while a large one, particularly if infected, may need drainage and treatment with antibiotics
3.	Intestinal obstruction, paralytic ileus and peritonitis	The client should be hospitalized if she is not already in hospital. Keep the patient on nil orally put nasogastric suction, IV fluids and give antibiotics and analgesics, as indicated. Refer to higher centre, if required
4.	Tetanus	A rare complication. If tetanus is detected, the patient must be transferred to a proper centre for treatment immediately.
5.	Incisional hernia	A rare complication that needs surgical treatment.

Conditions not Attributable to Sterilization Procedure

1. Menstrual irregularities (for example menorrhagia, scanty period) — Sometimes occur but these are not complications of sterilization. Reassurance and treatment according to the cause is required in most cases.
2. Chronic pelvic inflammatory disease — It usually presents itself as pelvic pain and requires treatment with bed rest, antibiotics and analgesics. However, one should keep in mind ectopic pregnancy and should be ruled out.
3. Psychological problems (for example, depression) — Discussion of problem, clarification of the role of sterilization and answering questions are important.
4. Failure of the operation, leading to pregnancy — The client should be advised to report to the facility immediately after missed periods. The client should be offered MTP or be medically supported throughout the pregnancy. She should be offered repeat surgery, as indicated. Ectopic pregnancy must be ruled out as tubectomy predisposes to this condition.

Unforseen Complications and Scenarios that can be Encountered with Tubal Sterilization

1. *Tubo-ovarian masses:* These may cause difficulty in mobilizing the tubes and if dissection is attempted, can result in excessive bleeding.
2. *Dense adhesions due to previous surgeries:* If tubes are embedded in thick adhesions, they are best left alone as dissection of adhesions can cause hemorrhage or postoperative infections.
3. *PID or pelvic tuberculosis:* This may cause a plastered pelvis or frozen pelvis with inaccessible tubes.
4. *Highly vascular tubes:* With large vascular or venous formations, it may be difficult to get an avascular portion of the tube and there is more likelihood of hemorrhage.
5. *Congenital absence of tubes:* This is rare. By tracing over the fundus, absence of tubes can be detected. Counselling of client is important and postoperative ultrasound and/or hysterosalpingogram may be advised for confirmation.
6. *Tubal pathology:* Cases with hydrosalphinx or pyosalphinx, edematous tubes, haemorrhagic corpus luteum, ectopic pregnancy or malignancy should be documented and referred to a higher centre.
7. *Malignancy:* Malignancy of tubes, ovaries and uterus if found, should be documented. Tubectomy can be done if feasible but referral to a proper centre is mandatory.
8. *Unsuspected pregnancy:* Patient should be counseled about the presence of the unsuspected pregnancy and what her options are. Separate consent should be obtained for MTP. Pregnancy test may be done and, if possible, an ultrasound examination is also recommended. If she is willing, tubectomy can be done but proper documentation and follow-up should be carried out.

Failure of Sterilization

Effectiveness varies slightly depending on how the tubes are blocked but pregnancy rates are low with all techniques. The failure rate of laparoscopic sterilization is similar to minilap sterilization at approximately 1 pregnancy per 100 women year in the first year. Failure rate increases beyond 10 years of surgery and reaches 2 per 100 women years. Failure may be due to abnormalities of the fallopian tubes; procedural errors and reopening of the tube (recanalization) during the healing process.

In cases where surgeon is unable to identify the tube on one side and thereby could not occlude/ligate it, he/she should document it on the case sheet and inform the client accordingly that the sterilization procedure has not been successful. This documentation on the case sheet should also be countersigned by the client or their thumb impression taken. In such cases, sterilization certificate should not be issued even if she resumes her menstrual cycle. Such cases where sterilization certificate has not been issued are not eligible for compensation for 'failure' under FPIS (Family Planning Indemnity Scheme).

The presence of early, undetected pregnancy at the time of the procedure may be perceived as a failure and must be ruled out carefully. Such cases where the client is subsequently found to be pregnant on examination are not eligible for compensation for 'failure' under FPIS.

In case of missed menstrual period, the clients are advised to report to the healthcare facility within 2 weeks for confirmation about the failure of her sterilization procedure. She should be offered MTP and repeat sterilization procedure or be medically supported throughout the pregnancy if she so wishes. Ectopic pregnancy must be ruled out as female sterilization predisposes to this condition.

BIBLIOGRAPHY

1. Arjun Adlakha (April 1997), Population Trends: India (PDF), U.S. Department of Commerce, Economics and Statistics Administration, Bureau of the Census, archived from the original (PDF) on 10 October 2013, retrieved 5 December 2009
2. GN Ramu (2006), Brothers and sisters in India: A study of urban adult siblings, University of Toronto Press, ISBN 978-0-8020-9077-5
3. India and Family Planning: An Overview (PDF), Department of Family and Community Health, World Health Organization, archived from the original (PDF) on 21 December 2009, retrieved 2009-11-25
4. Marian Rengel (2000), Encyclopedia of Birth Control, Greenwood Publishing Group, ISBN 978-1-57356-255-3.
5. Population growth (annual %) data.worldbank.org. Retrieved 28 March 2018.
6. Rabindra Nath Pati (2003). Socio-cultural dimensions of Reproductive Child Health. APH Publishing. p. 51. ISBN 978-81-7648-510-4.
7. Singh, Susheela; Shekhar, Chander; Alagarajan, Manoj et al (1 January 2018). "The incidence of abortion and unintended pregnancy in India, 2015". The Lancet Global Health. 6 (1): e111-e120. doi:10.1016/S2214-109X(17)30453-9. ISSN 2214-109X.

Acknowledgements

The regulations, guidelines and complications are compiled in whole from the Government of India Reference Manual for Female Sterilization, November 2014. This manual is published by the Family Planning Division, Ministry of Health and Family Welfare, GOI. The authors acknowledge the same with regards to the manual, appendix and consent forms.

ANNEXURE I

Medical Record & Check List for Sterilization

A checklist is to be filled by the doctor before conducting sterilization procedure for ensuring the eligibility and fitness of the client for sterilization.

(To be filled before commencing the operation)

Name of Health Facility: ....

Beneficiary Registration No. ....

Date..............................

A. Eligibility Checklist

Client is within eligible age	Yes............... No....................
Client is ever married	Yes............... No....................
Client has at least one child over one year of age	Yes............... No....................
Lab investigations (Hb, urine) undertaken are within normal limits (7.0 gm/dl or more)	Yes............... No....................
Medical status as per clinical observation is within normal limits	Yes............... No....................
Mental status as per clinical observation is normal	Yes............... No....................
Local examination done is normal	Yes............... No....................
Informed consent given by the client	Yes............... No....................
Explained to the client that consent form has authority of a legal document	Yes............... No....................
Abdominal/pelvic examination has been done in the female and is Within Normal Limits	Yes............... No....................
Infection prevention practices as per laid down standards	Yes............... No....................

B. Menstrual History (for female clients)

Cycle Days	
Length	
Regularity	Regular..
	Irregular...
Date of LMP (DD/MM/YYYY)	................/................./...................

C. Obstetric History (for female clients)

Number of Spontaneous Abortions	
Number of Induced Abortions	
Currently Lactating	Yes.................... No....................
Amenorrheic	Yes.................... No....................
Whether Pregnant	Yes.................... No.................... If Yes (no. of weeks pregnancy)..................................
No. of Living Children	Total No..
Last Child birth (Date/Month/Year)	................../................/..................

D. Contraceptive History

Have you or your spouse ever used contraception?	Yes.................... No....................
Are you or your spouse currently using any contraception or have you or your spouse used any contraception during the last six months? (✓) Tick the option	• None.. • IUCD.. • Condoms...................................... • Oral Pills...................................... • Any Other (specify)....................

E. Medical History

Recent medical Illness	Yes.................... No....................
Previous Surgery	Yes.................... No....................
Allergies to medication	Yes.................... No....................
Bleeding Disorder	Yes.................... No....................
Anemia	Yes.................... No....................
Diabetes	Yes.................... No....................
Jaundice or liver disorder	Yes.................... No....................
RTI/STI/PID	Yes.................... No....................
Convulsive disorder	Yes.................... No....................
Tuberculosis	Yes.................... No....................
Malaria	Yes.................... No....................
Asthma	Yes.................... No....................
Heart Disease	Yes.................... No....................
Hypertension	Yes.................... No....................
Mental Illness	Yes.................... No....................
Sexual Problems	Yes.................... No....................
Prostatitis (Male sterilization)	Yes.................... No....................
Epididymitis (Male Sterilization)	Yes.................... No....................
H/O Blood Transfusion	Yes.................... No....................
Gynecological problems (Female Sterilization)	Yes.................... No....................
Currently on medication (if yes, specify)	Yes.................... No....................

Comments ....

F. Physical Examination

BP……………………………………Pulse……………………………Temperature……………………

Lungs	Normal………………… Abnormal…………………
Heart	Normal………………… Abnormal…………………
Abdomen	Normal………………… Abnormal…………………

G. Local Examination (Strike out whichever is not applicable)

1. Male Sterilization

Skin of Scrotum	Normal………………… Abnormal…………………
Testis	Normal…………………Abnormal…………………
Epididymis	Normal…………………Abnormal…………………
Hydrocele	Yes………………………No…………………………
Varicocele	Yes………………………No…………………………
Hernia	Yes………………………No…………………………
Vas Deferens	Normal…………………Abnormal…………………
Both Vas Palpable	Yes………………………No…………………………

2. Female Sterilization

External Genitalia	Normal…………………Abnormal…………………
PS Examination	Normal…………………Abnormal…………………
PV Examination	Normal…………………Abnormal…………………
Uterus Position	A/V…………………………R/V………………………… Mid position………………Not determined……
Uterus size	Normal……………Abnormal Size…………
Uterus Mobility	Yes………No (Restricted or Fixed) ………………
Cervical Erosion	Yes…………………………No……………………………
Adnexa	Normal…………………Abnormal…………………

Comments ……………………………………………………………………………………………………
……

H. Laboratory Investigations

Hemoglobin level	…………………………………………………………Gms%
Urine: Albumin	Yes………………… No………………………
Urine- Sugar	Present…………… Absent
Urine test for Pregnancy	Positive: ………… Negative
Any Other (specify)	……………………………………………………

Name: …………………………………………   Signature of the Examining Doctor

Date: …………………………………………   **Hospital Seal** ………………………………………

I. Preoperative Preparation

Fasting	Yes.............................. duration................hours
	No......................
Passed urine	Yes/No.......................
Any other (specify)	

J. Anaesthesia/Analgesia

Type of anaesthesia given (✓) Tick the option	• Local only • Local and analgesia • General, no intubation • General, intubation • Any other (specify)
Time Drug name Dosage Route	....

Signature of anaesthetist in case of regional or general anaesthesia

K. Surgical Approach (Strike out whichever is not Applicable)

Male sterilization

Local anaesthesia	Lignocaine 2%...............................cc Other
Technique	Conventional...................NSV..............................
Type of incision Conventional NSV	Single vertical................... Double vertical................... Single puncture
Material for occlusion of vas	2-0 Silk..............................2-0 Catgut...........................
Fascial interposition	Yes No................................ If no, give reasons. ....
Length of vas resected	....Cm
Suture of silk for conventional vasectomy	Silk..Other...........................
Surgical notes	
Any other surgery done at time of sterilization?	Yes No................................. If yes give details...................
Specify details of complications and management	

Name: .... Signature of the operating surgeon

Date: ....

Female sterilization	
Local anaesthesia	Lignocaine % Other

Timing of procedure
(✓) Tick the option used
	• 24 hours—7 days post-partum
	• Interval (42 days or more after delivery or abortion)
	• With abortion, induced or spontaneous
	  * Less than 12 weeks
	  * More than 12 weeks
	  * Any other (specify)

Technique
(✓) Tick the option used
	• Minilap
	  * With C section
	  * With other surgery
	• Laparoscopy
	  * SPL/DPL

Method of occlusion of fallopian tubes
(✓) Tick the option used
	• Modified Pomeroy Laparoscopy:
	  * Ring
	  * Clip

Details of gas insufflation Pneumoperitoneum created (CO_2/Air)	Yes ....No....................
Insufflator used	Yes ....No....................
Specify details of complications and management	

Name: ....   Signature of the operating surgeon

Date: ....

L. Vital Signs: Monitoring Chart (For Female Sterilization)

*Sedation: 0—Alert 1—Drowsy 2—Sleeping/arousable 3—Not arousable

Event	Time	Sedation*	Pulse	Blood Pressure	Respiratory Rate	Bleeding	Comments (Treatment)
Preoperative (every 15 min after premedication)							
Intra-operative (continuous)							
Post-operative 1. Every 15 min for first hour and longer if the patient is not stable/awake	15 min 30 min 45 min						
2. Every 1 hour until 4 hours after surgery	1hr 2hrs 3hrs 4hrs						

Name and Signature of attending nurse ....

M. Post-Operative Information

Passed urine	Yes	....	No.............................
Abdominal distension	Yes	....	No.............................
Patient feeling well	Yes	....	No.............................
If no, please specify			

N. Instructions For Discharge

Male sterilization client observed   Yes ....No ....
for half an hour after surgery

Female sterilization client observed   Yes ....No ....
for four hours after surgery

Post-operative instructions given verbally   Yes ....No ....

Post-operative instructions given in writing Yes ....No ....

Patient counselled for postoperative instructions   Yes ....No ....

Comments..
....

Name: ....   **Signature of the discharging doctor**

ANNEXURE II

Post Operative Instruction Card

Name and type of hospital/facility	
Client's name	
Father's name	
Husband's name/Wife's Name	
Address	
Contact number (if available)	
Date of operation	/ / (D/M/Y)
Type of operation	Minilap/Post-partum/Laparoscopic (SP/DP)/ Conventional Vasectomy/NSV

1. Follow-up:
   a) After 48 hours, first contact is established
   b) On the 7th day for stitch removal
   c) **Female Sterilization:** After one month or after first menstrual period, whichever is earlier
      Male Sterilization: After 3 months, for semen examination for sperm count
   d) In an emergency, as and when required to the nearest health facility
2. Medication as prescribed:
3. Return home and rest for the remainder of the day.
4. **Female Sterilization:** - Resume only light work after 48 hours and gradually return to full activity in two weeks following surgery.
5. **Male Sterilization:** - Scrotal support or snug undergarment for 48 hours.
   - Resume normal work after 48 hours and return to full activity, including cycling, after one week following surgery.
6. Resume normal diet as soon as possible.
7. Keep the incision area clean and dry. Do not disturb or open the dressing.
8. Bathe after 24 hours following the surgery. If the dressing becomes wet, it should be changed so that the incision area is kept dry until the stitches are removed.
9. **Sexual intercourse:**
   Vasectomy/ Tubectomy does not interfere with sexual pleasure, ability or performance.
   Female Sterilization: - In the case of interval sterilization (Minilap and Laparoscopic), the client may have intercourse one week after surgery or whenever she feels comfortable thereafter.
   - In the case of post partum sterilization (after caesarian or normal delivery), the client may have intercourse two week after surgery or whenever she feels comfortable.
10. Report to the doctor or clinic if there is excessive pain, fainting, fever, bleeding or pus discharge from the incision or if the client has not passed urine, not passed flatus and experiences bloating of the abdomen.
11. Contact health personnel or a doctor in case of any doubt.

12. **Female Sterilization:** Return to the facility if, there is any missed period/no periods, with in 2 weeks to rule out pregnancy.
13. **Male Sterilization:** Return to the facility after three months for semen examination to see if azoospermia has been achieved. If semen still shows sperm return to facility every month till 6 months.

Follow-up report

Follow up	Time after surgery	Date of follow-up	Complications, if any	Action Taken
1st	48 hours			
2nd	7th day			
3rd	1 month after surgery or after the first menstrual period, whichever is earlier (Female Sterilization)			
	After 3 months for semen examination (Male Sterilization)			
Emergency				

Comment..

....

Result of Semen Examination:..

Name: ....   Designation:..

                                        Signature of the person filling out the report

Chapter 20

Criteria for Selection of Patients for Tubal Ligation

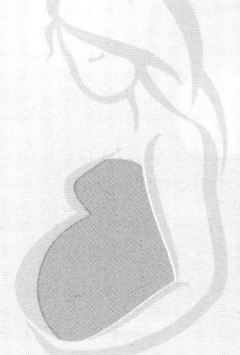

○ Devki Potwar ○ Asha Dalal

Sterilization is a surgical procedure that is intended to be permanent and special care must be taken to assure that every client makes a voluntary, informed choice of the method. Transcervical methods of female sterilization are not addressed in these recommendations.

There is no medical condition that would absolutely restrict a person's eligibility for sterilization, although some conditions and circumstances will require that certain precautions are taken, including those where the recommendation is assigned as Category C (caution), D (delay) or S (special). For some of these conditions and circumstances, the theoretical or proven risks may outweigh the advantages of undergoing sterilization. Where the risks of sterilization outweigh the benefits, long-term, highly effective contraceptive methods are a preferable alternative. Decisions in this regard will have to be made on an individual basis, considering the risks and benefits of sterilization versus the risks of pregnancy, and the availability and acceptability of highly effective, alternative methods.[1]

Timing of the Surgical Procedure[1]

- **Interval sterilization** should be performed within 7 days of the menstrual period (in the follicular phase of the menstrual cycle)
- **Postpartum sterilization** should be done after 24 hours up to 7 days of delivery.
- **Sterilization with medical termination of pregnancy (MTP)** can be performed concurrently.
- **Sterilization following spontaneous abortion** can be performed provided the client fulfils the medical eligibility criteria.
- **Laparoscopic tubal ligation** should not be done concurrently with second trimester abortion and in the postpartum period.

A number of studies have reported that the incidence of regret and dissatisfaction is increased when sterilization has been performed concomitantly with caesarean section. Regret has also been shown to increase after postpartum sterilization associated with vaginal delivery.[2]

All clients should be carefully counselled about the intended permanence of sterilization and the availability of alternative, long-term, highly effective methods. This is of extra concern for young people.[1]

Case Selection/Eligibility Checklist[1]

The following should be looked for (self-declaration by the client will be the basis for compiling this information)

1. Client is within eligible age (client should be below the age of 49 years and above the age of 22 years)
2. Client is ever married
3. Client has at least one child over one year of age.
4. Lab investigations (Hb, urine) undertaken are within normal limits (7.0 gm or more)
5. Medical status as per clinical observation is within normal limits
6. Mental status as per clinical observation is normal.
7. Local examination done is normal
8. Informed consent given by the client
9. Explained to the client that consent form has authority of a legal document.
10. Abdominal/pelvic examination has been done in the female and is within normal limits.

It is important to consider a woman's past surgical and medical history in the decision regarding surgical approach. A laparoscopic approach may be best avoided in women who have a history of multiple abdominal surgeries, intra-abdominal adhesive disease, repaired abdominal wall hernias, morbid obesity or contraindications to general anaesthesia.[3]

The Medical Eligibility Criteria for Female Surgical Sterilization procedures outlined by WHO (2015) serve as guidelines for case selection based on the clinical findings of the client.[1]

However, the final selection of the case selection criteria mentioned above and guided by the medical eligibility criteria.

Explanation for A, C, D and S are stated below:

A—Accept: There is no medical reason to deny sterilization to a person with this condition.

C—Caution: The procedure is normally conducted in a routine setting, but with extra preparations and precautions.

D—Delay: The procedure is delayed until the condition is evaluated and/or corrected. Alternative temporary methods of contraception should be provided.

S—Special: The procedure should be undertaken in a setting with an experienced surgeon and staff, the equipment needed for providing general anaesthesia, and other backup medical support. To meet these conditions, the capacity to decide on the most appropriate anaesthesia regimen is also needed. Alternative temporary methods of contraception should be provided if referral is required or if there is otherwise any delay.

Criteria for Selection of Patients for Tubal Ligation

A—Accept : There is no medical reason to deny sterilization to a person with this condition.
1. Mild pre-eclampsia
2. Past ectopic pregnancy
3. Smoking and age <35 years
4. History of high blood pressure during pregnancy (where current blood pressure is measurable and normal)
5. History of DVT/PE
6. Family history of DVT/PE in first-degree relatives
7. Along with major/minor surgery without prolonged immobilization
8. History of known thrombogenic mutations (e.g. Factor V Leiden; prothrombin mutation; protein S, protein C, and antithrombin deficiencies)
9. Superficial venous disorders (varicose veins/superficial venous thrombosis)
10. Known dyslipidaemias without other known cardiovascular risk factors
11. Migraine headaches or non-migrainous (mild or severe) headaches
12. Vaginal bleeding patterns [irregular pattern without heavy bleeding, heavy or prolonged bleeding (includes regular and irregular patterns)]
13. Benign ovarian tumours (including cysts)
14. Severe dysmenorrhoea
15. Gestational trophoblastic disease (decreasing or undetectable β-HCG levels)
16. Cervical ectropion
17. Cervical intraepithelial neoplasia (CIN)
18. Breast disease (undiagnosed mass, benign breast disease, family history of cancer, past history of breast cancer and no evidence of current disease for 5 years)
19. Past pelvic inflammatory disease (PID) (assuming no current risk factors for STIs, with subsequent pregnancy)
20. Vaginitis (including *Trichomonas vaginalis* and bacterial vaginosis)
21. Increased risk of STIs
22. High risk of HIV
23. Asymptomatic or mild HIV clinical disease (WHO stage 1 or 2)
24. Uncomplicated schistosomiasis
25. Non-pelvic tuberculosis
26. Malaria
27. History of gestational diabetes
28. Simple goiter
29. Current aymptomatic gall bladder disease or past history of cholecystectomy
30. History of pregnancy related or past-COC related cholestasis
31. Viral hepatitis (carrier or chronic)
32. Mild compensated cirrhosis
33. Liver tumours—benign (focal nodular hyperplasia)

Extra preparations and precautions need to be taken if tubal ligation is to be considered in the following conditions (C—Caution):
1. Young women
2. Obesity ≥30 kg/m² body mass index (BMI)
3. Hypertension, adequately controlled. Elevated blood pressure levels (properly taken measurements), systolic 140–159 mmHg or diastolic 90–99 mmHg.
4. History of ischaemic heart disease
5. Stroke (history of cerebrovascular accident)
6. Uncomplicated valvular heart disease (the woman requires prophylactic antibiotics)
7. Epilepsy
8. Depressive disorders
9. Current breast cancer
10. Uterine fibroids (with or without distortion of the uterine cavity)
11. Past pelvic inflammatory disease without subsequent pregnancy
12. Schistosomiasis (fibrosis of the liver): Liver function may need to be evaluated
13. Diabetes without vasculopathy
14. Hypothyroidism
15. Liver tumours—benign adenomas, malignant hepatomas
16. Anaemias—thalassaemia, sickle-cell disease
17. Iron deficiency anaemia (Hb ≥7 to <10 g/dl)
18. Diaphragmatic hernia
19. Kidney disease
20. Severe nutritional deficiencies
21. Previous abdominal or pelvic surgeries

Procedure should not be performed if the patient has the following conditions (D—DELAY):
1. Pregnancy
2. Postpartum (after 7 days to less than 42 days)
3. Severe pre-eclampsia/eclampsia
4. Prolonged rupture of membranes, 24 hours or more
5. Puerperal sepsis, intrapartum or puerperal fever
6. Severe antepartum or postpartum or post-abortal haemorrhage
7. Severe trauma to the genital tract (cervical or vaginal tear at time of delivery/abortion)
8. Post-abortal sepsis or fever
9. Acute haematometra
10. Acute DVT/PE
11. Along with major surgery with prolonged immobilization
12. Current ischaemic heart disease
13. Unexplained vaginal bleeding (the condition must be evaluated before the procedure is performed)
14. Gestational traphoblastic disease (persistently elevated β-HCG levels or malignant disease)

15. Cervical cancer (awaiting treatment)
16. Endometrial cancer, ovarian cancer
17. Current PID
18. Current purulent cervicitis or chlamydial infection or gonorrhea
19. Current symptomatic gall bladder disease
20. Acute viral hepatitis
21. Iron-deficiency anaemia (Hb < 7 g/dl)
22. Local infection
23. Acute bronchitis, pneumonia
24. Systemic infection or gastroenteritis

Special Conditions (S—Special)

1. If exploratory surgery or laparoscopy is conducted during uterine rupture or perforation, and the patient is stable, then repair of the problem and tubal sterilization may be performed concurrently if no additional risk is involved.
2. Multiple risk factors for arterial cardiovascular disease (such as older age, smoking, diabetes, hypertension and known dyslipidaemias)
3. *Hypertension:* Systolic ≥ 160 mmHg or diastolic ≥ 100 mmHg (single reading of blood pressure level is not sufficient to classify a woman as hypertensive.)
   Elevated blood pressure should be controlled before surgery. There are increased anaesthesia-related risks and an increased risk of cardiac arrhythmia with uncontrolled hypertension. Careful monitoring of blood pressure intraoperatively is particularly necessary in this situation.
4. Vascular disease
5. Deep vein thrombosis (DVT)/pulmonary embolism (PE) and established on anticoagulant therapy
6. Complicated valvular heart disease (pulmonary hypertension, risk of atrial fibrillation, history of subacute bacterial endocarditis) : These women are at high risk for complications associated with anaesthesia and surgery. If the woman has atrial fibrillation that has not been successfully managed or current subacute bacterial endocarditis, the procedure should be delayed.
7. Rheumatic diseases [systemic lupus erythematosus (SLE)]: For all categories of SLE, classifications are based on the assumption that no other risk factors for cardiovascular disease are present.
   a. Positive (or unknown) antiphospholipid antibodies
   b. Severe thrombocytopenia
   c. Immunosuppressive treatment
8. Endometriosis
9. *Severe or advanced HIV clinical disease (WHO stage 3 or 4):* The presence of an AIDS-related illness may require that the procedure be delayed.
10. Pelvic tuberculosis

11. Diabetes with nephropathy/retinopathy/neuropathy and/or diabetes lasting more than 20 years duration.
12. Hyperthyroidism
13. Severe decompensated cirrhosis
14. Coagulation disorders
15. Chronic asthma, bronchitis, emphysema, lung infection
16. Fixed uterus due to previous surgery or infection
17. Abdominal wall or umbilical hernia: Hernia repair and tubal sterilization should be performed concurrently, if possible.

To conclude: A targeted medical history, physical examination and laboratory investigations need to be completed to ascertain eligibility for surgery. With proper counseling and informed consent, most women can have female sterilization safely.

REFERENCES

1. Medical Eligibility Criteria for contraceptive use, World Health Organization, Fifth edition, 2015
2. Faculty of Sexual and Reproductive Healthcare Clinical Guidance, Male and Female Sterilisation, Clinical Effectiveness Unit, September 2014. (ISSN 1755-103X)
3. Schmidt E, Diedrich J, et al. Glob. Libr.Women's med., 2014 (ISSN: 1756-2228)

MTP and Tubal Ligations—Problems at Rural Areas of India

○ Gajanan Velhal ○ Sneha Shirodkar

For more than 48 years, following the enactment of the Medical Termination of Pregnancy (MTP) Act of 1971, women in India have been entitled to legal abortion services in registered facilities and by certified providers. Women have the right to access abortions across a range of situations. Consent of the husband or guardian is not required for adult women (Aged 18 and above). With these liberal conditions, the MTP Act was intended to reduce the incidence of illegal and unsafe abortions. However, most women continue to obtain abortion services outside of registered settings, and/or from uncertified and often unqualified providers more so in rural areas.[1] Amendment (2003) in the MTP rules allows certified practitioners to provide medical abortion from his/her clinic, even if it may not be an approved site, provided he/she has access to a site approved under MTP Act. The law requires that for the purpose of access, the provider should display a Certificate to this effect from the owner of the approved site. The providers should comply with the requirements of MTP Act.[2]

Sterilization (female tubectomy) is the most commonly used permanent contraceptive method worldwide. Sterilization operations are skilled procedures and therefore warrant extra care and caution.

Global Scenario

- Over a span of 4 years, from 2010 to 2014, about 56 million induced (safe and unsafe) abortions occurred worldwide each year, which amounts to 35 induced abortions per 1000 women aged between 15–44 years. One-fourth of all the pregnancies ended in an induced abortion, more in developing countries as compared to developed countries.[3]
- In developing countries, about 25 million unsafe abortions took place during these 4 years, and out of these, 8 million were carried out in the least-safe or dangerous conditions. More

than 50% of all the estimated unsafe abortions globally were in Asia. About 75% of the abortions that occurred in Africa and Latin America were unsafe. Each year between 4.7% and 13.2% of maternal deaths can be attributed to unsafe abortions.[4]
- According to WHO, every eight minutes a woman die due to complications arising from unsafe abortions in developing countries making it a leading cause of maternal mortality (13%).[5] Around 7 million women are admitted to hospitals every year in developing countries for complications associated with unsafe abortions.[6]
- The annual cost of treating major complications from unsafe abortion is estimated at US $553 million.[7]
- In developed countries, 30 women died for every 100 000 unsafe abortions as against 220 in developing countries and 520 in Sub-Saharan Africa region. Africa region accounts for 29% of all unsafe abortions, and 62% of unsafe abortion-related deaths.[4]
- Forty per cent of the world's women have access to legal induced abortions "without restriction as to reason, within gestational limits." Maternal mortality seldom results from safe abortions. Legal abortions performed in the developed world are among the safest procedures in medicine. In the US, the risk of maternal death from abortion is 0.6 per 100,000 procedures, making abortion about 14 times safer than childbirth (8.8 maternal deaths per 100,000 live births). The risk of abortion-related mortality increases with gestational age, but remains lower than that of childbirth.[8]
- China has the highest number of sterilized population (70 million), followed by India (>45 million) in the world.[9] Global data shows approximately 2–3/1000 failures following female sterilization with minor variation country-wise. However, there is a possibility of underreporting as follow-up is often a challenge.[10] According to the international sources, with tubectomy, the risk of failure (becoming pregnant again) is roughly one in 200, the risk of postoperative complication is one in 100 and the risk of death is three in 100,000. Even when tubal occlusion operation are competently performed with all technical precautions, intrauterine pregnancy occurs subsequently in 0.05% cases.[11]

National Scenario

Unsafe abortions contribute to eight percent of maternal deaths in India. In absolute numbers, close to 10 women die due to unsafe abortions each day.[1] While abortion has been legal in India since 1971, available research shows that 56% of the 6.4 million abortions that take place in the country are unsafe.[2] It is unfortunate that women continue to face severe complications which are totally preventable through just ensuring easy access to safe abortion services. Abortion in India is controversially the cause of Gendercide. In many parts of India, daughters are not preferred and hence sex-selective abortion is commonly practiced, resulting in an unnatural male to female population sex ratio.

Female sterilization is the mainstay of contraceptive methods in India. Every year over four million female sterilization operations are done in the country.[12] Abdominal TL is the most common procedure adopted in rural areas because of lack of trained professionals for laparoscopic TL procedures.

In India, public sector health infrastructure network includes 729 district hospitals, 5510 community health centres (CHCs) and 25650 primary health centres (PHCs). In general, in

India, a few public sector health facilities provide abortion services. Women's access to safe abortion services from public sector facilities is limited by a range of health system and community-level factors. MTP and TL (especially laparoscopic TL) services are rarely available at the Primary Health Centre (PHC) level, most PHCs and even some Community Health Centres (CHCs) lack trained staff and the required equipment and supplies for providing MTP and TL or do not have the necessary certification.[1] In Karnataka, only 25% of PHCs have the infrastructure, and personnel to offer safe abortion services. Access to certified providers is better in urban areas, but the safety and quality of care differ little.[13]

The training of Medical Officers, working at different levels itself is not comprehensive. It focuses only on Dilation and Curettage (D and C) and Electrical Vacuum Aspiration (EVA) and excludes Manual Vacuum Aspiration (MVA) and Medical Methods of Abortion (MMA). Many of those that provide abortion services, continue to use Dilation and Curettage (D and C) for first trimester abortions, a method internationally recognized as inappropriate in general, and only to be used when MVA or medical methods of abortion are unavailable. Nearly 50 per cent of all abortions occur in rural India, where only 25% of government facilities offering abortion are located.[13]

Women seeking to terminate their pregnancies are forced to resort to unsafe methods, particularly when access to legal abortion is restricted.

Despite abortion being legal, following factors limit availability and utilization of services by women[14]

- Social factors
- Policy factors
- Economic factors and
- Physical access to services

Social Factors

1. Ignorance and lack of awareness that abortion is legal
2. Social stigma attached to abortion
3. Gender discrimination and low status of women, inability to take decisions regarding sexual and reproductive issues
4. Involvement of multiple decision makers for women undergoing abortions
5. Clandestine and greedy ways of some traditional healers and health workers
6. Sexual assault and child abuse leading to unwanted pregnancies
7. Lack of male responsibility
8. Women do not go to male service providers

Policy Factors

1. Legal aspect of abortion not disseminated adequately
2. Low and improper use of contraceptives for family planning, contraceptive failure, etc.
3. Limited number of qualified providers for safe abortion and policies that limit full use of mid-level providers

4. Lack of promotion of place where safe and legal services can be accessed
5. Inadequate equipment and supplies at public health centers
6. Insisting on acceptance of a particular contraceptive method during abortion care
7. Weak referral linkages

Economic Factors

1. Poverty and economic hardships
2. Trained providers in private sector charge heavily

Physical Access to Services

1. Limited availability of qualified providers in rural/peripheral areas
2. Inadequate equipment and supplies at public health facilities in rural/peripheral areas

Government Initiatives

There have been concerted efforts by the Government of India to increase access to safe abortion services at the PHCs. As early as 2000, the National Population Policy (NPP) (Ministry of Health and Family Welfare), noted the provision of safe abortion services as an important strategy for reducing maternal deaths. Recognizing the need to increase access to safe abortion, particularly in rural areas, the policy recommended expanding abortion services to the PHC level. Notably, in an attempt, the provider base for services in general (National Rural Health Mission, 2005), added a new cadre of service providers, including doctors trained in the Ayurveda and Homoeopathy branches of medicine (Ministry of Health and Family Welfare, 2005). The rules and regulation governing the MTP Act were amended in May 2003 to specify that Medical Abortion (MA) could be provided by certified providers in unregistered facilities, as long as they had access to a registered facility for backup. As a result, medical abortion can now be provided at the PHC level, provided that backup surgical facility at a higher level is readily available for referral. Furthermore, the Ministry of Health and Family Welfare has specific strategies to increase access to safe abortion services both at the community and facility levels. *At the community level*, strategies include spreading awareness on issues related to safe abortion services. *At the provider level*, training of Auxiliary Nurse Midwives (ANMs) and Accredited Social Health Activists (ASHAs) to provide confidential counseling is advocated; ANMs, ASHAs and Anganwadi Workers (AWWs) are expected to counsel and refer women as well as provide post-abortion care. At the facility level, the aim is to ensure the availability of quality MVA technologies at all CHCs and First Referral Units (FRUs), and at least half of all 24/7 PHCs, and to encourage the provision of quality MTP services by the private and NGO sectors. Guidelines to provide MVA up to eight weeks of gestation at the PHC level have also been prepared, thus further paving the way for increased access to safe abortion services nationwide (Ministry of Health and Family Welfare).

Recognizing the urgent need to enable rural women to acquire accessible and high quality abortion services, a number of *organizations*–Ipas (coordinating partner), Action Research and Training for Health (ARTH), the Centre for Enquiry into Health and Allied Themes (CEHAT), the Family Planning Association of India (FPAI), the Federation of Obstetric and

Gynecological Societies of India (FOGSI), International Maternal and Child Health (IMCH)-Uppsala University, the Population Council and the Society of Midwives, India (SOMI), came together in 2006 to form the Consortium for Safe Abortions in India. The goal of the Consortium is to increase access to legal, safe and comprehensive abortion services, including post-abortion family planning, in the public health system, and especially among the rural poor. One of its key activities was to develop a comprehensive and evidence-based abortion care model suitable for rural women in different settings. The model, which aimed at addressing both facility based and community-based barriers, focused on enabling public sector sites to offer comprehensive abortion care services and simultaneously, to build awareness at woman and community levels about the legality of abortion and the availability of safe abortion services in the public sector.[15]

The Government has established *MTP training centers* in each state and specifies a training protocol to ensure the thorough safe abortion training of government practitioners. As per GOI guidelines, MTP training was being conducted for a period of 12 working days. However, in view of the feedback received from various sources, the hands-on training experience obtained in 12 days was not found adequate. It has been decided to fix the duration of MTP training to 18 days for MBBS doctors and 4 days for Obstetric and Gynecology specialist. Manual Vacuum Aspiration (MVA), Medical abortion have been included in the syllabus of this training.

Considering that 73 per cent of abortions in India occur in the first trimester, providers should be encouraged to use MVA within eight weeks or MMA within the first seven weeks of gestation.[2]

Improving access to comprehensive abortion care in India with focus on expanding provider base—a policy brief—the intent to "diversify the categories of healthcare providers (for provision of reproductive and child health services)", and to "strengthen and expand safe abortion services including training mid-level providers" is clearly articulated in the National Population Policy of India, 2000. **WHO's 2015 Guidelines**—"Health worker roles in providing safe abortion care and post-abortion contraception"—suggest following legal and policy changes required to expand evidence-based recommendations on the range of healthcare providers who can effectively and safely perform various interventions for provision of safe abortion and post-abortion care

The MTP Act permits only allopathic doctors (with specialization in Obstetrics and Gynecology or general practitioners who have undergone a pre-defined certification training) to provide abortion services. The WHO 2015 Guidelines recommend that a range of healthcare providers, including doctors of complementary systems of medicine, nurses and Auxiliary Nurse Midwives (ANMs), in addition to general physicians and Obs-Gynaec specialists, can safely and effectively perform first trimester abortions, using either vacuum aspiration or medical methods. Studies conducted in India too, have found that abortion care can safely and effectively be provided by a range of providers, including nurses and AYUSH practitioners. Experts recommended expanding the provider base for first trimester abortions to overcome the acute shortage of trained physicians and specialists that restricts access to Comprehensive Abortion Care (CAC) services. In the public sector, there is a 13% and 77% shortfall of medical officers (MBBS) and specialists (Ob-Gyn) respectively. Research studies have compared Manual

Vacuum Aspiration (MVA) and Medical Methods of Abortion (MMA) services provided by trained nurses and ayurvedic doctors with the services provided by allopathic doctors and found the services by non-allopathic doctor cadres to be not only equally efficacious, but also equally acceptable by women. The experts felt that the simplicity and safety of current abortion technologies for the first trimester permit a wider range of healthcare providers to be trained to offer abortion care in the first trimester. Given the increased reliance on MMA, as well as the limited monitoring and supervision in healthcare provision, the experts felt that the non-physician cadres should initially be permitted to perform first trimester abortions using MMA only. This may be expanded later to include VA, or other technologies as may emerge. India has close to 70,000 nurses and 2,20,000 ANMs working in the public sector alone. Additionally, 40% of the primary care facilities engage AYUSH doctors as staff. Expanding the provider base for abortion provision will significantly increase the pool of trainable providers. Availability of trained cadres like nurses and ANMs will also ensure that even the most peripheral facilities are functional and services for first trimester abortion are available. It is also recommended to permit all approved facilities where a skilled provider is available, including PHCs, to offer first trimester abortion services (i.e. up to 12 weeks). Permitting PHCs with trained providers to offer CAC services up to 12 weeks will improve geographical access to abortions for women by bringing services closer to their doorsteps. This is especially critical in the rural context where detection of pregnancy and decision to terminate are often delayed. Clear directions, in this respect, towards implementation of these guidelines are not given so far, but are under consideration.[16]

Pathfinder International has been working in India since 1999 with programs in urban slums and rural areas of five states across India, including Delhi, Bihar, Rajasthan, Maharashtra, and Karnataka. Pathfinder believes that reproductive healthcare is a basic human right and that when women and men are given control over their reproductive lives, they are able to significantly improve the health and welfare of their families and communities. Pathfinder also works to ensure safe abortions where they are legal and to provide quality care for the thousands of women who have experienced unsafe abortions.[17]

The problem of unsafe abortion in India may be attributed both to poor medical care and to widespread ignorance and misunderstanding among women about safety and quality of care. Of central importance is the inadequate training in abortion procedures offered to Indian medical students, the majority of whom are not qualified to perform any abortions. Those who are legally qualified to perform abortions have not received training in the relatively new techniques of Manual Vacuum Aspiration (MVA) and Medical Methods of Abortion (MMA), which are far simpler, safer, and more affordable for early abortion than the widely known and used dilation and curettage. They also are inadequately prepared in infection prevention and in counselling women in post-abortion contraception that could reduce the probability of future unwanted pregnancies and consequent abortions.

Between June 2000 and June 2006, Pathfinder International successfully undertook the Improved Access to Safe Abortion Care (IASAC) project; an innovative program designed to improve reproductive health and reduce maternal deaths and complications resulting from unsafe abortion in seven northern districts in the state of Karnataka, India.[17]

Unsafe abortions are a priority area for the Government and efforts need to be strengthened to ensure that comprehensive abortion care services are implemented across the country within the framework and provisions of the Medical Termination of Pregnancy Act (the MTP Act), 1971. The Government enacted the Pre-Natal Diagnostic Techniques (Regulation and Prevention of Misuse) Act in 1994 to address sex determination. The Act was amended in 2003 to broad base the coverage and was renamed Pre-Conception and Pre-Natal Diagnostic Techniques (Prohibition of Sex Selection) Act. These two Acts are designed to address different issues, however, there are unavoidable interlinkages between these across the health system: at policy, planning as well as implementation levels which pose challenges in simultaneously addressing gender biased sex selection while protecting women's access to safe, legal abortion services. Although the reasons for the skewed sex ratio stems from multiple deep-rooted social and cultural issues, the most common reason given to explain it, is the easy availability of ultrasound technologies and abortions in the country. In many places, an instant reaction based on this misunderstanding has led to restrictions on access to abortion services—especially second trimester abortions—seen as an easy solution to fix the problem of sex selection. Such reactions have increased the challenges faced by women in accessing safe abortion services. Very often the practice of sex selection is linked to access to legal abortion. Calculated on basis of actual girls born as compared to the number that should have been born if the sex ratio at birth was normal (around 952), the estimated missing female births out of the total births is 5.7 lakhs or 4.6%.[6] If this number of missing female births is juxtaposed against the estimated number of total abortions (64 lakhs), it can be estimated that of all the abortions in the country, only nine percent are likely to be sex selective. This provides evidence that restrictions on abortion will not be effective or efficient in preventing sex selection.[18]

Women Centered Comprehensive Abortion Care (WCAC)

Basically we need WCAC which includes a range of medical and related health service that support women in exercising their sexual and reproductive rights.

A women centered module for abortion care comprises three key elements:
1. Choice
2. Access
3. Quality

Choice: In its broadest sense, it means the 'right and opportunity' to select between options implying thereby that there should be no interference in a woman's right to make choices about her body and health.

With regards to pregnancy and abortion, choice also refers to women's right to determine
- When to become pregnant
- Whether to continue with or terminate a pregnancy
- Freedom to select available abortion procedures, contraceptives, trained providers, facilities, etc.

Access: It is the medical and ethical responsibility of appropriate professionals to provide abortion care for legal indications.

Barriers to Access
- Non-availability of trained, technically competent, approved personnel within easy reach or in close community
- Insufficient numbers of approved personnel and facilities
- High expenses, long distance and too much time spent in seeking services
- Some providers display attitudes that may be disrespectful, abusive or coercive, which discourage women and limit their access
- Cultural factors like denial of opportunity for education, mobility, decision making and financial dependency on men also act as deterrents to access
- Subtle factors like preference for male child, excessive influence of mother-in-law, pressure to bear more children, also limit access to services
- Women may hesitate to take services from male personnel
- Some women may be afraid to ask questions or make decisions in presence of other health workers

Quality: A quality of care framework for abortion consists of a woman having choices and access to services that are of high quality. High quality abortion care includes many factors and varies from situation to situation given the local context and available resources.

Barriers to Quality
- Lack of adequate attention from service personnel to individuals and social circumstances of women seeking abortion care
- Inadequate effort, time and skill devoted for proper counseling
- Slow pace in adopting new and safer technological advancements. This holds true for laparoscopic sterilization
- Absence and non-compliance of standard clinical and procedure protocols
- Inadequate training and system support in use of protocols
- Limited counseling for post-abortion contraceptive services and lack of choices for clients
- Weak referral linkages and little coordination with other clinical facilities
- Attitudes and perceptions of healthcare staff, at times, compromise sensitive handling of emotions and anxieties and have difficulty in maintaining privacy and confidentially.

Need to Promote Rights-based Approach
Despite all the attention to human right and the progress made, women continue to face discrimination in many spheres of life in relation to men. More evident is the threat of mortality and morbidity arising out their reproductive roles and choices in the areas of marriage, sexual relationships, conception, contraception and abortion. A rights-based approach puts reproductive health in the broader context of social justice applying principle of ethics and values, and national obligations and commitments made for more effective for human health/reproductive health programs and services. Getting women their due or gender equality with a priority to serving poor and unreached population are the key consideration of a rights-based approach. Service providers are made to feel accountable for women's health and respect

their right to health and life by giving support in accessing gender-sensitive and comprehensive service for pregnancy, abortion and childbirth. Men in the family and communities are made to recognize and respect women's right to life and health by taking responsibility for behaviors effecting women and be supportive in removing barriers women face in utilizing timely services.

Health workers play a critical role in helping women exercise their human and sexual and reproductive rights. By being aware of the rights-based approach, health service providers can:
- Provide more women-sensitive service
- Advocate for better reproductive health services on behalf of women
- Influence policymaker to strengthen health service by way of access and quality
- Collaborate with NGOs and other groups to address community and family beliefs and practices as well as influence attitudes of men.

Models are needed that incorporate the private sector in the provision of abortion in rural areas, and ensure that the services provided are of good quality.[14]

It has been estimated that the incidence of unsafe abortion could be reduced by up to 75% (from 20 million to 5 million annually) if modern family planning and maternal health services were readily available globally.[19]

Reducing the unmet needs, making abortion services accessible to women at an affordable cost and of high quality, promotion of public–private partnership models for provision of MTP and TL services, increasing number of trained medical professional at all levels of healthcare delivery system and creating awareness on a wider scale to generate demands for decentralized services, would go long way to decrease unsafe abortions in the country in near future.

REFFERENCES

1. Report of Maternal Health Division, Department of Family Welfare, Ministry of Health and FamilyWelfare Government of India. Guidelines for Operationalising a Primary Health Centre for Providing 24-Hour Delivery and Newborn Care under RCH-II 2005. New Delhi, India. SRS office of registrar general. Special bulletin on maternal mortality in India 2007–2009.
2. RCH Phase II , http://www.maha-arogya.gov.in /programs/nhp/rch/trgsafeabortion.htm (Accessed on 23/08/2019)
3. https://www.who.int/news-room/fact-sheets/detail/preventing-unsafe-abortion(Accessed on 23/08/2019)
4. Ganatra B, Gerdts C, Rossier C, Johnson Jr B R, Tuncalp Ö, Assifi A, Sedgh G, Singh S, Bankole A, Popinchalk A, Bearak J, Kang Z, Alkema L. Global, regional, and subregional classification of abortions by safety, 2010–14: estimates from a Bayesian hierarchical model. The Lancet. 2017 Sep (Accessed from https://www.thelancet.com/pdfs/journals/lancet/PIIS0140-6736(17)31794-4.pdf)
5. World Health Organization. Unsafe abortion: global and regional estimates of the incidence of unsafe abortion and associated mortality in 2003. 5th ed. Geneva: World Health Organization. 2008,56
6. Singh S, Maddow-Zimet I. Facility-based treatment for medical complications resulting from unsafe pregnancy termination in the developing world, 2012: a review of evidence from 26 countries. BJOG 2015; published online Aug 19. DOI:10.1111/1471-0528.13552. (Accessed on 23/08/2019, from https://www.ncbi.nlm.nih.gov/pubmed/26287503)

7. Vlassoff et al. Economic impact of unsafe abortion-related morbidity and mortality: evidence and estimation challenges. Brighton, Institute of Development Studies, 2008 (IDS Research Reports 59).
8. Abortion options for rural women: Case studies from villages of Bokaro district, Jharkhand. Abortion Assessment Project-India, Lindsay Barnes, CEHAT, Research Centre of Anusandhan Trust, September 2003.
9. Srividya V, Jayanth Kumar, Family Planning Practices Prior to the Acceptance of Tubectomy: A Study Among Women Attending a Maternity Home in Bangalore, India J Clin Diagn Res. Aug 2013;7(8):1640–1643 (http://www.ncbi.ncbi.gov/pmc/articles/PMC3782919/, accessed on 26/08/2019).
10. Guidelines for Operationalising a Primary Health Centre for Providing 24-Hour Delivery and Newborn Care under RCH-II 2005. Report of Maternal Health Division, Department of Family Welfare, MOH and FWi, Government of India. New Delhi, India. SRS office of registrar general. Special bulletin on maternal mortality in India 2007–2009.
11. Vipul A, Hemlata C, Shirish S et al, 'Ectopic tubular pregnancy in post tubectomy death 'Rev Esp Med Legal .2011;37 (2):67–71.
12. Maternal and Child Health, Community Solution Exchange for the Maternal and Child Health Joy Elamon and Meenakshi Aggarwal, Dec.2010, SRUSTI, Orissa ftp://ftp.solutionexchange.net.in /public /mch / cr /cr-se-mch -07101001.pdf (Accessed on 26/08/2019).
13. http://www.pathfinder.org/publications-tools/pdfs/Imroved-Access-to-Safe-Abortion-Care-Karnataka-India.pdf (Accessed on 25/08/2019).
14. Women centered Comprehensive Abortion Care (Trainers manual), Ipas India County office, New Delhi, 2010.
15. Increasing access to safe abortion in rural Maharashtra: Outcomes of a Comprehensive Abortion care model, Shireen Jejeebhoy, AJ fancies Zavier, Rajib Acharyam Shveta Kalyanwala, Population Council 2011.
16. Improving Access to comprehensive abortion care in India with focus on expanding provider base—A policy brief, Ipas www.ipasdevelopmentfoundation.org
17. Unsafe Abortions, http://www.icmr.nic.in /annual / nirrh / L%20Chapter%206%20109%20-%20114.pdf (Accessed on 27/08/2019).
18. Guidelines ensuring access to safe abortions and addressing gender biased sex selection, MOHFW, GOI, February 2015.
19. https://en.wikipedia.org/wiki/Abortion_in_India

Chapter 22

Medicolegal Issues and Informed Consent Format in Sterilization Operation

○ Meenakshi Deshpande

The Development of Standards on Sterilization Services is an important step in ensuring the provision of quality services in the Reproductive and Child Health Program of the Government of India for addressing the large unmet need in terminal methods. The Ministry of Health and Family Welfare (MOHFW) has revised and updated the standards/manuals/guidelines and directed the states to adhere to the same to ensure quality of service provision. FP manuals and guidelines have been widely disseminated and can be freely accessed at the National Health Mission (NHM) website.[6]

These are a few guidelines from Government of India, Ministry of Health and Family Welfare.

Basic Qualification Requirement of Provider

- *Female:* Minilap services—trained MBBS doctor
- Laparoscopic sterilization—DGO, MD (Obst. and Gynae.), MS (Surgery) (trained in laparoscopic sterilization)
- *Male:* Conventional vasectomy and no-scalpel vasectomy (NSV)—trained MBBS doctor
- The state should constitute a districtwise panel of doctors for performing sterilization operations in government institutions and accredited private/NGO centres based on the above criteria.
- Only those doctors whose names appear on the panel should be entitled to carry out sterilization operations in the government and/or government-accredited institutions.
- AYUSH doctors are not permitted to conduct the same.
- A provider empanelled in one state/district is eligible to perform surgeries in other states/districts of India.

- The panel should be updated quarterly. **ICOG-FOGSI recommends laparoscopic sterilization should be performed by a gynecologist with DGO/MD/MS qualification, without the need for additional certification of training.**

The Hon'ble Supreme Court of India has given certain directives in its Order dated 1.3.2005 in Civil Writ Petition No. 209/2003 (Ramakant Rai V/s Union of India) and dated 14.9. 2016: 4 inter alia, directed the Union of India and States/UTs for ensuring enforcement of Union Government's Guidelines for conducting sterilization procedures and norms for bringing out uniformity with regard of sterilization procedures by:

1. Creation of panel of doctors/health facilities for conducting sterilization procedures and laying down of criteria for empanelment of doctors for conducting sterilization procedures.
2. Laying down of checklist to be followed by every doctor before carrying out sterilization procedure.
3. Laying down of uniform proforma for obtaining of consent of person undergoing sterilization, giving postoperative instructions and discharge cards.
4. Setting up of Quality Assurance Committee for ensuring enforcement of pre and postoperative guidelines regarding sterilization procedures.

Case Selection (See Chapter 20 for Details)

1. Clients should be married (including ever-married).
2. Female clients should be below the age of 49 years and above the age of 22 years. Male clients should ideally be below the age of 60 years.
3. The couple should have at least one child whose age is above one year unless the sterilization is medically indicated.
4. Clients or their spouses/partners must not have undergone sterilization in the past (not applicable in cases of failure of previous sterilization).
5. Clients must be in a sound state of mind so as to understand the full implications of sterilization.
6. Mentally ill clients must be certified by a psychiatrist, and a statement should be given by the legal guardian/spouse regarding the soundness of the client's state of mind.

Informed Consent

The following steps must be taken before the client signs the consent form:
- Clients must be informed of all the available methods of family planning and made aware that for all practical purposes this operation is a permanent one.
- Clients must make an informed decision for sterilization voluntarily. Consent for the sterilization operation should not be obtained under coercion or when the client is under sedation.
- Clients must be counseled whenever necessary in the language they understand.
- Clients should be made to understand what will happen before, during, and after the surgery, its side effects, and potential complications.

The following features of the sterilization procedure should be explained to the client: It is a permanent procedure for preventing future pregnancies.

- It is a surgical procedure that has a possibility of complications, including failure, requiring further management.
- It does not affect sexual pleasure, ability or performance.
  - It does not affect the client's strength or his ability to perform normal day-to-day functions.
  - After vasectomy, it is necessary to use a back-up contraceptive method until azoospermia is achieved (usually this takes three months).
  - Sterilization does not protect against RTIs, STIs, and HIV/AIDS.
- A reversal of this surgery is possible but the reversal involves major surgery and its success cannot be guaranteed.
- Clients must be encouraged to ask questions to clarify their doubts, if any.
- Clients must be told that they have the option of deciding against the procedure at any time without being denied their rights to other reproductive health services.

Recommended Consent Form

The GOI has developed this 'consent form' in consultation with all stakeholders. This Consent Form filled by the person at the time of enrolling himself/herself for sterilization operation shall be proof of coverage

Client must herself/himself sign the consent form for sterilization before the surgery
I, Smt/Shri ...., hereby give consent for my sterilization operation. I am married and my husband/wife is alive. My age is .... years and my husband's/wife's age is .... years. We have .... male and .... female living children. The age of my youngest living child is .... years.

I am aware that I have the option of deciding against the sterilization procedure at any time without sacrificing my rights to other reproductive health services. I have decided to undergo the sterilization/re-sterilization operation on my own without any outside pressure, inducement or force. I declare that I/my spouse has not been sterilized previously (may not be applicable in case of re-sterilization). I am aware that other methods of contraception are available to me. I know that for all practical purposes this operation is permanent. I also know that there are standards for female and male sterilization services—some chances of failure of the operation for which the operating doctor and the health facility will not be held responsible by me or by my relatives or by any other person whomsoever.

I am aware that I am undergoing an operation that carries an element of risk. The eligibility criteria for the operation have been explained to me, and I affirm that I am eligible to undergo the operation according to the criteria.

I agree to undergo the operation under any type of anaesthesia that the doctor/health facility thinks suitable for me and to be given other medicines as considered appropriate by the doctor/health facility concerned.

If, after the sterilization operation, I/my spouse experience (s) a missed menstrual cycle, then I/my spouse shall report within two weeks of the missed menstrual cycle to the doctor/health facility and may avail of the facility to get an MTP done free of cost.

In case of complications following the sterilization operation, including failure, I will accept the compensation as per the existing provisions of the Government of India Family Planning

Insurance Scheme as full and final settlement. If I/my wife get (s) pregnant after the failure of the sterilization operation and if I am not able to get the foetus aborted within two weeks, then I will not be entitled to claim any compensation over and above the compensation offered under the Family Planning Insurance Scheme from any court of law in this regard or any other compensation for the upbringing of the child.

I agree to come for follow-up visits to the hospital/institution/doctor/health facility as instructed, failing which I shall be responsible for the consequences, if any.

I understand that vasectomy does not result in immediate sterilization.

*I agree to come for semen analysis three months after the operation to confirm the success of the sterilization surgery (azoospermia), failing which I shall be responsible for the consequences, if any. (*Applicable in cases of male sterilization) I have read the above information. The above information has been read out and explained to me in my own language, and it has been explained to me that this form has the authority of a legal document.

Name and signature/thumb impression of the acceptor
....

Signature of witness: ....
Full name..
Full address..

#(Only for those beneficiaries who cannot read and write) Applicable in cases where the client cannot read and where the above information has been read out.

Shri/Smt .... has been fully informed about the contents of the Informed Consent Form in his/her own/local language.

Signature of counsellor** Full name .... Full address .... I certify that I have satisfied myself that: 1) Shri/Smt ....is within the eligible age group and is medically fit for the sterilization operation. 2) I have explained all clauses to the client and also explained that this form has the authority of a legal document. 3) I have filled out the medical record-cum-checklist and followed the standards for sterilization procedures as laid down by the Government of India.

....
Signature of operating doctor (Name and address) Seal
Signature of medical officer in-charge of the facility (Name and address) Seal

Medicolegal Issues

- In order to avoid any litigation/allegation of coercion or lack of understanding of conditions elaborated in the consent form, there is a provision of signature of witness along with clients'signature/thumb impression.

- As per the guidelines, consent of spouse is not required for sterilization and the signed consent of client suffices. The same may be communicated to the spouse. However, the GoI encourages joint counseling of couples, although it is not mandatory.
- For mentally unsound 'ever-married' client, a certificate from a psychiatrist indicating their unsound mental status is required. Thereafter, the legal guardian can provide consent, if the client is otherwise fit to undergo surgery.
- If a client refuses to undergo sterilization operation in the operation theatre even after signing the 'Consent form', the client cannot be forced to undergo sterilization
- Documentation of the refusal should mandatorily be done in the case sheet with a witness. However, it is preferable to have the client's signature/thumb impression too in these cases.

Certificate of Sterilization

A certificate of sterilization should be issued after one month of the surgery or after the first menstrual period by the Medical Officer of the facility. And after semen report has come azoospermic in males.

Sterilization certificate one should check:
1. Name of beneficiary is same as filled in on consent form.
2. Date of sterilization is mentioned under specific column.
3. Certificate issued should have signature and date of issuing authority.
4. Sterilization Certificate is in proper format as prescribed by the State and having Registration Number and date.

Failure of Operation Leading to Pregnancy

- This may be due to either technical deficiency in the surgical procedure or spontaneous re-canalization.
- To detect failure leading to pregnancy at the earliest, the client should be advised to report to the facility immediately after missed periods.
- The client should be offered MTP and repeat sterilization surgery or should be medically supported throughout the pregnancy if she so wishes.
- Ectopic pregnancy must be ruled out as tubectomy predisposes to this condition.
- Each case of sterilization failure should be reported to the District Quality Assurance Committee. The District Quality Assurance Committee will conduct a preliminary investigation and report to the State Quality Assurance Committee.

National Family Planning Indemnity Scheme (NFPIS)

With effect from 01.04.2013, it has been decided that States/UTs would process and make payment of claims to acceptors of sterilization in the event of death/failures/complications/Indemnity cover to doctors/health facilities.

The states/UTs would make suitable budget provisions for implementation of the scheme through their respective state/UT Programme Implementation Plans (PIPs) under the National

Rural Health Mission (NRHM) and the scheme is renamed "Family Planning Indemnity Scheme".

Claims arising out of Sterilization Operation Amount (Rs.)

SECTION 1
a. Death at hospital/within seven days of discharge—₹2,00,000
b. Death following sterilization (8th–30th day from discharge)—₹50,000
c. Expense for treatment of medical complications—₹25,000
d. Failure of sterilization—₹30,000

SECTION 2
e. Doctors/facilities covered for litigations up to 4 cases per year including defense cost 2,00,000 (per case)

Requirement of documents for claims under the scheme: Based on the following documents, claims shall be processed by the insurer under different sections of the scheme:

1. *Death following sterilization (Section IA and IB):*
    a. Claim form-cum-medical certificate in original duly signed and stamped by the CMO/CDMO/CHMO/CDHMO/DMO/DHO/Joint Director designated for this purpose at district level.
    b. Copy of consent form duly attested by CMO/CDMO/CHMO/ CDHMO /DMO/DHO/Joint Director designated for this purpose at district level.
    c. Copy of Sterilization certificate duly attested by CMO/CDMO/CHMO/CDHMO/DMO/DHO/Joint Director designated for this purpose at district level.
    d. Copy of death certificate issued by Hospital/Municipality or authority designated duly attested by the CMO/CDMO/CHMO/CDHMO/DMO/DHO/Joint Director designated for this purpose at district level.

2. *Failure of sterilization (Section IC):*
    a. Claim form-cum-medical certificate in original duly signed and stamped by the CMO/CDMO/CHMO/DMO/DHO/Joint Director designated for this purpose at district level.
    b. Copy of consent form duly attested by CMO/CDMO/CHMO/CDHMO/DMO/DHO/Joint Director designated for this purpose at district level.
    c. Copy of sterilization certificate duly attested by CMO/CDMO/CHMO/CDHMO/DMO/DHO/Joint Director designated for this purpose at district level.
    d. Copy of any of the following diagnostic reports confirming failure of sterilization duly attested by CMO/CDMO/CHMO/CDHMO/DMO/DHO/Joint Director designated for this purpose at district level:

A. *In case of tubectomy these reports may be:*
   1. Urine test report
   2. MTP report
   3. Per abdominal diagnosis
   4. USG report
   5. In extreme cases birth certificate in case of full-term pregnancy

B. *In case of vasectomy*—semen test report
3. *Complication arising due to sterilization (Section ID):*
    a. Claim form-cum-medical certificate in original duly signed and stamped by the CMO/CDMO/CHMO/CDHMO/DMO/DHO/Joint Director designated for this purpose at district level.
    b. Copy of consent form duly attested by CMO/CDMO/CHMO/CDHMO/DMO/DHO/Joint Director designated for this purpose at district level.
    c. Copy of Sterilization certificate duly attested by CMO/CDMO/CHMO/CDHMO/DMO/DHO/Joint Director designated for this purpose at district level.
    d. Original bills/receipts/cash memos along with original prescription and case sheet confirming treatment taken for complication due to sterilization.

Leave with Wages for Tubectomy Operation

- *Section 9A in The Maternity Benefit Act, 1961:* In case of tubectomy operation, a woman shall, on production of such proof as may be prescribed, be entitled to leave with wages at the rate of maternity benefit for a period of two weeks immediately following the day of her tubectomy operation.
- *Section 10 in The Maternity Benefit Act, 1961:* Leave for illness arising out of pregnancy, delivery, premature birth of child, miscarriage, medical termination of pregnancy, tubectomy operation: A woman suffering from illness arising out of pregnancy delivery, premature birth of child (miscarriage, medical termination of pregnancy or tubectomy operation) shall, on production of such proof as may be prescribed, be entitled, in addition to the period of absence allowed to her under Section 6, or, as the case may be, under Section 9, to leave with wages at the rate of maternity benefit for a maximum period of one month.

Some FAQs

How do we define the term ever married in the case selection criteria?

The term 'ever married' refers to a female/male client married at least once in their lifetime (irrespective of their current marital status).

Can life saving anesthesia skills (LSAS) trained doctors be utilized for administering anaesthesia during sterilization?

LSAS trained doctors are authorized to provide anesthesia only in cases of caesarian sections and not for stand alone sterilization procedures; however, in case of sterilization concurrent with caesarian section LSAS trained providers can administer anesthesia.

Can sterilization be provided to live-in couples?

No, either of the couple should be 'ever married' before they can be considered for provision of sterilization services in the public/accredited private health facilities.

If a woman delivers at home, is she entitled and eligible for postpartum sterilisation (PPS)?

Yes, she is entitled and eligible for postpartum sterilization up to seven days of delivery, provided the correct date of delivery is communicated to the provider. In case the date of delivery is disputable and the seven days' criteria are doubtful, then the woman should be motivated to undergo sterilization after six weeks (interval sterilization).

Can a sterilization procedure be performed on a client who is not in the eligible couple list of that area?

Yes, provided the client fulfills all the criteria for undergoing a sterilization procedure. As per GOI guidelines, no client can be denied services if they fulfill the eligibility criteria.

Can PPS be offered to women immediately after birth of her first child?

No, PPS cannot and should not be offered to women immediately after the birth of her first child. As per the GOI guidelines, the age of the child should be at least one year before a sterilization procedure can be considered.

Can a widow with one or no children be offered sterilization services on demand?

Any client who is ever married can be offered sterilization services on demand. The services cannot be provided to the widow if she has no children. In case she has a child under 1 year of age, then the procedure should be delayed till the child attains the age of 1 year.

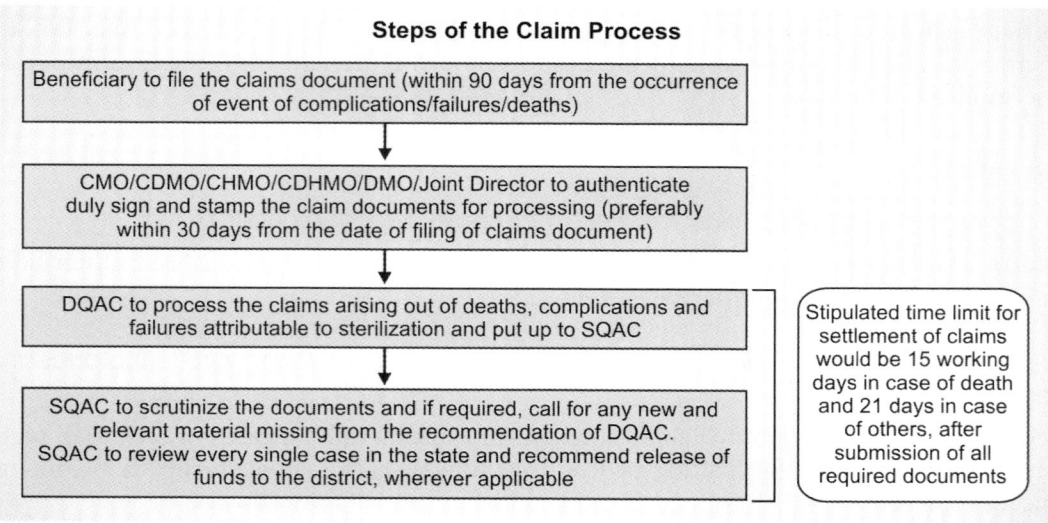

Fig. 22.1: Steps of the claim process. Abbreviations: FP: Family Planning; NHM: National Health Mission; CMO: Chief Medical Officer; CDMO: Chief District Medical Officer; DMO: District Medical Officer; DHO: District Health Officer; QAC: Quality Assurance Committee; SQAC: State Quality Assurance Committee; DQAC: District Quality Assurance Committee

BIBLIOGRAPHY

1. https://mohfw.gov.in/sites/default/files/ Family Planning annual report 2015-16.
2. http://nhm.gov.in
3. http://www.fogsi.org/wp-content/uploads/fogsi-focus/Female_Sterilization.pdf
4. https://www.k4health.org/toolkits/permanent-methods/male-and-female-sterilization-guidelines-india-ministry-health
5. https://www.slideshare.net/LifecareCentre/govt-of-india-guidelines-2014on-standards-of-female-sterilisation-dr-sharda-jain-life-care-centre
6. Standard and Quality Assurance in Sterilization services, FAQs frequently asked questions, March 2016: Family Planning Division, Ministry of health and Family Welfare Government of India.

Section IV

Infertility Practice

23. ICMR Guidelines and Practice of Infertility
24. Ethics in Infertility Practice
25. Surrogacy
26. Regulatory Aspects of Assisted Reproduction
27. Setting Up an IUI Clinic

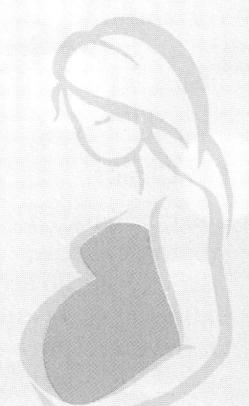

Chapter 23

ICMR Guidelines and Practice of Infertility

○ S Krishna Kumar

INTRODUCTION

Infertility is a burgeoning problem that causes intense mental agony and trauma that cannot be quantified in scientific terms. There are no detailed figures of the extent of infertility prevalent in India but the incidence is estimated to be between 10 and 15%. Out of a population of 1000 million Indians, an estimated 25% (250 million individuals) may be conservatively estimated to be attempting parenthood at any given time; approximately 13 to 19 million couples are likely to be infertile in the country at any given time.

Most types of infertility such as reproductive tract infections (RTIs) and genital tuberculosis are preventable and amenable to treatment. About 8% of infertile couples, however, need serious medical intervention involving the use of advanced ART (assisted reproductive technologies) procedures such as IVF (*in vitro* fertilization) or ICSI (intracytoplasmic sperm injection). The successful practice of ART requires considerable technical expertise and expensive infrastructure.

Infertility has far-reaching societal implications. Therefore, with the rapidly increasing use of ART in our country, it is imperative to ensure safety and have safeguards against possible misuse. Scientific societies around the world, such as the ASRM, ESHRE and IFFS, have drawn up guidelines for the safe and ethical practice of ART. The European Union and the Governments of several countries such as Australia, the UK and the USA have taken steps to accredit and supervise the performance of infertility clinics.

At present here are neither guidelines nor a legislation in regard to the practice of ART in India. The ICMR (Indian Council of Medical Research) has put forth a set of guidelines for ART clinics in India. These have been drafted after extensive consultations held at both the ICMR and other national institutions, with scientists, medical practitioners, lawyers, social scientists and activists. The guidelines are meant to ensure that ART clinics in India are accredited, regulated and supervised to assure the patients as well as the public that our ART clinics offer services that are at par with those available anywhere in the world.

There are many stipulations on various aspects of ART, starting from basic treatment up to and including third party reproduction including donor egg IVF and surrogacy. Only the most relevant aspects from the point of view of general gynaecologists treating infertility will be covered here. Extensive discussions on surrogacy are beyond the scope of this document.

ART Clinics

The guidelines layout basic minimum requirements for ART clinics including the embryology laboratory areas. A well-designed ART clinic of level 2 or level 3 should have a non-sterile and a strictly sterile area. The space requirement includes a reception area, a waiting room for the patients, a consulting room for the gynaecologist, examination area with privacy, clinical laboratory, store room, record room, autoclave room, semen collection room, separate andrology laboratory, clean room for IUI, operation theatre, etc. Some of the spaces could be combined as long as there is no compromise in the quality of service. However, the space for the sterile area cannot be combined with those for the non-sterile area and *vice versa*.

Evaluation of the Couple

Husband

- Physical examination, both systemic and local
- Semen analysis including both morphological and functional tests. An abnormal finding on a repeat semen examination warrants full-scale investigation by an appropriate specialist
- Screening for infections including syphilis, HBV, HCV and HIV, and their appropriate management
- Appropriate endocrinological investigations and therapy

Wife

- Physical examination, both systemic and local
- Detection and timing of ovulation by basal body temperature (BBT), cervical mucus studies, ultrasonography, premenstrual endometrial biopsy, histopathological examination and serum progesterone estimation in the mid-luteal phase
- Assessment of tubal patency by hysterosalpingography, sonosalpingography, or laparoscopy
- Screening for local factors including cervical mucus-related problems and lower genital tract infections
- Assessment of uterine cavity by hysteroscopy
- Screening for reproductive tract infections including syphilis, chlamydia, tuberculosis, HBV, HCV and HIV, and appropriate management
- Appropriate endocrinological investigations and therapy

AIH/AID/IUI/IUI-D

AIH/AID is a technique which consists in placing in the interior of the vagina a sample of unprocessed semen. IUI/IUI-D involves the processing of semen in the laboratory so as to yield pure, activated sperm, devoid of seminal plasma, which are then directly placed into the uterus.

AID and IUI-D is an ethically acceptable procedure provided there is a medical indication and psychological confirmation for its use. Anonymity and screening of the donor must be confirmed and only frozen sperm samples that have passed appropriate quarantining for infectious diseases such as HIV, hepatitis B and C, and syphilis should be used. AID involves the placing of a donor's semen into the interior of the vagina.

Common Indications for AID/IUI-D

- Husband has non-obstructive azoospermia.
- Husband has a hereditary genetic defect.
- The couple has Rh incompatibility.
- The woman is isoimmunized and has lost previous pregnancies and intrauterine transfusion is not possible.
- Husband has severe oligozoospermia and the couple does not wish to undergo any of the sophisticated ART procedures such as intracytoplasmic sperm injection (ICSI).

The possible risk of transmission of diseases from the donor to the future child constitute drawbacks that must be brought to the notice of the patients. It is necessary to obtain informed consent of both the partners after they are counseled about the possible psychological conflict they may face later in their life with the knowledge that one of them is not the biological parent of their child.

In vitro Fertilization and Embryo Transfer (IVF and ET)

The technique of IVF consists of bringing about the fertilization of the oocyte and the spermatozoa in the laboratory. IVF involves induction of ovulation in order to obtain multiple oocytes, thus making available more embryos with which higher pregnancy rates can be achieved. Serial monitoring of ovarian follicular growth by ultrasonography indicates the response to ovarian stimulation. At the appropriate moment of follicular growth, the follicles are aspirated to obtain the oocytes. These are mixed with appropriately capacitated spermatozoa from the husband (or donor sperm) and kept in an incubator for fertilization.

Embryos are transferred into the uterine cavity between days 2 and 5 after oocyte aspiration. If implantation ensues, pregnancy can be confirmed by 14 to 16 days after embryo transfer by determining the presence of hCG in a blood sample. The success rate of IVF is approximately 30–40%.

Common Indications

- Tubal disease with bilateral blocks
- Severe male factor
- Multiple failed IUIs
- PCOS
- Endometriosis
- Unexplained infertility

Intracytoplasmic Sperm Injection (ICSI)

The incidence of fertilization with sub-optimal semen is much lower in contrast to normal semen samples. A sizeable number of couples are not suitable for IVF because their sperm count is far below 10 million/ml with less than 30% sperm being motile. Alternate methods have to be used to facilitate fertilization. These include partial zona dissection (PZD), sub-zonal insemination (SUZI), and intracytoplasmic sperm injection (ICSI). ICSI is the most widely accepted choice of treatment for male factor infertility. It can be carried out with fresh or frozen-thawed ejaculated or epididymal/testicular motile or live spermatozoa.

Indications

ICSI with Ejaculated Sperm

- Severe male-factor infertility
- Fertilization failure after standard IVF treatment
- Number of spermatozoa in the ejaculate too low for IVF

ICSI with Microsurgical Epididymal Sperm Aspiration (MESA/PESA)

- Congenital bilateral absence of the vas deferens (CBAVD)
- Failed vaso-epididymal anastomosis
- Failed vasovasal anastomosis
- Obstruction of both ejaculatory ducts
- An ejaculation because of spinal cord injury
- Retrograde ejaculation

ICSI with Testicular Sperm Aspiration (TESA)

- Extensive scarring, rendering MESA/PESA impossible
- Germ cell hypoplasia (hypospermatogenesis)
- Germ cell aplasia with focal spermatogenesis
- ICSI can also be performed with oocytes which have been cryopreserved/vitrified.

Oocyte Donation and Embryo Donation

Oocyte donation requires stimulating a healthy young woman to generate eggs which are retrieved, using the husband's semen for fertilization and transferring the resultant embryo to the infertile female partner. Embryo donation utilizes donated eggs and donor sperm. Donors should be healthy (as determined by medical and psychological examination, screening for STDs, and absence of HIV antibodies) women in the age group of 18–35 years.

Indications

- Gonadal dysgenesis
- Premature ovarian failure
- Iatrogenic ovarian failure (due to ovarian surgery, radiation, or chemotherapy)

- Carriers of autosomal recessive disorders
- *Women who have attained menopause:* Ovum/embryo donation can be carried out in menopausal women with no surviving child and desiring to have a child. The endometrium of a menopausal woman has the ability to respond to sex hormones and provide a receptive environment for the implantation of an embryo. Various protocols are now available to prepare the endometrium of the recipient for OD or ED with estrogens and progestogens until the placenta takes over the function of maintaining the gestation.

CODE OF PRACTICE

Confidentiality

Any information about couples and donors must be kept confidential. No information about the treatment of couples provided under a treatment agreement may be disclosed to anyone other than the accredited authority, except with the consent of the person(s) to whom the information relates, or in a medical emergency concerning the patient, or a court order. It is the patient's right to decide what information will be passed on and to whom, except in the case of a court order.

Information

All relevant information must be given to the patient before a treatment is given. Thus, before starting treatment, information should be given to the patient on the limitations and results of the proposed treatment, possible side-effects, the techniques involved, comparison with other available treatments, the availability of counselling, the cost of the treatment, the rights of the child born through ART, and the need for the clinic to keep a register of the outcome of a treatment.

Consent

No treatment should be given without the written consent of the couple for all possible stages of treatment, including the possible freezing of supernumerary embryos. A standard consent form recommended by the accreditation authority should be used by all ART clinics. Specific consent must be obtained from couples who have their gametes or embryos frozen, in regard to what should be done with them if he/she dies, or becomes incapable of varying or revoking his or her consent.

Counseling

The ICMR guidelines clearly stipulate the presence of a qualified counsellor to be attached to the ART clinic as part of the team. Couples seeking registered treatment must be given a suitable opportunity to receive proper counseling about the various implications of the treatment. No one is obliged to accept counseling but it is generally recognized as being beneficial, and couples should be encouraged to go through it. Besides offering psychological and emotional support, it is the role of the clinician and counsellor to discuss the specific complications which may be encountered during the treatment of the infertile couple.

Use of Gametes and Embryos

No more than three oocytes or embryos may be placed in a woman in any one cycle, regardless of the procedure/s used, excepting under exceptional circumstances which should be recorded. No woman should be treated with gametes or with embryos derived from the gametes of more than one man or woman during any one-treatment cycle.

Storage and Handling of Gametes and Embryos

The 'highest possible standards' in the storage and handling of gametes and embryos in respect of their security, and in regard to their recording and identification, should be followed.

Research

The accreditation authority must approve all research that involves embryos created *in vitro*.
- No human embryo may be placed in a non-human animal
- All research projects must be approved by the Institutional Ethics Committee before submission to the accreditation authority.

Responsibilities of the Clinic

- To give adequate information to patients.
- To explain to the patient the rationale of choosing a particular treatment and indicate the choices the patient has (including the cheapest possible course of treatment), with advantages and disadvantages of each choice.
- To help the patient exercise a choice, which may be best for him/her, taking into account the individual's circumstances.
- To maintain records in an appropriate proforma to enable collation by a national body.
- To keep all information about donors, recipients and couples confidential and secure.
- The information about the donor (including a copy of the donor's DNA fingerprint if available, but excluding personal information) should be released by the ART clinic after appropriate identification, only to the offspring and only if asked by him/her after he/she reaches the age of 18 years, or as and when specified and required for legal purposes, and never to the parents (excepting when directed by a court of law).
- To maintain appropriate, detailed record of all donor oocytes, sperm or embryos used, the manner of their use (e.g. the technique in which they are used, and the individual/couple/surrogate mother on whom they are used). These records must be maintained for at least ten years after which the records must be transferred to a central depository to be maintained by the ICMR.
- To have the schedule of all its charges suitably displayed in the clinic and made known to the patient at the beginning of the treatment.
- To ensure that no technique is used on a patient for which demonstrated expertise does not exist with the staff of the clinic.
- To be totally transparent in all its operations. The ART clinics must, therefore, let the patient know what the success rates of the clinic are in regard to the procedures intended to be used on the patient.
- To have all consent forms available in English and local language(s).

Information to be given to Patients

Information must be given to couples seeking treatment, on the following points:
- The basis, limitations and possible outcome of the treatment proposed, variations in its effectiveness over time, including the success rates with the recommended treatments obtained in the clinic as well as around the world.
- The possible side-effects and the risks of treatment to the women and the resulting child, including the risks associated with multiple pregnancy.
- The need to reduce the number of viable foetuses, in order to ensure the survival of at least two foetuses.
- Possible disruption of the patient's domestic life which the treatment may cause.
- The techniques involved, including the possible deterioration of gametes or embryos associated with storage, and possible pain and discomfort.
- The cost (with suitable break-up) to the patient of the treatment proposed and of an alternative treatment, if any (there must be no other "hidden costs").
- To make the couple aware, if relevant, that a child born through ART has a right to seek information about his genetic parent/surrogate mother on reaching 18 years, excepting personal information.
- The advantages and disadvantages of continuing treatment after a certain number of attempts.
- Pamphlets (one-page on each technique in all local languages and English) which give clear, precise and honest information about the procedure recommended to be used will help the couple make an informed choice.

Prohibited Scenarios

- A third party donor of sperm or oocytes must be informed that the offspring will not know his/her identity.
- There is no bar to the use of ART by a single woman who wishes to have a child, and no ART clinic may refuse to offer its services to the above. The child thus born will have all the legal rights from the woman.
- The ART clinic must not be a party to any commercial element in donor programmes or in gestational surrogacy.
- A surrogate mother carrying a child biologically unrelated to her must register as a patient in her own name.
- The birth certificate shall be in the name of the genetic parents.
- All the expenses of the surrogate mother during the period of pregnancy and postnatal care relating to pregnancy should be borne by the couple seeking surrogacy.
- The surrogate mother would also be entitled to a monetary compensation from the couple for agreeing to act as a surrogate; the exact value of this compensation should be decided by discussion between the couple and the proposed surrogate mother.
- An oocyte donor cannot act as a surrogate mother simultaneously.
- A third-party donor and a surrogate mother must relinquish in writing all parental rights concerning the offspring and vice versa.

- No ART procedure shall be done without the spouse's consent.
- The accepted age for a sperm donor shall be between 21 and 45 years for the ovum donor between 18 and 35 years.
- Sex selection at any stage after fertilization, or abortion of foetus of any particular sex should not be permitted, except to avoid the risk of transmission of a genetic abnormality.
- No ART clinic shall offer to provide a couple with a child of the desired sex.
- Collection of gametes from a dying person will only be permitted if the widow wishes to have a child.
- Use of sperm donated by a relative or a known friend of either the wife or the husband shall not be permitted.
- The clinic and the couple, shall have the right to have the fullest possible information from the semen bank on the donor such as height, weight, skin colour, educational qualification, profession, family background, freedom from any known diseases or carrier status (such as hepatitis B or AIDS), ethnic origin, and the DNA fingerprint (if possible), before accepting the donor semen (except personal identity).
- It will be the responsibility of the semen bank and the clinic to ensure that the couple does not come to know the identity of the donor.
- Semen from two individuals must never be mixed before use, under any circumstances.
- The consent on the consent form must be a true informed consent witnessed by a person who is in no way associated with the clinic.

COMPLICATIONS

Precautions in Ovarian Stimulation

It is important that ART procedures aimed to facilitate the bringing together of oocytes and spermatozoa should occur when the oocyte is ready to fertilize. It is very difficult to predict when ovulation will occur and whether the oocytes released will be fertilizable. Therefore, follicular development is induced by administering clomiphene citrate (CC) and or human menopausal gonadotropin (hMG) prepared from menopausal urine, or follicle stimulating hormone (FSH), followed by human chorionic gonadotropin (hCG) for the induction of ovulation just when the ovarian follicle has ripened and grown to its optimal size as determined by ultrasonography. Insemination can be carried out *in vivo*, or the oocyte aspirated and subjected to *in vitro* fertilization or ICSI.

Ovarian stimulation should be carried out with the utmost caution to avoid ovarian hyperstimulation syndrome (OHSS). Basal blood levels of FSH and LH should be estimated on day 1 or 2 of the menstrual cycle. LH levels higher than FSH are indicative of the women having polycystic ovaries; such women are prone to develop multiple follicles when stimulated and OHSS. It is important to carefully monitor their ovarian response ultrasonographically.

Multiple Gestation

The reported incidence of multiple gestation ranges from 20 to 30%. Incidence of twin pregnancies in the range of 10–20% may have to be accepted as inevitable, but specific efforts must be made to reduce the incidence of triplets and higher order multiple births. Therefore, not more than three oocytes should be transferred for GIFT and not more than three embryos for IVF-ET at one sitting, excepting under exceptional circumstances (such as elderly women, poor implantation, advanced endometriosis or poor embryo quality) which should be recorded; the remaining embryos, if any, may be cryopreserved and if required, transferred at a later cycle.

Ectopic Pregnancy

Ectopic pregnancy rates could be as high as up to 8% for ART procedures. A high index of suspicion and early detection could help to reduce the morbidity and mortality associated with ectopic gestations in these situations.

Spontaneous Abortion

Spontaneous abortion rates range from 20 to 35%. Abortion rates rise with increasing age of the mother and in multiple pregnancies, especially with three or more foetuses. In cases where more than two foetuses are present, selective embryo reduction should be advised. It is essential that the advantages of embryo reduction (better chances of the survival of other foetuses and the fact that they are likely to be born nearer term and with better birth weight) and disadvantages (the possibility that there might be an increased risk of abortion following the procedure) must be explained to the couple, and their informed consent taken before embryo reduction is attempted.

Preterm Labour and Preterm Birth

There is a higher risk of premature/low birth weight delivery following ART, especially in the presence of multiple gestation.

Indiscriminate Use of ICSI

- ICSI has been claimed to be a panacea for severe male infertility. However, there are some concerns in regard to the use of ICSI. Although ICSI has revolutionized the treatment for male infertility, its widespread use has raised medical concerns about the transfer of genetic defects to future generations.
- There is a higher than normal frequency of sex chromosome abnormalities in children born of ICSI procedures compared with normal population. Besides, infertile men carrying chromosome micro-deletions pass this defect to ICSI-born sons. During ICSI, the process of fertilization is dramatically changed. Because ICSI bypasses a part of the process of natural selection and certain early developmental mechanisms, concerns have been expressed about the possible reproductive health risk(s) to the offspring.

Possible Misuse of ART—Sale of Embryos and Stem Cells

- There is a growing interest in embryonic stem cells because of their potential use for developing spare organs or replacing defective tissues such as parts of the brain destroyed

due to Alzheimer's disease, or pancreatic cells in diabetic patients. The range of their potential use is limited only by one's imagination.
- ART clinics are the only source of embryonic stem cells. Spare embryos are either frozen or returned to the infertile couple for replacement during a later cycle, or donated to another infertile couple, or discarded after five years using a suitable protocol.
- Therefore, sale or transfer of human embryos or any part thereof, or of gametes in any form and in any way, i.e. directly or indirectly—to any party outside the country must be prohibited. Within the country, such embryos or gametes could be made available to bonafide researchers only as a gift, with both parties (the donor and the recipient) having no commercial transaction, interest or intent.

BIBLIOGRAPHY

- BN Chakravorty, et al. National Guidelines for Accreditation, Supervision and Regulation of ART Clinics in India. Indian Council of Medical Research, National Academy of Medical Sciences, 2005.
- Bonduelle M, et al. Incidence of chromosomal aberrations in childern born after assisted reproduction through intracytoplasmic sperm injection. Human Reproduction, 1998;13:781–2.
- Brinsden PR (Ed.). A Textbook of in vitro Fertilization and Assisted Reproduction. The Parthenon Publishing Group, New York and London, 1999.
- Chakravarty BN. Legislation and Regulations Regarding the Practice of Assisted Reproduction in India. J. Assisted Reprod. Genetics, 2001;18:10–14.
- Cram DS et al. Y chromosome analysis of infertile men and their sons conceived through intracytoplasmic sperm injection: Vertical transmission of deletions and rarity of de novo deletions. Fertil. Steril., 2000;74:909–15.
- de Wert G. M. Ethics of intracytoplasmic sperm injection: Proceed with care. Human Reproduction, 1998 (Suppl); 219–227.
- Gianaroli L et al. ESHRE guidelines for good practice in IVF laboratories. Committee of the Special Interest Group on Embryology of the European Society of Human Reproduction and Embryology. Human Reproduction, 2002;15:2241–6.
- Human Fertilization and Embryology Act, London 1990.
- Human Fertilization and Embryology Authority. Code of Practice, HFEA, London, 1993.
- S. Oehninger and R G Gasolen: Should ICSI be the treatment of choice for all cases of in vitro conception? No, not in light of the scientific data. Human Reproduction 2002;17: 2337.
- The Assisted Reproductive Technologies (Regulation) Rules. Ministry of Health and Family Welfare, Govt of India, Indian Council of Medical Research, 2010.
- The Ethics Committee of the American Fertility Society. Ethical Considerations of the New Reproductive Technologies. Fertil. Steril., 1994 (Suppl. 5);62:1215–55.
- The Prenatal Diagnostic Techniques (Regulation and Prevention of Misuse) Act, Government of India, 1994.
- The Transplantation of Human Organs Act, Government of India, 1994.
- World Health Organization (WHO) Laboratory Manual for the Examination of Human Semen and Sperm-Cervical Mucus Interaction. Cambridge University Press, Cambridge, 1999.

Chapter 24

Ethics in Infertility Practice

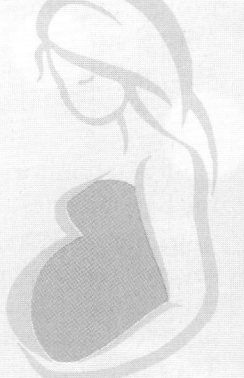

○ Preeti Bhandari

INTRODUCTION

One of the greatest medical achievements in the 20th century was the introduction and development of assisted reproductive technologies. Many years of effort were finally rewarded by the announcement in 1978 by Edwards and Steptoe of the birth of Louise Brown, the first child born after IVF treatment. Following the breakthrough, the new technique rapidly spread throughout the world. However, the techniques of assisting human reproduction are also having an impact on human relationships, which have become more complicated, regulated and litigated, and is raising issues of concern amongst practitioners regarding their liabilities.[1]

Basic Ethical Issues—Indian Scenario

Most developing countries, like India are struggling to provide a basic minimum of care. They are confronted with immense problems of overpopulation, poverty and deprivation of the most basic goods like clean drinking water and food, which also affect the general health of the population. The question then becomes whether governments should not spend their money trying to resolve these problems rather than embarking on expensive high-technology programmes for non-life-threatening conditions like infertility.

According to the main ethical theory, one should do whatever maximizes happiness or well-being. More well-being would be created or more unhappiness avoided by providing assisted reproductive technology (ART) to couples in developing countries. However, it is not clear to what extent these negative consequences of infertility in developing countries justify the provision of infertility treatment.

INDIAN REGULATORY FRAMEWORK OF ART

In September 1995, an organization called The MARCH (The Medically Aware and Responsible Citizens of Hyderabad) was established in Hyderabad to bring together members of the medical profession, the emerging drug industry, members of the staff of research laboratories interested in problems that may relate to medical and healthcare, under the same platform, to discuss key issues of major importance in the area by meeting once every month and then pursuing the decisions taken at this meeting.

It was through the initiatives of the MARCH that the national system of accreditation of clinical laboratories in the country, which is administered by the National Accreditation Board for Laboratories (NABL), came about.

In the year 2000, some members of the MARCH brought to the notice of the group that several unethical practices were going on in infertility clinics in the city and the state. Following this, Indian Council of Medical Research (ICMR) set up a committee on 20th April 2001 to work out a system for the accreditation, supervision and regulation of ART clinics in India. The first meeting of this committee was held on 14th May 2001 at the Institute for Research in Reproduction of the ICMR in Mumbai.[2]

Finally, a document titled 'National Guidelines for Accreditation, Supervision and Regulation of ART Clinics in India' was finalized by ICMR in 2004 and approved by the Ministry of Health and Family Welfare with very minor administrative modifications.

A. Oocyte Cryopreservation

Women and their reproductive choices are always a welcome subject for ethical concern. Whether it is oocyte donation or surrogacy, one of the recurring questions is always this: Should women be allowed to engage in practices that may cause them physical or psychological harm, or should these practices be prohibited in the name of women's well-being and the moral high ground. Also whether we should protect women's autonomous decision to cryopreserve their oocytes, just in case they have no good oocytes left by the time they are ready to reproduce.

While the option for cancer patients to freeze oocytes in the face of treatments that may render them infertile is generally considered in a positive light, offering the same option to healthy women is met with rather more suspicion and reluctance, both by practitioners and policy makers. First, there are a number of fundamental objections: Oocyte cryopreservation is still experimental; it is unnatural; it represents an unwarranted medicalization of reproduction; risks for mother and child rise as the age of the mother rises, etc. A number of ethicists have done the exercise of addressing these objections and of weighing them against the benefits of social freezing: Increased gender equality; increased control over reproductive destiny; more time to find a suitable partner, to complete education and to achieve financial and psychological stability before embarking on parenthood.

Although some fertility centres in the USA and Europe offer ovarian tissue and/or oocyte freezing to healthy women fearing the loss of natural fertility, there is international consensus within the main professional bodies that this is premature, given the experimental status of these techniques. It is felt that as long as their efficiency and safety are still the subject of research, ovarian tissue and oocyte freezing should only be offered to women facing possible fertility loss due to necessary medical treatment or disease. However, many in the field do expect that the further development of these techniques will lead to their being routinely used for 'non-medical reasons' as well.[3] These reasons may include the incompatibility of normal— age childbearing and the pursuit of other life or career plans, or simply not yet having found a suitable partner with whom to start a family.[4]

In its recently updated statement on 'Ovarian tissue and oocyte cryopreservation' the Practice Committee of the American Society for Reproductive Medicine (ASRM) concludes that both ovarian tissue and oocyte cryopreservation are still to be regarded as experimental techniques that should be offered only in a proper research setting aimed at clarifying present uncertainties concerning efficiency and safety.[5]

With regard to ovarian tissue, the ASRM Practice Committee statement seems to rule this out: in view of the 'present potential risk-to-benefit ratio', ovarian tissue cryopreservation should not be offered 'as a means to defer reproductive aging'.[5] A similar statement was made by the Task Force on Ethics and Law of the European Society of Human Reproduction and Embryology (ESHRE), saying that ovarian tissue cryopreservation may presently only be offered if there is an 'immediate threat to fertility'.[6] With regard to oocytes, the view of both committees is that as long as cryopreservation is to be regarded as research, it would be too early to 'recommend' (Practice Committee) or 'encourage' (Task Force) the procedure to those without a medical indication. Although this leaves room for cryopreserving oocytes from healthy women who present themselves as voluntary research subjects, the Practice Committee stresses that this would be in spite of their not being 'appropriate candidates', unlike women requiring medical treatment.

B. Disposal of Surplus Embryos

In order to be effective and economical, ART programs often aim for fertilization of more embryos than will be implanted in women for whose pregnancy the embryos are created. Disposal of surplus embryos raises legal and ethical concerns. Non-consensual donation of embryos also raises legal and ethical concerns. Disposal embryos is ethically disconcerting, particularly to those who believe that protected human life commences at conception.

ICMR has given certain strict guidelines regarding this,
- Couples must give specific consent to storage and use of their embryos. The Human Fertilization & Embryology Act, UK (1990), allows a 5-year storage period which India would also follow.
- Consent shall need to be taken from the couple for the use of their stored embryos by other couples or for research, in the event of their embryos not being used by themselves. This consent will not be required if the couple defaults in payment of maintenance charges after two reminders sent by registered post.
- Research on embryos shall be restricted to the first fourteen days only and will be conducted only with the permission of the owner of the embryos.
- No commercial transaction will be allowed for the use of embryos for research.

C. Access of ART to Postmenopausal Women

A range of objections have been made for allowing these women access to ART, including concerns about their ability to care for the child, the risk of birth defects and the unnaturalness of extending child bearing capacity beyond the menopause.

D. Pre-implantation Genetic Diagnosis

Pre-implantation genetic diagnosis (PGD) is a promising genetic and reproductive technology that was developed during the mid-1980s in the United Kingdom, as an extension or alternative to prenatal diagnoses (PND).[7] It offers hope to couples at a high risk of transmitting genetic disorders to their offspring, and also to those suffering from recurrent pregnancy loss and repetitive IVF failure.

This growing trend towards the use of such technologies in eugenics, wherein children are elected or designed based on parents' wishes, has heightened the need for definite statutory guidelines to regulate practice. Also, the adoption of PGD to screen embryos for non-medical traits like gender, intelligence, and height may greatly alter the process of natural reproduction and the growth of the offspring.[8] All these developments in genetic testing have opened up a Pandora's box, with serious and challenging moral, ethical, and social concerns.

Unintended consequences, or adverse effects for both individuals and the society could occur due to reproductive genetic technologies such as PGD; some of them have the potential to aggravate social inequities and injustices.[9]

Some of the ethical and social concerns associated with PGD include the following:
- **Embryo status:** There is an ongoing debate as to the kind of recognition meted out to the embryo, i.e. if it should be offered the same respect as to that of a fetus or child or adult. With some agreeing on its importance, the rejection of embryos and its subsequent destruction is morally objectionable and unacceptable. Others contradict the above by suggesting that embryos are too rudimentary to grant them individual rights.[8] Hence, PGD embryos have lesser moral value than a fetus and are ethically preferred for disposal over termination of pregnancy after PND.
- **Extent of use:** The controversy regarding the extent of PGD use exists; where some opine that it should be restricted to serious medical purposes, while others support its adoption to a wide array of conditions, inclusive of those that are not requested for PND (like late-onset disorders).
- **Carrier embryos:** A few tests executed during PGD have the potential to identify disease afflicted as well as the carrier embryos. Some couples may not prefer the carrier embryos even though the child would most probably be healthy, in order to avert the future generations to be affected. A 2006 report by the Human Genetics Commission (HGC), an advisory board to the UK government, recommends that the choice of embryo should be left to the parents if both the carrier and unaffected embryos are of equal quality.[10]
- **Designer babies:** PGD has the potential to impact the reproductive choices in the future,[10] wherein couples can select particular features like appearance, behavioral traits, sex, or sexual orientation of the unborn child.

- **Gender selection:** PGD could be adopted for sex selection, when parents want to replace the loss of a child, due to accident or illness, or balance the sex ratio of their family. Some support the concept of bestowing the couples with the freedom to select the sex of their child, while others feel that this might change the balance of the future society. HFEA has prohibited the use of PGD for selecting sex for non-medical reasons. ASRM echoes the views of HFEA and indicates that the use of PGD for elective cases is unethical.[11] However, ASRM stipulates that the physicians can offer the option of pre-conceptive techniques for gender selection under specified conditions, provided they are safe and effective.[10]
- **Savior siblings:** The use of PGD for selecting savior siblings is one of the most controversial issues surrounding the technology. Initially HFEA had approved the use of PGD to obtain a human leukocyte antigen (HLA) match for existing children with genetic diseases, while also ensuring that the savior child would be genetically unaffected.

The 'slippery slope' argument: A 2007 report, based on the public survey in US, by the Genetics and Public Policy Center showed that majority of Americans support genetic testing to promote better health, both for themselves and their families, and also for medical research purposes. However, most of them also expressed concern and distrust over the probable discrimination that could occur. There is widespread speculation that PGD could be adopted for non-medical reasons, which in turn may diminish the support for its use in serious medical conditions. If such an assumption materializes, it could initiate a 'slippery slope'.

PGD supporters disagree on this, since the entire assumption is based on the hypothesis that the bottom of the slope is objectionable or adverse, and furthermore, if the bottom is superior to the top, it would be ethically correct to slide down the slope quickly. They further propose that the formation of appropriate guidelines would restrict the use of PGD for serious medical conditions only.

Indian scenario: Embryo biopsy is a procedure in which one or more blastomeres are removed from the embryo for PGS (Preimplantation Genetic Screening) to improve implantation rates, or for PGD (Preimplantation Genetic Diagnosis) to rule out genetic disorders; it must not be used for sex determination/selection unless medically indicated.[12]

E. Donor Insemination

A sperm donor may be classified as a donor or as a father. The former is generally anonymous and relinquishes all parental claims and responsibilities, while the later is known to the mother and assumes parental responsibilities. While most donors recruited by sperm banks are anonymous and legally relinquish parental rights and responsibilities, a few sperm banks allow children, with the consent of the donor, to initiate contact with their genetic father at a specified age.

When the sperm donor is known as in cases where individuals such as a gay man and a lesbian-decide to co-parent a child, it is very important that all parties be clear as to the legal obligations and consequences of the co-parenting arrangement. Since alternative families are not acknowledged in most jurisdictions, co-parenting may carry with it considerable legal risks.

Other issues involved in artificial insemination include health considerations, such as access to the donor's medical history and genetic heritage, and the emotional impact on the children of artificial insemination of not knowing their fathers or growing up in non-traditional families.

Indian perspective: In Indian mythology there are umpteen evidences of donor insemination. However, Delhi State was the first state to legalize the donor insemination, vide Delhi Artificial Insemination Act (human) 1995. Otherwise, it has remained uncharted area with no proper control. According to the ICMR guidelines, a child born through AID is presumed to be the legitimate child of the couple, born within wedlock, with consent of both the spouses, and with all the attendant rights of parentage, support and inheritance. Sperm donor shall have no parental right or duties in relation to the child, and their anonymity shall be protected.

The importance of limiting the number of donor offspring from a single sperm donor relates to preventing accidental consanguinity between the donor and off-spring. Different countries have their own guidelines for limiting the number of donor offspring depending upon the size of the country's population, density of population and mobility of population. In a country like China, each sperm donor can only impregnate five women through donor insemination or *in vitro* fertilization (IVF), whereas the ASRM recommends a limit of 25 children per population of 800,000 for a single donor. In the United States, there is no federal or state law limiting sperm donation. ASRM has recommended that all institutions, clinics and sperm banks should maintain sufficient records, which allows a limit to be set for the number of pregnancies for which a single donor is responsible. The Human Fertilization and Embryology Authority (HFEA) is United Kingdom's independent regulating authority overseeing the use of gametes and embryos in fertility treatment and research. It categorically states that gametes (or embryos created using gametes) from an individual donor should not be used to produce children for more than 10 families (refer to Chapter 26 for details of Regulatory Aspects of Assisted Reproduction).

F. Semen Banks

- An ART clinic or any other suitable independent organization may set up a semen bank. If set up by an ART clinic it must operate as a separate identity.
- The bank will ensure that all the requirements for a sperm donor are met and a suitable record of all donors is kept for 10 years after which, or if the bank is wounded up during this period, the records shall be transferred to ICMR repository.
- A bank may advertise suitably for sperm donors, who may be appropriately compensated financially.
- The semen bank shall not supply semen of one donor for more than ten successful pregnancies. The bank must be run professionally and must have facilities for cryopreservation of semen, following internationally accepted protocols.
- Semen samples must be cryopreserved for at least 6 months before first use, at which time the semen donor must be tested again for HIV and hepatitis B and C.
- The bank must ensure confidentiality with regard to the identity of the semen donor.
- All semen banks will require accreditation.

G. Surrogacy and Third Party Reproduction

With regards to third party reproduction (TPR), regulations are required in the areas of quality control and monitoring, safety, record keeping, inspection and licensing, consent, the identification and obligations of mothers and fathers, and requirements for donor screening. Carefully thought out laws and guidelines are important. TPR could be a legal nightmare in cases going wrong. Couples considering it must seek legal help before contracting with a donor or surrogate. The law involved in surrogacy is a contract law, but it is an emotional issue. In a class stratified society, where the surrogate contractors are bound to have more power and resources, the possibility of economic exploitation of the surrogate has to be prevented.

ICMR Ethical Considerations in Gestational Surrogacy[13]

- A child born through surrogacy must be adopted by the genetic (biological) parents.
- Advertisements regarding surrogacy should not be made by the ART clinic. The responsibility of finding a surrogate mother, through advertisement or otherwise should rest with the couple or registered agency.
- Legal papers regarding the contract agreement should be made by a lawyer.
- Payments to surrogate mothers should cover all genuine expenses associated with the pregnancy. Documentary evidence of the financial arrangement for surrogacy must be available. The ART centre should not be involved in this monetary aspect.
- A relative, a known person, as well as a person unknown to the couple may act as a surrogate mother for the couple. In the case of a relative acting as a surrogate, the relative should belong to same generation as the woman desiring the surrogate. The consent of the surrogate's spouse is essential in all cases.
- A surrogate mother should not be over 45 years of age.
- The surrogate mother must relinquish in writing all parental rights concerning the offspring and vice versa.

Surrogacy Regulation Bill, 2019[14]

The Cabinet approved the introduction of Surrogacy (Regulation) Bill, 2019 that aims to prohibit commercial surrogacy in India. The Bill proposes to regulate surrogacy in India by establishing a National Surrogacy Board at the central level and state surrogacy boards and appropriate authorities in the states and union territories. The purpose of the Bill is to ensure effective regulation of surrogacy, prohibit commercial surrogacy, and allow ethical surrogacy. India has emerged as a surrogacy hub for couples from other countries and there have been reports concerning unethical practices, exploitation of surrogate mothers, abandonment of children born out of surrogacy, and rackets involving intermediaries importing human embryos and gametes. The 228th report of the Commission of India has recommended prohibiting commercial surrogacy and allowing altruistic surrogacy by enacting suitable legislation.

Once the Bill is enacted by Parliament, the central government shall notify the date of the commencement of the Act. Consequently the National Surrogacy Board will be constituted. The states and union territories shall constitute state surrogacy boards. While commercial surrogacy will be prohibited, including sale and purchase of human embryos and gametes, ethical surrogacy for needy couples will be allowed on fulfillment of stipulated conditions. It will also prevent exploitation of surrogate mothers and children born through surrogacy.

REFERENCES

1. Dickens BM. Legal developments in assisted reproduction. Int J Gynaecol Obstet 2008;101: 211–5.
2. Bhargava PM, Donor Egg IVF: Its Regulation in India. In: Donor Egg IVF, 1st Edition, Allahbadia G (Editor) Jaypee Brothers, New Delhi, 2009; 391.
3. Homburg R, van der Veen F, Silber SJ. Oocyte vitrication-Women's emancipation set in stone. FertilSteril 2009;91:1319-20.
4. Nowak R. Egg freezing. A reproductive revolution. New Scientist 2007;21 March:8–9.
5. Practice Committee of the American Society for Reproductive Medicine and the Practice Committee of the Society for Assisted Reproductive Technology. Ovarian tissue and oocyte cryopreservation. FertilSteril 2008;90:S241–46.
6. Shenfield F, Pennings G, Cohen J, Devroey P, Sureau C, Tarlatzis B. Task force 7: ethical considerations for the cryopreservation of gametes and reproductive tissues for self use. Hum Reprod 2004;19:460–2.
7. Pre-implantation Genetic Diagnosis: Ethical Guidelines for Responsible Regulation. International Center for Technology Assessment. Last accessed August 5, 2009.
8. Dahl E. Ethical issues in new uses of pre-implantation genetic diagnosis: should parents be allowed to use pre-implantation genetic diagnosis to choose the sexual orientation of their children? Human Reprod. 2003 Jul;18(7):1368–9.
9. RHTP statement on development and use of prenatal genetic testing and preimplantation genetic diagnosis. Reproductive Health Technologies Project. Last accessed August 5, 2009.
10. Human Genetics Commission. Making Babies: reproductive decisions and genetic technologies. Last accessed August 5, 2009.
11. Reproduction and responsibility: The Regulation of New Biotechnologies. The President's Council on Bioethics. Last accessed August 5, 2009.
12. The Assisted Reproductive Technologies (regulation) Rules, 2010 Ministry of Health and Family Welfare Govt. Of India, New Delhi. Part 6; 6.12.
13. Indian Council of Medical Research (ICMR) ART (Regulation) Bill on surrogacy 2010.
14. https://www.indiatoday.in/india-today-insight/story/surrogacy-bill-2019-whose-womb-is-it-1595195-2019-09-04

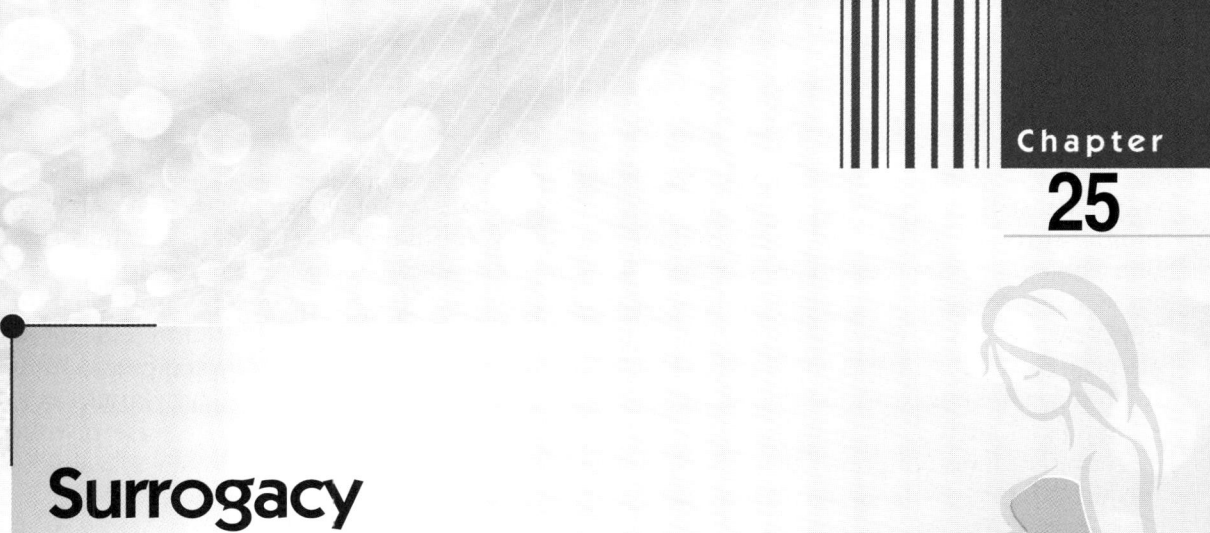

Chapter 25

Surrogacy

○ Kaushal Kadam ○ Hitesha Ramnani ○ Kalika Joshi

INTRODUCTION

Surrogacy is an important method of assisted reproduction. The word "surrogate" is rooted in Latin "Subrogare" (to substitute), which means "appointed to act in the place of." Surrogacy implies that a woman becomes pregnant and gives birth to a child with the intention of giving away this child to another person or couple, commonly referred to as the 'intended' or 'commissioning' parents. A surrogate mother is the woman who carries and gives birth to the child and the intended parent is the person who intends to raise the child.

Types of Surrogacy

There are two main types of surrogacy: Traditional and Gestational. *Traditional surrogacy* arrangement is believed to have happened about 2000 years before the birth of Christ and was mentioned in the Old Testament of the Bible. Sarah and Abraham were unable to conceive and Sarah hired her maiden Hagar to carry a child for her husband. Subsequently Hagar gave birth to a son, Ishmael, for Sarah and Abraham. Nowadays traditional (also called genetic or partial) surrogacy is the result of artificial insemination of the surrogate mother with the intended father's sperm. This means that the surrogate mother's eggs are used, making her a genetic parent along with the intended father.

Gestational or IVF surrogacy (also called *host or full surrogacy*) is defined as an arrangement in which an embryo from the intended parents, or from a donated oocyte or sperm, is transferred to the surrogate's uterus. In gestational surrogacy, the woman who carries the child (the gestational carrier) has no genetic connection to the child. This is the kind of surrogacy practice currently allowed in India.

Surrogacy may also be Commercial or Altruistic. **Altruistic surrogacy** is where a surrogate mother agrees to gestate a child for intended parents without being compensated monetarily. She may only be reimbursed for medical costs directly related to the pregnancy and for loss of income due to the pregnancy. **Commercial surrogacy** is an option in which intending parent offers a financial incentive to secure a willing surrogate. This medical procedure is legal in several countries including India where due to excellent medical infrastructure, high international demand and ready availability of surrogates it is reaching industry proportions. Commercial surrogacy, however, is a controversial method of conception because people, governments and religious groups have questioned the ethics of involving money in a child's birth.

Indications for Surrogacy

There are a myriad of underlying medical indications where surrogacy is the only option or a potential option available for family building. The major indications that would need a gestational carrier include:

i. Absent uterus (congenital; MRKH syndrome or post-hysterectomy)
ii. Structurally scarred uterus or other uterine anomalies
iii. Recurrent pregnancy losses (RPL; 2 or more unexplained pregnancy losses)
iv. Repeated implantation failure (RIF; 3 or more failed IVF embryo transfers)
v. Maternal medical conditions where pregnancy could pose a significant health risk (heart and renal conditions)
vi. Maternal medications used to treat a disease, which are potentially teratogenic
vii. Biological inability to conceive a child (Same-sex male couples or single men).

Legislation in Different Countries

Commercial Surrogacy is legal in Ukraine, Georgia, Israel, Russia, India and California, USA. Many other states of the USA allow altruistic surrogacy only. Altruistic surrogacy is also practiced in Australia, Canada and New Zealand and some parts of Europe like, UK, The Netherlands, Belgium and Greece. Surrogacy is officially not allowed in Austria, Bulgaria, Denmark, Finland, France, Germany, Italy, Malta, Norway, Portugal, Spain and Sweden. European countries like Poland and the Czech Republic currently have no laws regulating surrogacy.

Overview of the Process

Although, the process of surrogacy involves the standard medical aspect of IVF and gestational surrogate co-ordination, there are also the ethical, psychosocial and legal aspects to it that make the process much more complex. A brief overview to the process consists of:

i. The recruitment of a gestational surrogate (GS)
ii. Screening (medical and psychosocial) of the surrogate
iii. Counseling of the intended parents (IP) and GS
iv. Co-ordination of the cycles of IPs and GC (gestational carrier)

v. Legal contract between IPs and GC

vi. Monitoring of the pregnancy and antenatal care of surrogate

vii. Delivery of the surrogate

viii. Postpartum psychological and legal aspects for both

All of these require a multidisciplinary approach that involves unique and tight collaboration between fertility physician(s), fertility clinic support staff, agency facilitators, psychosocial counselors, lawyers, the GC, the IPs, an obstetrician and the hospital where the delivery takes place.

Recruitment and Screening of Surrogate

The Indian government had drafted legislation, earlier floated in 2008, finally framed as ART Regulation draft bill 2010 and 2014. As per this, the age of the surrogate mother should be 23–35 years, (25–35 years, Surrogacy Regulation Bill 2019) and she should not have delivered more than 5 times including her own children. She should have one child of minimum 3 years old and not less than 2 years interval between 2 deliveries. Surrogate mother would not be allowed to undergo embryo transfer more than 3 times. No woman shall act as a surrogate mother more than once in her lifetime (Surrogacy Regulation bill 2019). If the surrogate were a married woman, the consent of her spouse would be required before she may act as surrogate. In the case of a relative acting as a surrogate, the relative should belong to the same generation as the women desiring the surrogate. No woman shall act as a surrogate mother by providing her own gametes.

A surrogate should be screened for STD, communicable diseases and should not have received blood transfusion in last 6 months. A medical and psychological fitness is to be obtained from a Registered Medical Practitioner. Routine blood tests should involve complete infectious disease screen, Pap smear, ECG, X-ray, abdominal and pelvic ultrasound to rule out any pre-existing conditions.

All the expenses including insurance of surrogate, medical bill and other reasonable expenses related to pregnancy and childbirth should be borne by intended parents. A surrogacy contract should include life insurance cover for surrogate mother.

Counseling of IPs and GC

Separate counseling is mandatory for every set of IPs and GC. Issues that could develop before, during and after the pregnancy are explored during the counseling session. Counseling for the surrogate must involve discussions regarding her coping strategies, potential attachment to the developing fetus that is not genetically related to her. Her attitude towards multiple pregnancies, fetal reduction or even a pregnancy loss should be explored. End of pregnancy issues regarding the birth plan and plans around relinquishing the baby as well as the future relationship between the GC, the IPs and the potential offspring must be reviewed. IPs should be counseled regarding multiple gestations, antenatal complications as well as anomalous fetus and pregnancy termination. Financial liabilities should also be explained in details.

Legal Agreement

All parties sign a contract or a legal agreement after obtaining independent legal advice. Each party has their attorney to ensure their legal interests are represented and protected. Documents to be taken from the IPs include copy of their passports or Aadhar card and marriage certificate. Documents from potential GC include copy of Aadhar card/election card, marriage certificate, and proof of address and death certificate of spouse in case of a widow or divorce certificate in case of a divorcee. Birth certificate of her children to confirm she has her own child.

Cycle Co-ordination of GCs and IPs

The embryo transfer into a Gestational Surrogate could be fresh or a frozen embryo transfer. The surrogate is likewise prepared from day 2 of her menses when she is started on estradiol valerate tablets to prepare her endometrium. Once the endometrial lining has reached 8 mm, she is then started on progesterone that is given for 3 to 5 days prior to doing the embryo transfer. In cases where her cycle needs co-ordination with that of her IP, the surrogate may be given progesterone only or an oral contraceptive pill to co-ordinate her menses with that of the IP. Progesterone support is continued for 15 days after which a pregnancy test is done.

Concerns about Surrogacy Arrangements

A major concern with respect to surrogacy arrangements has been for the health of surrogate mother, the welfare of the child and the family created by the birth of the new baby. There have been worries regarding possible exploitation or coercion of women to act as gestational carriers (GC). Additionally, the surrogate mother is exposed to risks of obstetric complications because of multiple gestations. There has also been concern that psychological reactions may occur postpartum in relation to surrendering the child, as the carrier may develop emotional attachments to the child she has carried. However, a recent study conducted by a team from Cambridge University on Indian surrogates from our clinic, Corion Fertility Clinic in Mumbai concluded that though the surrogates did experience higher levels of depression post-delivery after handing the baby, but there were no long-term issues regards the same.

Psychosocial Concerns with Surrogacy

Sixteen studies, eight cohort studies, six case series and two qualitative studies including between 8 and 61 surrogate mothers, examined psychological outcome. No serious psychopathology among the surrogate mothers was noted. Socially, the surrogates are able to improve their quality of life with the compensation they received from the surrogacy arrangement.

No major differences in the parents' psychological states or mother–child interactions were observed in groups made up of commissioning mothers, mothers who had received oocyte donation and mothers who had conceived naturally. The mothers and fathers of children born through surrogacy had similar marital satisfaction as parents in gamete donation families.

Ethical Concerns with Surrogacy

The prime ethical concern raised in the whole system of surrogacy is regarding the concern about exploitation, commodification, and/or coercion when women are paid to be pregnant and deliver babies, especially in cases where there are large wealth and power differentials between intended parents and surrogates. Also as per report by Center for Social Research, "the majority of the surrogates are uneducated, housemaids sometimes engaged in construction work. They are often persuaded in such deals by their spouse/middleman (Surrogate Agents) for earning easy money".

Additionally, with the involvement of money, surrogacy is understood as more of an economic transaction than a motherly act. Motherhood becomes commercialized, which is contrary to the values of society in India.

Some other concerns include questions like, what could be the relationship between genetic mother, gestational mother, and social mother? Is it possible to socially or legally accept multiple motherhoods?

Current Surrogacy Practice in India

Presently, in India, we do not have any law regulating the process of surrogacy. Commercial surrogacy in India was allowed in 2002. However, as per a notification passed by our Ministry of Health and Family Welfare, in November 2015, surrogacy was banned for all foreign nationals including those holding OCI (Overseas Citizenship of India) and POI (Person of Indian Origin) cards. Currently, surrogacy is allowed for Indian nationals only. The Surrogacy (Regulation) Act 2016, was approved by the Union Cabinet and passed in the lower house with amendments in December 2018 but is still awaiting approval from the Rajya Sabha and has not come into force as an Act. The Assisted Reproductive Technologies (Regulation) Bill, 2014 is also awaiting parliamentary approval. In such a scenario, it is appropriate to function as per the ICMR Guidelines and Assisted Reproductive Technologies (Regulation) Bill 2010 as directed by notification from the Ministry of Health and Family Welfare.

ADDENDUM

In November 2019, the Government referred the Surrogacy bill to a 23 member select committee of Rajya Sabha. The propsed bill, recommends a ban on commercial surrogacy and allows only altruistic surrogacy.

Salient Features

i. *ICMR Guidelines*

- Surrogacy by assisted conception should normally be considered only for patients for whom it would be physically or medically impossible/undesirable to carry a baby to term.
- The responsibility of finding a surrogate mother, through advertisement or otherwise, should rest with the couple, or a semen bank.
- A surrogate mother should not be over 45 years of age. Before accepting a woman as a possible surrogate for a particular couple's child, the ART clinic must ensure (and put on record) that the woman satisfies all the testable criteria to go through a successful full-term pregnancy.

- In the case of a relative acting as a surrogate, the relative should belong to the same generation as the women desiring the surrogate.
- No woman may act as a surrogate more than thrice in her lifetime.

ii. *The Assisted Reproductive Technologies (Regulation) Bill, 2010*
- The Bill attempts to regulate the functioning of ART clinics to ensure that the services provided are ethical and that the medical, social and legal rights of all those concerned are protected.
- The bill details procedures for accreditation and supervision of infertility clinics (and semen banks) handling spermatozoa or oocytes outside of the body, or dealing with gamete donors and surrogacy.
- All expenses, including those related to insurance if available, of the surrogate related to a pregnancy achieved in furtherance of assisted reproductive technology shall, during the period of pregnancy and after delivery as per medical advice, and till the child is ready to be delivered as per medical advice, to the biological parent or parents, shall be borne by the couple or individual seeking surrogacy.
- The birth certificate issued in respect of a baby born through surrogacy shall bear the name(s) of individual/individuals who commissioned the surrogacy, as parents.
- The person or persons who have availed of the services of a surrogate mother shall be legally bound to accept the custody of the child/children irrespective of any abnormality that the child/children.
- A couple or an individual shall not have the service of more than one surrogate at any given time.

iii. *Surrogacy (Regulation) Act, 2016*
- This Act bans commercial surrogacy and allows altruistic surrogacy only.
- The intending couple should be in possession of a certificate of essentiality issued by the appropriate authority, which is a certificate of proven infertility in favour of either or both members of the intending couple from a District Medical Board;
- An order concerning the parentage and custody of the child to be born through surrogacy, should be passed by a court of the Magistrate of the first class or above, on an application made by the intending couple and the surrogate mother.
- An insurance coverage of such amount as may be prescribed in favor of the surrogate mother for a period of sixteen months covering postpartum delivery complications from an insurance company.
- The surrogate mother should be in possession of an eligibility certificate.
- An eligibility certificate for intending couple—the age of the intending couple is between 23 and 50 years in case of female and between 26 and 55 years in case of male on the day of certification.
- The intending couple are married for at least five years and are Indian citizens
- The intending couple must not have any surviving child biologically or through adoption or through surrogacy earlier.

CONCLUSION

"Surrogacy is a Human Victory over Nature". Gestational surrogacy gives hope to individuals and couples who could not otherwise build a family outside of adoption. Surrogacy involves complex connections and is therefore controversial. Major concern with respect to surrogacy arrangements regarding the surrogate mother, the welfare of the child and the family created by the birth of the new baby. With the involvement of money, surrogacy is understood as more of an economic transaction than a motherly act. If surrogacy is viewed as 'care work' being done then surrogacy will become a noble deed. Physicians rendering this service should behave responsibly and practice it safely and ethically. The surrogacy Bill attempts to safeguard the rights of the surrogate, prevent their exploitation and protect the rights of the child born out of this arrangement. The medical fraternity is looking forward to the government allowing commercial surrogacy, regulating it and allowing suitable compensation and ensuring it is practised in licensed clinics that are monitored by independent bodies.

BIBLIOGRAPHY

1. ART Regulation draft bill 2010. [Last accessed on 2012 May 2]. Available from: http://icmr.nic.in/guide/ART%20REGULATION%20Draft%20Bill1.pdf
2. Blake L, Casey P, Jadva V, Golombok S. Marital stability and quality in families created by assisted reproduction techniques: a follow-up study. Reprod Biomed Online 2012;25:678–83.
3. Brunet L, Carruthers J, Davaki K, King D, Marzo C, Mccandless JA. A Comparative Study on the Regime of Surrogacy in EU Member States. 2013
4. Committee on Ethics. ACOG committee opinion number 397, February 2008: Surrogate motherhood. Obstet Gynecol 2008;111:465–70.
5. Deomampo D. Defining parents, making citizens: nationality and citizenship in transnational surrogacy. Med Anthropol 2015;34:210–225.
6. FIGO Committee Report: Surrogacy. Int J Gynaecol Obstet 2008;102:312–313. Fischer S, Gillman I. Surrogate motherhood: attachment, attitudes and social support. Psychiatry 1991;54:13–20.
7. Jadva V, Murray C, Lycett E, MacCallum F, Golombok S Surrogacy: The experiences of surrogate mothers. Hum Reprod. 2003;18:2196–204.
8. Insights into Different Aspects of Surrogacy practices. Nayana Hitesh Patel, Yuvraj Digvijaysingh Jadeja: J Hum Reprod Sci. 2018 Jul-Sep; 11(3):212–18.
9. Shenfield F, Pennings G, Cohen J, Devroey P, de Wert G, Tarlatzis B. ESHRE Task Force on Ethics and Law 10: surrogacy. Hum Reprod 2005;20:2705–2707.
10. Surrogate-Mother-Praiseworthy or Stigmatised: a qualitative study on perceptions of surrogacy in Assam, India. Anna Arvidsson , Polly Vauquline, (Global Health Action, 2017 (Vol. 10, 1328890 https://doi.org/10.1080/16549716.2017.1328890)
11. Surrogacy: Outcomes for surrogate mothers, children and the resulting families—a systematic review Viveca Soderstrom-Anttila, Ulla-Britt Wennerholm, et al. Human Reproduction Update, Vol.22, No.2 pp. 260–276, 201
12. Surrogacy Regulation Bill 2019 Available from: https://hrln.org/wp-content/uploads/2019/08/Surrogacy-Regulation-Bill-2019.pdf
13. Van Zyl L, van Niekerk A. Interpretations, perspectives and intentions in surrogate motherhood. J Med Ethics 2000;26:404–9.
14. Zegers-Hochschild F, Adamson GD, de Mouzon J, Ishihara O, Mansour R, Nygren K, Sullivan E, van der Poel on behalf of ICMART and WHO. The International Committee for Monitoring Assisted Reproductive Technology (ICMART) and the World Health Organization (WHO) Revised glossary on ART Terminology. Hum Reprod 2009;24:2683–2687.

Chapter 26

Regulatory Aspects of Assisted Reproduction

○ Nandita Palshetkar   ○ Hrishikesh D Pai   ○ Manisha T Kundnani

INTRODUCTION

Infertility is one of the highly prevalent medical problems affecting approximately 15% couples of reproductive age group. In a country like India, the problem is associated with enormous social implications too. In such situation, assisted reproduction is looked upon by many couples as modality of last resort to fulfill their dreams of parenthood. This escalated demand of assisted reproduction has led to mushrooming of ART clinics all across the country.

Assisted reproduction involves handling the gametes outside the body, also often involves semen or oocyte donation or the use of surrogate mother. Not only these techniques require enormous expertise and infrastructure, these are surrounded by many ethical, legal and moral issues. The common controversial issues include: Restriction of ART based on age or sexual orientation, fertilizing more embryos than required, use of donor gametes or embryos, surrogacy, discarding or donating excess embryos, preimplantation genetic screening of embryos, use of embryos for research and rights of children born after ART. Also, there are concerns that ART professionals are inclined to recommend IVF because of the financial gains associated with the treatment.

In view of the above, it thus becomes important to regulate the functioning of ART clinics to ensure safe and ethical practice, curbing commercialization. Such regulation and supervision becomes easier in the presence of established guidelines or laws. In India, ICMR has developed national guidelines for accreditation, supervision and registration of ART clinics, which has been accepted by Government of India. These guidelines were revised in 2010 (these guidelines are covered elsewhere in this book). All ART clinics are required to be registered by ICMR. Also, an ART Bill has been drafted which was revised in the year 2017 to regulate the functioning of the ART clinics and ART banks. A surrogacy bill draft was released in 2018.

ART Bill/ Draft, 2017

The ART bill was formulated in 2008, reviewed and redrafted in 2010, 2014 and recently in 2017. The ART (regulation) Bill, 2017 is an act to establish the National Board, the State Boards and the National Registry for the Regulation and Supervision of assisted reproductive technology clinics and banks. The bill aims to prevent any misuse and to promote safe and ethical practice of assisted reproductive technology services. The bill details the procedure for accreditation and supervision of infertility clinics and gamete banks, ensuring maximum benefit to the infertile couple but within a recognized framework of ethics and healthy medical practice.

The bill intends to establish a National Board for assisted reproductive technology and a National Registry to be called the National Registry of Assisted Reproductive Technology Clinics and Banks in India. All ART clinics and banks shall be registered under the national registry. The National Registry shall act as a central database in the country, through which details of all the assisted reproductive technology clinics and banks, including nature and types of services provided by them, outcome of the services and other relevant information can be obtained.

According to the Bill, no new ART clinic can start operating unless it has obtained a temporary registration to do so. The registration needs to be confirmed on accreditation by appropriate authority within 2 years of temporary registration. The registration must be renewed every 7 years. Existing ART clinics will also have to obtain a temporary registration within 6 months of notification of the accreditation authority, and permanent registration within 2 years of the notification.

However, presently in India we do not have any laws regulating the ART as the bill has not yet been passed and hence it does not have a binding force. In the current scenario, it is appropriate to function under the framework of ICMR guidelines.

Categories of Infertility Clinics

The ICMR Guidelines categorize the ART clinics into three levels depending upon the facilities and resources available:

Primary (Levels 1A and 1B) infertility clinic: These clinics involve in preliminary investigations and work up to find out cause and type of infertility. Procedures not involving handling of gametes outside the body can be carried out. These clinics do not require any registration.

Secondary (Level 2) infertility clinic: These clinics have facilities for artificial insemination with husband or donor semen sample and carry out procedures except those involving handling of oocytes outside the body. These clinics will require registration under the national authority.

Tertiary (Level 3) infertility clinic: These clinics involve in all kinds of diagnostic and therapeutic activities (except research on human embryos), and carry out all procedures involving handling of gametes outside the body and also cryopreservation of gametes and embryos. These clinics will require registration under the national authority.

Duties of the ART Clinic and Bank

Duties of an ART Clinic

- The ART clinic shall provide complete information and thorough counselling to the patients about the various treatment options available, advantages, disadvantages and cost of the procedures, their medical side effects, risks including the risk of multiple pregnancy, and the possibility of child adoption. The clinic should help the couple arrive at an informed decision that would be the best for them.
- As per the recent ART Bill draft 2017, no ART procedure should be done on a woman less than 18 and more than 45 years. Similarly, the upper and lower age for male partners are between 21 and 55 years.
- At the completion of treatment, all ART clinics should provide a discharge certificate to the couple stating the details of the ART procedure performed.
- Written informed consent should be taken at all stages of treatment from all the parties involved.
- Donor gametes and egg donors should be procured only from registered ART banks that have ensured that the donor has been medically tested for all infectious and communicable diseases.
- ART bank may advertise for gamete donors who may be compensated financially from the bank.
- The information about the couple and the gamete donors should be kept confidential and should not be disclosed to anyone other than a central database to be maintained by the National Registry except in a medical emergency at the request of the couple to whom the information relates, or by an order of a court.
- Embryos or gametes should not be cryopreserved without specific instructions and consent in writing in respect of what should be done with the gametes or embryos in case of death or incapacity of any of the parties.
- No embryos or gametes should be stored for more than 5 years.
- After 5 years, the embryo should be allowed to perish or donated to an approved research organization with the consent of the patients.
- If during the period of five years, one of the partners dies, the surviving partner can use the embryo for herself or for her partner, provided an appropriate consent was taken earlier.
- In case of death of both partners or if the patients fail to pay the fees, the ART clinic can either allow the embryos to perish or donate for research.
- A woman shall not be treated with gametes or embryos derived from more than one man or woman during any one treatment cycle.
- No mixing of semen samples should be done.
- Embryo splitting to increase the number of available embryos is prohibited.
- The collection of gametes from a person whose death is imminent shall only be permissible if such person's spouse intends to avail assisted reproductive technology to have a child.
- Ova derived from a foetus should not be used for any ART procedures.

Duties of an ART Bank

The general issues related to gamete donation including strict confidentiality, thorough counseling, written informed consent and appropriate storage and handling of gametes should be addressed. Proper counseling about the procedure involved and their implications should be provided to the gamete donors.

- The screening of gamete donors and surrogates; the collection, screening and storage of semen; and provision of oocyte donor and surrogates, shall be done by an ART bank registered as an independent entity and the bank should operate independently of any ART clinic.
- The ART banks shall have standard, scientifically established facilities and defined standard operating procedures for all its scientific and technical activities.
- ART bank may advertise for gamete donors who may be compensated financially from the bank.
- ART Banks must ensure that donors are free of any infectious or sexually transmitted disease, any communicable diseases and identifiable and common genetic disorders such as thalassemia.
- All necessary information in respect of a sperm or oocyte donor or a surrogate, including the name, identity and address of such donor or surrogate, should be recorded. All such information should be kept confidential.
- Donors must relinquish in writing all parental rights concerning to the off spring and vice versa.
- The highest possible standards should be followed in the storage and handling of gametes and embryos in respect of their security, and with regard to their recording and identification.
- No donor gamete shall be stored for a period of more than five years. After this period they can either be destroyed or donated for research after proper consents.
- Record of all the gametes received, stored and supplied, and details of the use of the gametes of each donor should be maintained by the ART bank.
- All records should be maintained for at least ten years, after which the records shall be transferred to a central database of the Department of Health Research, Government of India.
- If the ART bank closes before the expiry of the ten year period, the records should be transferred to the central database immediately.
- All ART banks shall ensure that all information about clients and donors is kept confidential and that information about gamete donation shall not be disclosed to anyone other than the central database of the Department of Health Research.

Sperm Donation

a. Sperm donor should be between 21 and 45 years of age, both inclusive. Semen analysis should be normal as per WHO standards.
b. Relevant information about the physical characteristics, age, education, blood group, etc. should be recorded.

c. ART bank should cryopreserve sperm donations for a quarantine period for at least six months before being released for use.
d. Sperm of a single donor should not be used for more than 75 times.
e. The sample supplied by the ART bank should be used by the ART clinic only once and for single recipient.
f. No mixing of semen sample is permitted.
g. Use of known donors is not permitted.
h. An ART bank can store semen sample obtained from the donor for exclusive use of the wife or partner of the donor.

Oocyte Donation (ART Bill 2010)

- Oocyte donors should be between 21 and 35 years, both inclusive.
- Eggs from one donor can be shared between two recipients only, provided that at least seven oocytes are available for each recipient.
- No woman shall donate more than six times in her life with not less than a three-month interval between oocyte pickups.

However, according to the recent ART Bill draft released in 2017, the egg donor can donate eggs only once in her lifetime, and maximum of seven eggs only can be retrieved.

Rights of the Children Born through Gamete Donation or Surrogacy

- In case of a married couple, a child born through ART shall be presumed to be legitimate child of the couple. The child will have legal right to parental support, inheritance and all other privileges.
- In case there is divorce/ separation of couple after ART but before birth, the child born shall be the legitimate child of the couple.
- If insemination is done in case of single woman, the child born shall have all legal rights and shall be the legitimate child of that woman.
- A child born to a woman with the stored sperm of her dead husband shall be considered as their legitimate child.
- The birth certificate of a child born through the use of assisted reproductive technology shall contain the name or names of the parent or parents, as the case may be, who sought such use.
- If a foreigner or a foreign couple seeks sperm or egg donation in India, the child even though born in India, shall not be an Indian citizen.
- A child may, upon reaching the age of 18, ask for any information, relating to the donor or surrogate mother, but such information excludes personal identification.
- Personal identification of the genetic parent or the surrogate can be released only in cases of life-threatening medical conditions which may require physical testing or samples of the genetic parent or parents or surrogate mother. However, such information cannot be released without the prior informed consent of the genetic parents or surrogate mother.

Record Keeping

All ART clinics should maintain detailed records of all the oocytes, sperms and embryos used, the manner and technique of use and in whom they were used (couple, surrogate). All records, charts, forms, reports, consent letters should be maintained. The records of all gametes received, stored and supplied and details of use of the gametes of each donor should also be maintained.

These records should be kept for a period of ten years, and after this period the records shall be transferred to a central database. If the clinic closes before ten years, these records should be transferred to the central database immediately.

Research on Embryos

Research should only be conducted on gametes and embryos that have been donated for such purpose only with the permission of Department of Health Research. No research should be conducted on human embryos unless such research is necessary in public interest. No work should be done related to human reproductive cloning. The sale of any gametes and embryos or their transfer to any country outside India, for research is absolutely prohibited.

Pre-implantation Genetic Screening

Pre-implantation genetic diagnosis shall be used only to screen the embryo for known, pre-existing, heritable or genetic disease. The embryos found to be abnormal by PGD can be destroyed or donated to the research laboratory for research purposes after proper consent from the couple.

Sex Selection

No ART clinic shall offer to provide a couple with a child of pre-determined sex nor should be involved in any techniques that increase the probability of having a child of particular sex. Any act at any stage of treatment to determine the sex of the child to be born will be considered a criminal offence. Any procedure to yield fractions enriched in sperms of X and Y variations should not be conducted. Identifying the sex of an *in vitro* embryo should only be done to prevent a sex-linked disorder or disease.

Restriction on Sale and Transfer of Gametes and Embryos

The sale and transfer of gametes and embryos, directly or indirectly, within and outside India is prohibited. However, patients own gametes or embryos can be transferred for personal use with the permission of the National Registry.

The Surrogacy Bill Draft, 2018

The surrogacy bill aims to constitute National and State Surrogacy Boards and appointment of appropriate authorities to regulate the practice and process of surrogacy in the country. According to the Bill, only clinics registered as surrogacy clinics shall conduct activities relating to surrogacy and surrogacy procedures.

Surrogacy should be performed only for valid indication for the same when either or both members of the couple is suffering from proven infertility; and it is done only for altruistic purposes with no commercial element. No one should involve in promoting and providing commercial surrogacy.

The **intending couple** should have the eligibility certificate issued by the appropriate authorities stating the essentiality of surrogacy. The intending couple should be married for at least 5 years and should not have any surviving child biologically or through adoption or through surrogacy earlier. The female partner's age should be between 23 and 50 years and male age should be between 26 and 55 years on the day of certification.

The **intended surrogate mother** should also have the eligibility certificate issued by the appropriate authority. Only a close relative of the intending couple can act as the surrogate mother. She should be a married woman between 25 and 35 years of age and should have a child of her own. The surrogate cannot provide her own oocytes. A woman can act as surrogate only once in her lifetime. A certificate of medical and psychological fitness for surrogacy and surrogacy procedures is required.

Any child born out of surrogacy procedure would be considered legal child of the intending couple and shall be entitled to all the rights and privileges available to a natural child under any law.

However, presently in India we do not have any laws regulating the surrogacy as the bill has not yet been passed and hence it does not have a binding force. In the current scenario, it is appropriate to function under the framework of ICMR guidelines.

BIBLIOGRAPHY

1. The ART Regulation Bill 2017.
2. The Assisted Reproductive Technologies (Regulation) Bill and the Assisted Reproductive Technologies (Regulation) Rules, 2010. Indian Council of Medical Research, New Delhi.
3. The Surrogacy Regulation Bill 2018 (as passed by Lok Sabha).
4. World Health Organization Laboratory Manual for the examination of human semen and sperm cervical mucus interaction.

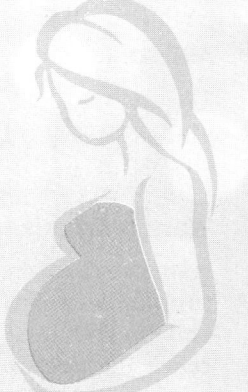

Chapter 27

Setting Up an IUI Clinic

○ Pratik Tambe ○ Shradda Agarwal

INTRODUCTION

According to a WHO estimate, the overall prevalence of primary infertility in India is between 3.9 and 16.8%, with nearly 27.5 million couples actively trying to conceive. Although the government had included infertility in ninth five year plan (1997–2002) in its comprehensive reproductive and child health package, our primary healthcare system is still not equipped to handle such a caseload. A survey by the ICMR found that most state funded health centres are ill-equipped to deal with cases of infertility. However, only 8% of infertile couples need advanced medical interventions involving use of ART procedures like IVF and ICSI which are expensive.

With the rapidly increasing use of ART, there is an increase in number of ART clinics and it has become compulsory to ensure the safety of patients taking treatment as well as to safeguard against their possible misuse. Recently ICMR and other national institutions, with scientists, medical practitioners, lawyers, social scientists and activists have prepared guidelines which are in the draft stage and will be enacted as law subject to approval from Parliament (ART Bill 2010).

What is ART?

ART comprises all techniques that attempt to obtain a pregnancy by manipulating the sperm or/and oocyte outside the body, and transferring the gamete or embryo into the uterus.

"Assisted Reproductive Technology Clinic" means any premise used for procedures related to Assisted Reproductive Technology. The following are the procedures are being followed by the ART clinics:

- Artificial insemination with husband's (AIH) semen
- Artificial insemination with donor (AID) semen

- Intra-uterine insemination using husband (IUI-H) semen
- Intra-uterine insemination using donor (IUI-D) semen
- Procedures related to *in vitro* fertilisation-embryo transfer (IVF-ET)

ART Bank

This refers to an organisation that is set up to supply sperm/semen, oocytes/oocyte donors and surrogate mothers to Assisted Reproductive Technology clinics or their patients. This chapter will focus on the ART regulations for setting up of an IUI clinic.

What is Intrauterine Insemination?

It involves introduction of sperm into the uterus of the woman using a special cannula. The prepared sperm are injected with a fine cannula to reach the uterine cavity and have a shorter distance of the two fallopian tubes and have a shorter distance to swim in order to reach the oocyte released at the time of ovulation. This differs from artificial insemination which consists of placing the husband's semen into the vagina (AIH) or with donor sperm (AID).

Intrauterine Insemination with either Husband's or Donor Semen (IUI-H or IUI-D)

IUI involves the processing of semen in the laboratory so as to yield pure, activated sperm, devoid of seminal plasma, which are then directly placed into the uterus. Common indications are:
1. Hostile uterine cervix that does not respond to medication. (Cervical hostility can be determined by doing tests such as the sperm–mucous interaction test or post-coital tests).
2. In cases where husband's sperm cannot be used such as
   a. Non-obstructive azoospermia
   b. The husband has a hereditary genetic defect
3. When the couples have Rh incompatibility. The women is iso-immunized and has lost previous pregnancies and intrauterine transfusion is not possible.
4. Husband has severe oligozoospermia and the couple does not wish to undergo any sophisticated ART such as ICSI.

Requirements for a Sperm Donor

1. The individual must be free of HIV and hepatitis B and C infections, hypertension, diabetes, sexually transmitted diseases, and identifiable and common genetic disorders such as thalassaemia.
2. The age of the donor must not be below 21 or above 45 years.
3. Semen analysis should be normal according to WHO standards.
4. The blood group and the Rh status of the individual must be determined and placed on record.
5. Other relevant information in respect of the donor, such as height, weight, age, educational qualifications, profession, colour of the skin and the eyes, record of major diseases including

any psychiatric disorder, and the family background in respect of history of any familial disorder, must be recorded in an appropriate proforma.

Patient Selection

Patient selection for referral and for ART should be based on the findings of basic investigations on the cause of infertility. These investigations should include the following:
- Physical examination, both systemic and local of both husband and wife.
- Detailed semen analysis; if any abnormality is detected, repeat tests should be done after suitable intervals.
- Screening for infections including syphilis, HBV, HCV and HIV for both partners.
- Detection and timing of ovulation by appropriate tests, for example, cervical mucus studies, ultrasonography, premenstrual endometrial biopsy, HSG, hysteroscopy and laparoscopy.

Patient selection for treatment of infertile couples can be categorised broadly into three groups: (1) Those with single defect in one of the partners; (2) those with multiple defects in one or both the partners; (3) no apparent defect in either partner (unexplained infertility).

Categories of Infertility Care Units

As per the current guidelines, infertility care units should be categorised into the four levels and authorised to offer treatments as described below. Level 1B, level 2 and level 3 infertility clinics should have a qualified gynaecologist and should maintain records as described in ART bill.

Primary (Level 1A) Infertility Care Units

These would be clinics where basic investigations are carried out and type and cause of infertility diagnosed. A primary infertility care unit or clinic could be a doctor's consulting room, such as a gynaecologist's or a physician's consulting room, or even a general hospital.

The gynaecologist or the physician in charge of a Level 1A infertility care unit should have an appropriate postgraduate degree and be capable of taking care of the above responsibilities. The responsibilities of a level 1A primary infertility care unit would be:
1. Completion of the basic investigations.
2. Treatment of minor anatomical defects like tough imperforate hymen.
3. Treatment of mild endometriosis after confirming its presence by diagnostic laparoscopy carried out by a competent surgeon.
4. Introduction of ovulation in non-ovulatory women (especially PCOS) with clomiphene citrate.
5. Treatment of oligozoospermia without asthenozoospermia.
6. Detecting infection of the reproductive tract using appropriate diagnostic tests.
7. Ability to carry out AIH.
8. Ability to carry out IUI using processed semen of husband or donor obtained from an accredited laboratory or semen bank which must maintain a record of complete details including the name, qualification and complete address of the gynaecologist/clinic requesting the processed semen and carrying out the IUI.

9. Referral of the couple to level 1B, level 2 or level 3 infertility care unit as appropriate, especially when the woman's age is more than 35, or when the couple has a multifactorial defect, or when patients with single treatable defect have not responded to conventional therapy.

In case a level 1A clinic is engaged in AIH and IUI it must maintain records of the use of the requisitioned semen and of all AIH and IUI done; these records will be liable to inspection by an appropriate Review Committee. A level 1A infertility care unit will not require an accreditation as per the guidelines.

Primary (Level 1B) Units Engaging Infertility Care and IUI

Infertility clinics falling into this category like those of level 2 and level 3 shall need accreditation. The IUI in such clinics must be done under the supervision of a gynaecologist with a postgraduate degree.

The following facilities should be present:
i. Immunological tests for infertility
ii. Sperm function tests like hypo-osmotic swelling test (HOST)
iii. Assessment of follicular growth and ovulation by serial transvaginal sonography (TVS).
iv. Hysteroscopy and laparoscopy.

Treatment Facilities in Level 1B Clinic

Facilities for semen preparation and certification and for intrauterine insemination (IUI), including an appropriate sterile area for IUI should be available. The facilities for investigation and for sperm preparation mentioned above could be shared with another accredited infertility clinic or semen bank (IUI procedures like wash and swim up technique and density gradient method).

Secondary (Level 2) Infertility Care Units

These units must have infrastructure for further in-depth investigation and extended treatment of infertility except where oocytes are handled outside the body.

Some of the investigations and treatment facilities required for Level 2 care units are detailed below:
i. Facilities for investigations as mentioned above for level 1B clinics.
ii. Provision for semen collection in men with a vibrator or an electro-ejaculator in functional erectile and ejaculatory problems.
iii. Conservative surgery either through a laparoscope, hysteroscope or via laparotomy. It should be possible to perform hysteroscopic cannulation of blocked tubes and resection of submucous myoma or uterine septum.
iv. Combined medical-surgical therapy by a co-ordinated team as in endometriosis or in some cases of polycystic ovaries (ovarian drilling).
v. Provision for extended treatment of infertility except for oocyte pick up and IVF, ICSI, etc.

Tertiary (Level 3) Infertility Care Units

Such units will have three functions to perform, viz. diagnostic and therapeutic at the highest level of specialisation and with the best of facilities and research.

Minimal Physical Requirements for an ART Clinic

A well-designed ART clinic of level 2 or level 3 should have a non-sterile and a strictly sterile area as detailed below. For level 1B infertility care units, a strictly sterile area will not be required. The space requirement will include a reception area, a waiting room for the patients, a consulting room for the gynaecologist, semen collection room, semen processing lab and a clean room for IUI.

The non-sterile area

1. A reception and waiting room for patients
2. *A room with privacy:* A room with privacy for interviewing and examining male and female partners independently is essential.
3. A general-purpose clinical laboratory
4. *Store room:* A well-stocked store for keeping essential stock. Facilities must be available for storing sterile (media, needles, catheters, Petri dishes and such items) and non-sterile material under refrigerated and non-refrigerated conditions as required.
5. *Record room:* Record keeping must be computerised as far as possible so that data is accessible retrospectively for analysis or when called upon by the supervisory agency. The records must be maintained for at least 10 years after which they are transferred to a central depository of ICMR.
6. Autoclave room
7. *Semen collection room:* This must be a well-appointed room with privacy and it should be located in a secluded area close to the laboratory. Such a facility must be available in-house rather than having the patient collect the sample and bring it to the laboratory for analysis as, in the latter case, semen quality and identity is likely to be compromised.

    Procedures for collection of semen as described in the WHO Semen Analysis Manual must be followed with special reference to the type of container used; these containers must be sterile, maintained at body temperature and nontoxic. This room must have a washbasin with availability of soap and clean towels. The room must also have a toilet and must not be used for any other purpose.
8. *Semen processing laboratory:* There must be a separate room with a laminar air flow for semen processing and examination of postcoital test smears, preferably close to the semen collection room. Good Laboratory Practice (GLP) guidelines as defined internationally must be followed. Care must be taken for the safe disposal of biological waste and other materials (syringes, glass slides, etc). Laboratory workers should be immunised against hepatitis B and tetanus.
9. *Clean room for IUI:* There must be a separate area/room with an appropriate table for intra-uterine insemination (IUI).

The sterile area
The operation theatre: This must be well-equipped with facilities for carrying out surgical endoscopy and transvaginal ovum pick-up. The operation theatre must be equipped for emergency resuscitative procedures. This is not mandatory for clinics restricting their practice to IUI procedures only.

Hormone and Other Assays

The infertility clinic must have ready access to laboratories that are able to carry out immunoassays of hormones (FSH, LH, prolactin, hCG, TSH, insulin, estradiol, progesterone, testosterone and DHEA) and tests such as for HIV and hepatitis B. Endocrine evaluation constitutes an essential diagnostic procedure to determine the cause of infertility.

Microbiology and Histopathology Laboratory

Maintenance: Each laboratory should maintain in writing, standard-operating manuals for the different procedures carried out in the laboratory.

A logbook should be maintained which records the temperature, carbon dioxide content and humidity of the incubators and the manometer readings of the laminar airflow. All instruments must be calibrated periodically (at least once every year) and a record of such calibration maintained.

Back-up Power Supply

Biomedical Waste Management

Fire exits and plan for evacuation
Since gametes need to have strict conditions for incubation, a back up power supply is essential to ensure that power outages do no influence consistency of results. As per existing regulations, biomedical waste management and fire safety measures need to be planned for and approved by the appropriate authority. Such licenses should be displayed when required and applications for renewal should take place well before the expiry date. The requisite number of fire extinguishers should be placed strategically and the evacuation plan clearly documented in case of a fire.

Essential qualifications of the ART team
The practice of ART requires a well-orchestrated teamwork between the gynaecologist, the andrologist and the clinical embryologist supported by a counsellor and a programme coordinator/director. The staff requirements given below would be mandatory for level 2 and level 3 clinics. In the case of small level 2 and level 3 clinics, the services of the andrologist, the clinical embryologist and/or the counsellor could be shared.

Gynaecologist

The minimal qualification for a gynaecologist in a Level 1B, Level 2 or Level 3 clinic is a post-graduate diploma or degree in gynaecology.

1. Should have knowledge of the practice and use of diagnostic methods for determining the cause of infertility.
2. Knowledge of the clinical aspects of reproductive endocrinology.
3. Competence/skills in gynecological ultrasonography

    The responsibilities of the gynaecologist would include the following:
    - Interviewing of the infertile couple initially.
    - Physical examination of the female.
    - Recommending appropriate tests to be carried out, interpreting them and treating medical disorders (infections, endocrine anomalies).
    - Carrying out laparoscopy or sonohysterosalpingography.
    - Advising the couple on planned relations in simple cases.
    - Carrying out AIH, AID, IUI, IVF or ICSI as the case may warrant, based on diagnostic evidence.

In case of male factor infertility, if the gynaecologist is confident and competent, he/she can treat such cases or refer them to the andrologist.

The treating doctor must be responsible for maintaining all records of diagnosis, treatment given and consent forms (*see* annexure). Before any treatment is given, it is advisable that the couple is referred to the counsellor, with all the details of the case, for proper advise and counselling.

Andrologist

In India it is the urologist with a postgraduate degree in urology that often takes on the task of treating male infertility. He should have additional training in diagnosis of various types of male infertility covering psychogenic impotence, anatomical anomalies of the penis which disable normal intercourse, endocrine factors that cause poor semen characteristics and/or impotence, infections, and causes of erectile dysfunction.

The responsibilities of the andrologist would include the following:
- Recording case histories.
- Prescribing appropriate diagnosis and treatment based on the diagnosis.
- Carrying out such surgical procedures as warranted by the diagnosis.
- Maintaining all the records, from the case history to the treatment given, and the patient consent forms (*see* annexure).

Clinical Embryologist

The clinical embryologist must be knowledgeable in mammalian embryology, reproductive endocrinology, genetics, molecular biology, biochemistry, microbiology and *in vitro* culture techniques. The biologist must also be familiar with ART. He must be either a medical graduate or have a postgraduate degree or a doctorate in an appropriate area of life sciences. He must be familiar with the principles and practice of semen analysis and cryopreservation of semen.

The responsibilities of the clinical embryologist include:
- To ensure that all the necessary equipments are present in the laboratory and are functional.
- To ensure that the records of the patients' treatment are maintained.

- To document the pathway of the gametes from both partners/embryos and their dates/growth sequence.
- To calibrate and maintain the equipment used in the laboratory at regular intervals.
- To maintain the logbook and records of temperature, CO_2, etc. on a daily basis.

Counsellors

Counsellors are an important adjunct to any infertility clinic. A person who has at least a degree (preferably a postgraduate degree) in social sciences, psychology, life sciences or medicine, and a good knowledge of the various causes of infertility and its social and gender implications.

Programme Co-ordinator/Director

The programme co-ordinator/director should have a postgraduate degree in an appropriate medical or biological science. In addition, he/she must have a reasonable experience of ART.

Responsibilities of an ART Clinic

1. To give adequate information to the patients regarding treatment, to explain the advantages and disadvantages of the procedure.
2. To give freedom to patients about choice of procedure.
3. To keep information about donors, recipients and couples confidential and secure.
4. Not to perform ART procedure in women less than 20 years of age.
5. Not to mix semen from two individuals.

Registration of ART Clinics

Clinics involved in any treatment involving use of gametes which have been donated or collected or processed *in vitro* should be regulated, registered and supervised by the state accreditation authority/state appropriate authorities in accordance with the National ART guidelines. This includes level 1B, level 2 and level 3 clinics.

The ART clinic must be registered under the following:
1. Shop and Establishment Act
2. PCPNDT Act
3. Biomedical Waste Management
4. NOC from Fire Safety department
5. ISO/FEQH/ASNH are desirable but not mandatory

Validity of Registration

Every certificate of registration shall be valid for a period of three years from the date of issue.

Consents, Agreements and Contracts for Conducting ART Procedures

As prescribed in Section 20 of the Act, the ART clinic shall obtain a written consent from the couple before conducting any ART procedure in a language that the couple understands. The couple's written consent for artificial insemination or intrauterine insemination with husband's semen or sperm shall be taken in Form E (*see* annexure). The couple's written consent for artificial insemination or intrauterine insemination with donor semen or sperm shall be taken in Form F (*see* annexure). Records are to be maintained and produced when required by the appropriate authority.

CONCLUSION

During the last two decades, there has been a marked increase in patient population in all infertility clinics in our country, but all infertility clinics may not be sufficiently equipped with the latest technology and expertise essential to offer the best possible. The above guidelines are meant to ensure that ART clinics in India are accredited, supervised and regulated to assure the patients that our clinics offer services at par with those available anywhere in this world. These will also help safeguard the interests of patients, donors, surrogates and the progeny born out of such treatments. Finally, it is imperative that the ART clinics and clinicians themselves follow these guidelines to avoid medicolegal issues.

ANNEXURES

Form E

Consent for Artificial Insemination or Intrauterine Insemination with Husband's Semen/Sperm (See Rule 15.1)

.... and ...., being husband and wife and both of legal age, authorize Dr .... to inseminate the wife artificially or intrauterine with the semen/sperm of the husband for achieving conception. We understand that even though the insemination may be repeated as often as recommended by the doctor, there is no guarantee or assurance that pregnancy or a live birth will result. We have also been told that the outcome of pregnancy may not be the same as those of the general pregnant population, for example, in respect of abortion, multiple pregnancies, anomalies or complications of pregnancy or delivery. The procedure carried out does not ensure a positive result, nor does it guarantee a mentally and physically normal child. This consent holds good for all the cycles performed at the clinic.

Endorsement by the ART Clinic

I/we have personally explained to .... and .... the details and implications of his/her/their signing this consent/approval form, and made sure to the extent humanly possible that he/she/they understand these details and implications.

Signed:................................. (Husband)
.... (Wife)
Name, address and signature of the Witness from the clinic
Name and address of the ART clinic   Dated:

Form F

Consent for Artificial Insemination or Intrauterine Insemination with Donor Semen (*see* Rule 15.1)

We, ………………………………………….. and ……………………………………………, being husband and wife and both of legal age, authorize Dr. …………………………………………… to inseminate the wife artificially or intrauterine with semen/sperm of a donor (ART bank's no. ……………………………….; obtained from …………………………………… ART bank with valid registration no. ……………) for achieving conception. We understand that even though the insemination may be repeated as often as recommended by the doctor, there is no guarantee or assurance that pregnancy or a live birth will result. We have also been told that the outcome of pregnancy may not be the same as those of the general pregnant population, for example, in respect of abortion, multiple pregnancies, anomalies or complications of pregnancy or delivery. We declare that we shall not attempt to find out the identity of the donor. I, the husband, also declare that should my wife bear any child or children as a result of such insemination(s), such child or children shall be as my own and shall be my legal heir(s). The procedure carried out does not ensure a positive result, nor does it guarantee a mentally and physically normal body. This consent holds good for all the cycles performed at the clinic.

Endorsement by the ART Clinic

I/we have personally explained to ……………. and ……………. the details and implications of his/her/their signing this consent/approval form, and made sure to the extent humanly possible that he/she/they understand these details and implications.

Signed: ………………………….. (Husband)
  ………………………….. (Wife)

Name, address and signature of the Witness from the clinic
Name and address of the ART clinic
Dated:

BIBLIOGRAPHY

1. ICMR Guideline. Chapter 4. Sample Consent Forms. https://icmr.nic.in/sites/default/files/guidelines/c.pdf
2. Ministry of Health & Family Welfare, Govt. of India. The Assisted Reproductive Technologies (Regulation) Bill 2010; Chapter 3: Code of Practice, Ethical Considerations and Legal Issues; 2010.

Section V

Women Rights

28. Protection and Safety Issues of Women and Children—An Update on Various Acts and Laws
29. Role of Women Commission in Domestic Violence
30. Policy Decisions for Women's Health
31. National Health Mission Welfare Programs for Women
32. Janani Suraksha Yojana (JSY)
33. Adoption
34. Government Policies Regarding Adolescent Reproductive Health
35. Lifestyle Modifications for Empowering Women
36. Medical Councils and Doctors: Medical Ethics Training—The Need of the Hour
37. Domestic Violence Act

Protection and Safety Issues of Women and Children—
An Update on Various Acts and Laws

○ Alka Kuthe

INTRODUCTION

"ll Stree Shaktiratulya Sada ll"

Globalization has presented new challenges for the realization of the goal of women's equality. On one side, woman is worshipped as Goddess and on the other side she is oppressed, suppressed, depressed, exploited and victimized by the male dominated society. A report of the United Nations say that "Women constitute half of the world population, perform nearly two-thirds of work hours, receive one-tenth of the world's income and own less than one-hundredth per cent of the world's property." [1] As far as India is concerned, the principle of gender equality is enshrined in the Indian Constitution in its Preamble, Fundamental Rights, Fundamental Duties and Directive Principles. The National Policy for The Empowerment of Women was passed in 2001. India has also ratified various international conventions and human rights instruments committed to secure equal rights of women. Key among them is the ratification of the Convention on Elimination of All Forms of Discrimination Against Women (CEDAW) in 1993. In spite of all these efforts, women still suffer from discrimination, exploitation and victimization.

Crimes against women occur every minute in India. Similar is the case with children. They are neglected, misused, mis-directed, sexually abused and many a times provoked to commit crime. Therefore they also need care, attention, love and sensitization about their legal rights and the laws which protect them.

Following is the list of the Laws which protect and offer safety to women and children.

Women-specific Legislations[2]

- The Dowry Prohibition Act, 1961 (28 of 1961)

- The Immoral Traffic (Prevention) Act, 1956, 1986
- Eve teasing and the Indecent Representation of Women (Prohibition) Act, 1986, Rules 1987
- The protection of women from Domestic Violence Act, 2005 and Rule 2006
- The Sexual Harassment of Women at Workplace (Prevention, Prohibition and Redressal) Act, 2013
- The Criminal Law (Amendment) Act, 1983, 2013

Women-related Legislations
- Code of Criminal Procedure, 1973
- The Indian Evidence Act, 1872 (yet to be reviewed)
- Indian Penal Code, 1860
- Information Technology Act, 2000, Amendment Act 2008, 2018

The Prenatal Diagnostic Techniques (Regulation and Prevention of Misuse) Act 1994, 1996
Preconception and Prenatal Sex Selection and Determination (Prohibition and Regulation) Act 2002, 2003, The Preconception and Prenatal Diagnostic Techniques (Prohibition of Sex Selection) Amendment 2012 (six months training) Rules 2014
- The Medical Termination of Pregnancy Act, 1971 (34 of 1971)
- The Surrogacy (Regulation) Bill, 2016
- The Factories Act, 1948
- The Equal Remuneration Act, 1976
- The Special Marriage Act, 1954
- Live in relationship
- The Employees Insurance Act 1948
- The Maternity Benefit Act 1961, (Amendment) Act, 2017
- National Commission for Women Act, 1990 (20 of 1990)

Child Specific/Related Laws
- Juvenile Justice (Care and Protection of Children) Act 2000, 2015
- Child Marriage Restraint Act 1976.
- POCSO Act 2012
- Prohibition of Child Marriage Act 2006
- Incest molestation, indecency and eve teasing
- Child trafficking and prostitution
- Child labor
- Drug abuse

Let us discuss women-specific legislations.

WOMEN-SPECIFIC LEGISLATIONS

1. The Dowry Prohibition Act, 1961

Dowry is one of the major challenges that our society continues to face and it is a common problem faced by married women. They may be harassed by their in-laws for dowry. To battle this social evil, the Dowry Prohibition Act, 1961 was enacted. Under the provisions of this Act, demand of dowry either before marriage, during marriage and or after the marriage is an offence. Minimum 5 years of imprisonment along with fine of ₹15000/- and/or the amount given in dowry whichever is higher.

Section 304-B IPC deals with dowry related death by which it is a punishable offence. It provides minimum 7 years to maximum life imprisonment. Section 302 is also applicable to such death and punishment can be extended to life imprisonment.

Section 498-A IPC deals with mental and physical torture for dowry provoking woman to commit suicide. It is a cognizable, non-bailable offence. Three years imprisonment is provided for this offence.

2. The Immoral Trafficking (Prevention) Act 1956, 1986

The Act, 1986, originally the suppression of immoral traffic in women and girls (SITA) 1956, is the central legislation dealing with trafficking in India. However, even though the name refers to immoral trafficking of persons, the ITPA's scope is limited to commercial, sexual exploitation or prostitution and penalizes those who facilitate and abet commercial exploitation, including clients and those who live off the earnings of prostitutes. It also provides for welfare measures towards rehabilitation of victims in the form of protective homes to be set up and managed by the state governments.

Specific Changes in the ITPA

i. The ITPA to be substituted with an overarching bill covering all aspects of trafficking.
ii. Definition of trafficking to follow Section 370, but with the addition of forced labor, brought under the purview of the new bill. The Parliamentary standing committees recommendation of adding the words, "inducement of religious and social nature" may also be added to the definition, to cover the Devdasi issue.
iii. Distinction to be made between sex work per se and commercial sexual exploitation following trafficking. It is therefore recommended by that the term "commercial sexual exploitation" and "trafficked victim" be clearly defined. Thus, distinction must be made between living "off" the wages and living "on" the wages of prostitute, as also recommended by the standing committee.
iv. The minimum punishment to be increased to 7 years for adult trafficking and 10 years for trafficking in children.
v. Deletion of Clause 8, which deals with soliciting is believed to lead to further harassment of the victim and should be replaced.
vi. Concept of "corrective" homes to be replaced with "rehabilitation homes".
vii. Creating a special fund for the welfare, rehabilitation, healthcare and education of women in prostitution and their children to overcome the severe resource constraint in this regard.

Other recommendations, some of which have been mentioned in the new trafficking of the persons (Prevention, protection and rehabilitation) Draft Act, 2017 as well, are:

viii. The punishment for dereliction of a duty.
ix. Applicability of punishment. If more than one law is involved, the law with the harsher punishment to prevail.
x. The provisions for hiding the identity of victims and the witness protection program.
xi. All offences made cognizable and nonbailable.
xii. Repatriation of cross-border victims provided for in the law.
xiii. Establishment of National Anti-Trafficking Bureau to coordinate and monitor all aspects of trafficking.

3. Eve Teasing and the Indecent Representation of Women (Prohibition) Act, 1986, Rules 1987

In 1986, The Indecent Representation of Women (Prohibition) Act was passed. It is an Act of the Parliament of India which was enacted to prohibit indecent representation of women through advertisement or in publications, writings, paintings, figures or in any other manner (Section 3 and Section 4). This law, as it is considered to be too narrow for this day and age, has undergone certain changes and an Amendment Bill was drafted in 2012 which broadened its scope.

Section 6: Penalty

Any person who contravenes the provisions of Section 3 or Section 4 shall be punishable on first conviction with imprisonment of either description for a term which may extend to two years and with fine which may extend to two thousand rupees and in the event of a second or subsequent conviction with imprisonment for a term of not less than six months but which may extend to five years and also with a fine not less than ten thousand rupees but which may extend to one lakh rupees.

Section 7

Offenses by Companies under this Act
Where any offence under this Act has been committed by a company and it is proved that the offence has been committed with the consent or convenience of or is attributable to any neglect on the part of, any director, manager, secretary or other officer shall be proceeded against and punished accordingly.

Section 8

Offences to be cognizable and bailable.
The 2012 amendment sought to widen the scope of the law by including new forms of communication such as the internet, satellite and cable television.

It proposed to expand the terms 'advertisement' and 'distribution' to include its new digital and electronic form or SMS, MMS.

Change in Definition

'Indecent representation of women' has been changed to "the depiction of the figure or form of a woman in such a way that it has the effect of being indecent or derogatory or is likely to deprave or affect public mortality".

For representing women indecently, the penalty for the first offence was increased to imprisonment of three years and a fine between ₹50,000 and ₹1 lakh. Earlier the punishment was two years and a fine of ₹2,000.

For a subsequent offence, the term of imprisonment shall be between two and seven years and a fine between ₹1 lakh and 5 lakh.

4. The Protection of Women from Domestic Violence Act, 2005 and Rule 2006

Domestic violence is a cognizable non-bailable offence. The Act provides for punishment for domestic violence committed by husband and his relatives and also provides legal assistance for women suffering from domestic violence. It also provides interim maintenance to women and also for compensation and damages. If the offence is proved but the offender does not obey court's order, then one year imprisonment along with fine of ₹20000/- is sanctioned under this Act. If the concerned protection officer does not fulfil the allocated responsibilities, then one year punishment and fine up to Rs. twenty thousand is provided under this Act.

5. Sexual Harassment of Women at Workplace (Prevention, Prohibition and Redressal) Act, 2013

In 1997 in a landmark judgment, the Supreme Court of India took a strong stand against sexual harassment of women in the workplace. Various forms of sexual harassment such as singing lewd songs, eve teasing, making sexual advances in spite of refusal, watching, capturing or sharing images and other media of a woman engaging in a private act without prior consent have all been criminalised by the Indian Penal Code.[3] There is an entire legislation dedicated to sexual harassment in the workplace—**Sexual Harassment of Women at Workplace (Prevention, Prohibition and Redressal) Act, 2013** to ensure women's safety at workplace.

Crimes against Women[4]

Rape is one of India's most common crimes against women and has been referred to by the UN's Human Rights Chief as a "national problem". According to a global poll conducted by Thomson Reuters, India is the "fourth most dangerous country" in the world for women. After Delhi gang rape case, the three-member committee headed by the former CJI (Chief Justice of India) Mr JS Verma submitted its report to the government on amendments to criminal laws and advocated for stricter anti-rape laws. Reform in anti-rape laws.

Criminal Law Amendment Act 1983[5]

The Criminal Law Amendment Act 1983 has made substantial changes in Section 375 and Section 376 of the IPC. Several new sections have been introduced therein, viz. Sections 376(A), 376(B), 376(C) and 376(D) of the IPC. These new sections have been introduced with the purpose to prohibit sexual abuse of woman of any age, who is in custody, care and control by various authorities.

Criminal Law Amendment Act 2013[5]

In consonance with the recommendations made by the Justice Verma Committee, in order to prevent violence against women comprehensive amendments were introduced in the Indian Penal Code, 1860, Code of Criminal Procedure, 1973 and the Indian Evidence Act, 1872 through the Criminal Law (Amendment) Act, 2013. The amendments sought to make provisions relating to violence against women more stringent. The key features are as follows:

a. New offences like acid attack, sexual harassment, voyeurism, disrobing a woman, stalking have now been incorporated into the Indian Penal Code. Enhanced punishment for crimes like rape, sexual harassment, stalking, voyeurism, acid attacks, indecent gestures like words and inappropriate touch, etc. has also been added.
b. Definition of rape has been widened to include non-penetrative sex as well.
c. Provisions for aggravated rape expanded to include rape committed by a person in a position of dominance, by a member of the armed forces deployed in an area, rape committed during communal or sectarian violence or on a woman incapable of giving consent.
d. Increased penalty for gang rape and causing serious injury to the victim resulting her to remain in a vegetative state.
e. Increased sentence for rape convicts, including life-term and death sentence.
f. Insertion of a new provisions casting a duty on all hospitals public, private run by the Central Government or State Government to provide first aid or medical treatment, free of cost to victims of any offence defined under Sections 326, 375 and 376 (acid attack and rape).
g. Further, Section 370 and 370A IPC provides for comprehensive measures to counter the menace of human trafficking including trafficking of children for exploitation in any form including physical exploitation or any form of sexual exploitation, slavery, servitude, or the forced removal of organs.

WOMAN-RELATED LEGISLATION

1. Code of Criminal Procedure, 1973

Under Section 125, Code of Criminal Procedure, a woman has got right to maintenance despite nationwide protest against such a move.

2. Indian Evidence Act, 1872

Sections 113(a), 113(b) and 114(c) provide for presumptions as to abetment of suicide by a married woman within 7 years of marriage, as dowry death of a woman and as to absence of consent of woman for sexual intercourse.

3. Indian Penal Code, 1860

Sections 292, 293 and 294 provide for punishment for sale and exhibition of obscene books and for obscene act in public place. Section 304-B deals about murder of women in connection with demand of dowry. Sections 312 to 318 deal about punishment for causing miscarriage. Section 354 provides punishment for outraging the modesty of any women, Sestion 366 deals about kidnapping for marriage against her will. Section 366-A deals about procuration of minor girls for sexual purpose. Section 376 deals about punishment for rape. Section 494 protects women from bigamy. Section 497 deals about protection of married women from adultery. Section 498-A of Indian Penal Code deals about subjecting women to cruelty by her husband or relatives and Section 509 provides punishment for uttering words and gesture or act intended to insult the modesty of a woman. Sections 375 and 376(2) of The Indian Penal Code criminalise rape. These sections spell out 7 years' and 10 years' imprisonment, respectively, as the punishment for rape. The key feature of these sections is the requirement for consent by the woman in question for the act not to be considered as rape. Thus, as a parent it is important that you explain the concept of consent to your daughters at an early age. Intercourse with a woman of unsound mind or a girl below 16 years of age is considered to be rape irrespective of consent being given. Domestic violence is considered to be a criminal offence according to Section 498-A of the Indian Penal Code. Certain provisions in the Indian Evidence Act and the Criminal Procedure Code also deal with this issue.

4. The Information Technology Act, 2000 (also known as ITA-2000, or the IT Act)[6]

The Information Technology Act, 2000 (also known as ITA-2000, or the IT Act)[6] is an Act of the Indian Parliament (No 21 of 2000) notified on 17th October 2000. It is the primary law in India dealing with cybercrime and electronic commerce.

Amendment Act 2008, 2018: Online harassment of women is prohibited under Section 67 of the Information Technology Act. Section 67 A—Punishment for publishing or transmitting material containing sexually explicit act or conduct, etc. in electronic form shall be punished on first conviction with imprisonment for a term which may extend to five years and with fine which may extend to ten lakh rupees and in the event of second or subsequent conviction with imprisonment which may extend for a term of seven years and fine which may extend to 10 lakh rupees

The IT Amendment Act was passed by the Indian Parliament in October 2008 and came into force a year later. The Amendment was made to address issues that the original bill failed to cover and to accommodate further development of IT and related security concerns since the law was enacted.

The Information Technology (Amendment) Act, 2018[7] shall come into force on such date, as the Central Government may, by notification in the Official Gazette, appoint.

Not just worldwide, in India too a number of children lost their lives while attempting Blue Whale tasks.Thus the Amendment Bill 2018 aims to provide adequate safeguards against dangerous gaming resources and online material that militate against our cultural values and ethos.

5. The Prenatal Diagnostic Techniques (Regulation and Prevention of Misuse) 1994,1996

The PCPNDT Act 2002, 2003, The Preconception and Prenatal Diagnostic Techniques (Prohibition of Sex Selection) Amendment 2012 (Six months Training) Rules 2014.

The Act prohibits the misuse of antenatal diagnostic tests for the purpose of sex determination which may lead to the abortion of female fetuses. These Acts also prohibit advertising of such use of these tests; require all facilities using them to be registered and prohibit persons conducting such tests to reveal the sex of the fetus. No Genetic Counseling Centre/Genetic Laboratory/Genetic Clinic and/or USG Clinic/Imaging Centre can function unless registered. One has to strictly follow the guidelines given as per the provisions of PCPNDT Act otherwise he/she is liable for punishment as prescribed in the Act.

6. The Medical Termination of Pregnancy Act, 1971

In India, the Medical Termination of Pregnancy Act, 1971 was enacted to safeguard woman's reproductive health. It came into effect into 1972, was amended in 1975 and 2002. The aim of the Act is to reduce the occurrence of illegal abortion and consequent maternal morbidity and mortality. Right now, it is not easy to terminate pregnancy in cases of rape and pregnancy above 20 weeks. It requires special permission from judiciary and a bit lengthy procedure. However, this Act is soon to be amended.

7. Surrogacy Laws in India[8]

In 2013, surrogacy by foreign homosexual couples and single parents was banned. In 2015, the Indian Government banned commercial surrogacy in India and permitted entry of embryo only for research purposes. In 2016, Surrogacy (Regulation) Bill was introduced and passed by Lok Sabha, proposing to permit only Indian heterosexual couples married for at least five years with infertility problems to access altruistic or unpaid surrogacy and thereby banning commercial surrogacy. The bill lapsed owing to the adjournment **sine die** of the parliament session. The Bill was reintroduced and passed by the Lok Sabha in 2019. The bill would require to be passed by Rajya Sabha, the upper house of Indian Parliament and Presidential assent before it becomes an Act and thereby a Law.

8. The Factories Act, 1948

The provisions of this Act provides for health, safety, welfare, and working hours for women working in factories.

9. The Equal Remuneration Act, 1976[9]

This Act prevents discrimination in terms of remuneration. It provides for payment of equal recompensation to men and women workers. Women in India have the right to earn as much as men and gender discrimination is also prohibited at the time of recruitment. Sections 4 and 5 of the Equal Remunerations Act, 1976 lay down the law regarding this.

10. Special Marriage Act, 1954

It is an Act of the Parliament of India enacted to provide a special form of marriage for the people of India and all Indian Nationals in foreign countries, irrespective of the religion or faith followed by either party. The Act originated from a piece of legislation proposed during the late 19th century. Marriages solemnized under Special Marriage Act are not governed by personal laws. The Special Marriage Act, 1954 replaced the old Act, 1872 which was found inadequate for certain desired reforms and Parliament enacted a new legislation.

11. Live-in Relationship

While Indian law does not criminalise pre-marital sex as long as it is between consenting adults, there are no laws regulating live-in relationships. However, courts have developed laws on this subject through decisions in cases to such an extent that the law against domestic violence applies to couples who are in live-in relationships and children born out of such relationships are treated as legitimate in certain circumstances.

12. The Employees State Insurance Act, 1948

The Act provides for insurance, pension and maternity benefits to women workers.

13. The Maternity Benefit Act, 1961

The Maternity Benefit Act, 1961 protects the employment of women during the time of her maternity and entitles her of a 'maternity benefit', i.e. full paid absence from work—to take care of her child. The Act is applicable to all establishments employing 10 or more persons. Facilitate 'Work from home'. It provides for maternity benefit with full wages for women workers.

The Act extends to the whole of India. However, the Act does not apply to any such factory/ other establishment to which the provisions of the Employees' State Insurance Act are applicable for the time being. Exception to this is woman employee who is not qualified to claim maternity benefit under Section 50 of that Act because her wages exceed ₹3000 or the amount so specified u/s 2(9) of the ESI Act. Or for any other reason, then such woman employee is entitled to claim benefit under this Act till she becomes qualified to claim maternity benefit under the ESI Act.

Cash Benefits

- 84 days leave with pay before/after delivery.
- A medical bonus of ₹1000/-
- Take the pay for 6 weeks after/before child birth within 48 hours of request
- In case of miscarriage or MTP, a woman shall, on production of the prescribed proof, be entitled to leave with wages at the rate of maternity benefit, for a period of 6 weeks immediately following the day of miscarriage or medical termination of pregnancy.
- **Leave for tubectomy** operation: In case of tubectomy operation, a woman shall, on production of prescribed proof, be entitled to leave with wages at the rate of maternity benefit for a period of 2 weeks immediately following the day of operation.
- **Leave for illness:** An additional paid leave with pay up to one month in case of illness arising out of pregnancy, delivery, premature birth of child, miscarriage or MTP or tubectomy operation (proof of illness).

Medical Bonus

Every woman entitled to maternity benefit shall also be allowed a medical bonus of Rs. 250, if no pre-natal confinement and post-natal care is provided for by the employer free of charge.

Penalties for Contravention of Act by Employer

For failure to pay maternity benefit, as provided for under the Act, the penalty is imprisonment up to one year and fine up to ₹5000. The minimum being 3 months and ₹2000 respectively.

For dismissal or discharge of a woman as provided for under the Act, the penalty is imprisonment up to one year and fine up to ₹5000. The minimum being 3 months and ₹2000 respectively.

Payment of Maternity Benefit in Case Death of a Woman (Section 7)

If a woman entitled to maternity benefit or any other amount under this Act, dies before receiving such maternity benefit or amount, the employer shall pay such benefit or amount to the person nominated by the woman in the notice given under Section 6 and in case there is no such nominee to her legal representative.

The Maternity Benefit (Amendment) Act, 2017[10] amends the Maternity Benefit Act, 1961. It has brought about certain groundbreaking laws which concern working women.[3] The amendment aims to provide the following

- 26 weeks paid maternity leave for the first two children [Section 5(3)]
- 12 weeks maternity leave for children beyond two
- 12 weeks leave for mothers adopting a child below the age of three months

The Act makes it mandatory for employers to provide crèche facilities either in office or in any place within 500 meters.

Working mothers will be permitted to make four visits during working hours to the crèche.

The employer may permit new mothers to work from home if it is possible to do so [Section 5(5)].

Woman's Health and Law

The National Commission for Women Act, 1992

The Act provides for setting up a statutory body, namely the National Commission for Women on 31st January 1992 (4), to take up remedial measures, and facilitates redressal of grievances and advise the Government on all policy matters relating to women. Its main area of activities includes review of the constitutional and legal safeguards for women, recommending remedial measures, facilitating redressal of grievances, undertaking studies and investigations, participation and advice in the planning processes and generally advising the Government on all matters of policy affecting the welfare and development of women in the country.

National Policy For The Empowerment of Woman was made in 2001[11] with the goal to bring about the advancement, development and empowerment of women. The policy prescriptions included **Social Empowerment of Women which lay down guidelines related to Health, Nutrition and Sanitation.**

Legislative Initiatives towards Empowerment of Woman[1]

The Fundamental Law of the land, namely Constitution of India guarantees equality for women. Let us have a look at some of the most important constitutional provisions pertaining to empowerment/protection and safety of woman.

Constitution of India, 1950

The Universal Declaration of Human Rights has declared that the woman belongs to a vulnerable group and it is a mandatory duty of every State party to protect the woman and to enact special statutes to uplift them.[12] The Constitution of India not only guarantees equality to women but also empowers the State to adopt measures to positive discrimination in favor of women. Article 14 embodies the idea of equality expressed in preamble.[13] While Article 15(1) prohibits the state from discriminating on the basis of religion, race, case, sex, or place of birth, Article 15(3) allows the state to make special provisions for women and children. Article 15 merely elaborates that same concept and acknowledges that women need special treatment for their upliftment. Article 16 provides equality of opportunity for all citizens in matters relating to employment or appointment to any office under the State. Article 39(a) urges the state to provide equal right to adequate means of livelihood to men and women. Article 39(d) provides for equal pay for equal work for both men and women. In pursuance of Article 42 of the Constitution, the Maternity Benefit Act has been passed in 1961. Article 44 enjoins the state to secure for the citizens a uniform civil code throughout the territory of India. Article 51A(e) says that it is the duty of the citizens to renounce practices that are derogatory to the dignity of women.

Child Specific/Related Laws

Here are a few basic laws related to child safety and protection.

1. *Juvenile Justice (Care and Protection of Children) Act, 2015*[14]

The Act has been passed by Parliament of India amidst intense controversy, debate and protest on many of its provisions by Child Rights fraternity. It replaced the Indian Juvenile delinquency law, Juvenile Justice (Care and Protection of Children) Act, 2000, and allows for juveniles in conflict with law in the age group 16–18, involved in heinous offences, to be tried as adults. The Act came into force from 15th January 2016. An Act to consolidate and amend the law relating to children alleged and found to be in conflict with the law and children in need of care and protection by catering to their basic needs through protection, treatment, social integration, by adopting a child-friendly approach in the adjudication and disposal of matters in the best interest of children and for their rehabilitation through processes provided, and institutions and bodies established, hereunder and for matters connected there with or incidental thereto.

Changes in Juvenile Justice Act, 2015

- The bill allows for juveniles 16 years or older to be tried as adults for heinous offences like rape and murder. Heinous offences are those which are punishable with imprisonment of seven years or more.

- The Act mandates setting up Juvenile Justice Boards and Child Welfare Committees in every district. Both must have at least one woman member each.
- The Act streamlines adoption procedures for orphan, abandoned and surrendered children. The existing Central Adoption Resource Authority (CARA) has been given the status a statutory body to enable it to perform its function more effectively, to frame the rules for adoption to be implemented by state and district level agencies.

As of 2019, Ministry of Woman and Child Development of Government of India is working towards bringing an amendment, primarily to remove courts from adoption process, to hand it over to Executive Magistrates/District Magistrates and to make child welfare committees administratively and judicially subordinate to the District Magistrate.

2. *The Child Marriage Restraint Act 1976*

The Act provides safeguards for girls from child marriage.

3. *The Prohibition of Child Marriage Act, 2006*[9]

The Prohibition of Child Marriage Act was made effective in 2007. This Act defines child marriage as a marriage where the groom or the bride is under age. Parents trying to marry under age girls are subject to action under this law since the law makes these marriages illegal. The Prohibition of Child Marriage Act, 2006 defines a 'child' as a boy under the age of 21 and a girl under the age of 18.

4. *Protection of Children from Sexual Offences Act, 2012 (POCSO Act)*

Notably sexual abuse is a global public health problem. It is a serious infringement of one's rights to health and protection. In order to address the problem of child sexual abuse cases through less ambiguous and more stringent legal provisions, The Protection of Children from Sexual Offences Act, popularly known as POCSO Act, was specially formulated by the Government on 20th June 2012. The Act has come into force with effect from 14th November, 2012 along with the Rules framed thereunder.

The POCSO Act, 2012 is a comprehensive law to provide for the protection of children from the offences of sexual assault, sexual harassment and pornography, while safeguarding the interests of the child at every stage of the judicial process by incorporating child-friendly mechanisms for reporting, recording of evidence, investigation and speedy trial of offences through designated special courts for the cause.

5. *Incest*

Sexual intercourse by a man within certain degree of blood relationship, i.e. between father and daughter, brother and sister, nephew and niece, and cousins, etc. is termed as incest. However, evolving definition is "The imposition of sexually inappropriate acts or acts with sexual overtones by one or more persons who derive authority through ongoing emotional bonding with that child." This definition expands the traditional definition of incest to include sexual abuse by anyone who has authority or power over the child. Incest *per se* is not a cognizable offence in India. However, any sexual relationship below 16 years of age (below

15 years in case of wife) without consent amounts to rape (Section 3 without consent amounts to rape) (Section 375 IPC) even if the offender is blood relative. Incestuous rape is the most common form of child sexual abuse.

6. Molestation, Indecency and Eve Teasing

Molestation, indecency and eve teasing are very common incidents in society. Adolescent girls have to face these misbehaviors in their routine social life. Most of the cases remain unreported to the police due to social stigma in our society. According to Section 294 of the Indian Penal Code 1860, whoever, to the annoyance of others does (a) any obscene act in any public place, (b) sings, recites or utters any obscene song, ballad or words, in or near any public place shall be punished.

7. Child Trafficking and Prostitution

Child prostitution and trafficking is the commercial sexual abuse of children. It is the sign of ultimate denial of human rights to adolescent. In spite of the number of legal provisions in India, e.g. Section 366-A IPC—abduction, kidnapping or seducing of minor girl, Section 372 and Section 373 IPC—selling and buying minor girls for prostitution and immoral traffic: They are still beyond control. In 1998, the Government of India (GOI) formulated the National Plan of Action to combat trafficking and sexual exploitation of women and children which prescribes an exhaustive set of guidelines to the central and state governments. The prohibition of "Trafficking" flows out of the Constitution of India (Article 23) and not merely through legislation. Article 34 of the Convention on the Rights of the Child requires State parties to undertake the responsibility to protect the child from all forms of sexual exploitation and sexual abuse. Article 35 of the same convention requires state parties to take appropriate national bilateral and multilateral measures to prevent the abduction of, the sale of or traffic of children for any purpose or in any form. Article 1(3), Article 1(4) of SAARC convention on preventing and combating trafficking of women and children for prostitution has also defined trafficking and traffickers respectively in broader sense.

8. Child Labor

India fosters the largest number of child labor in the world. The child labor (Prohibition and Regulation) Act, 1986 prohibits the engagement of children in certain employments and to regulate the conditions of work of children in certain other employments. Article 4 of the Universal Declaration of Human Rights, the International Bill of Human Rights (1948) adopted and proclaimed that "No one shall be held in slavery or servitude slavery and the slave trade shall be prohibited in all their forms."

9. Drug Abuse

Nowadays drug abuse has become global phenomenon. Teenagers feel it as a proof of maturation and entry to "pseudo-adulthood". It can also be a form of "rebellion against authority" and drug experimentation resulting in vicious cycle of drug abuse. The increasing trend of drug abuse in girls can be due to the misconception that "modern femity" means behaving or adopting male lifestyle. **The Cigarettes and Other Tobacco Products Act, 2003** prohibits sale of cigarette or other tobacco products to a person below the age of 18 years.

CONCLUSION

Both women and children belong to vulnerable class of society. Both require special attention, protection and care for their safe and healthy existence. Indian women have had an extremely difficult time, developing under the oppression of a male-dominated society, class and religion But now it is the time to break silence. Women are entitled to respect. Similarly parents and health providers should update themselves with child protection laws. There is a need for the society to change the mindset and the patriarchial views that have engulfed Indian mindsets since ages. Then only India would be better place specifically for women and children.

REFERENCES

1. Seyon R (Advocate): Legislative and judicial initiatives towards woman empowerment:Air Infotech:: http://www.airinfotech.in/article3.html (Accessed on 6th June 2019)
2. Laws and Acts: INDIA Women Welfare Foundation: http://www.womenwelfare.org/laws_acts.html: (Accessed on 10th June 2019)
3. Sushma Sosha Philip and Susan Philip: Laws every Indian girl must know: https://www.parentcircle.com/article/laws-every-indian-girl-must-know/2/ (Accessed on 5th October 2019)
4. Women in India: From Wikipedia, the free encyclopedia (Accessed on 10th June 2019)
5. Kuthe Alka: Issues in adolescence gynecology: Tiwari S, Badwa M, Tiwari M, Kuthe Alka, Editors: Textbook on Medico-legal Issues (Related to various specialties): 2nd edition-Jaypee Brothers Medical Publishers, New Delhi.2019: Pg 274–80.
6. Information Technology Act , 2000: Wikipedia.org (Accessed on 10th October 2019)
7. Information Technology (Amendment) Bill 2018 : Wikipedia.org (Accessed on 11th October 2019)
8. Surrogacy in India: Wilkipedia.org (Accessed on 21 th October 2019)
9. TanviDubey: Laws that protect womens rights: https://yourstory.com/2016/06/laws-that-protect-women-rights 1/(Accessed on 20th October 2019)
10. Maternity Benefit (Amendment Act, 2017): Wikipedia.org (Accessed on 7th October 2019)
11. Air India Etc. Etc vs Nergesh Meerza and Ors. Etc. Etc on 28 August, 1981. Empowerment Of Women.
12. Universal Declaraton on Human rights (UDHR:1948) (Accessed on 5th November 2019)
13. Arpan Sinha: Women protection and Changing laws: http://www.legalservicesindia.com/article/1818/Women-Protection-and-Changing-Laws.html 3/6 (Accessed on 12th November 2019)
14. Juvenile Justice (Care and Protection of Children Act 2015: www.slideshare.net (Accessed on 12th November 2019)

Chapter 29

Role of Women Commission in Domestic Violence

○ Mandakini Megh ○ Shomita Biswas ○ Preeti Deshpande

For long, the fairer sex has suffered at the hands of men, the exploitation ranges from physical to intangible abuse like mental and psychological torture. Women have been treated as child bearing machines, push-over, to nothing but animals at the hands of men. Domestic violence is one of the gravest and the most pervasive human rights violation. For too long now, women have accepted it as their destiny, perhaps, because of the justice system or the lack of it or because they are vulnerable, scared of being ostracized by their own or because speaking about domestic violence still remains a taboo for most women who suffer from it or for other reasons best known to them. Though women are legal citizens of India and have equal rights, as men, but India remains a male dominant society. From the time to time various acts were enforced to ensure women are protected.

DOMESTIC VIOLENCE

Violence against women is a serious problem in India. Overall, 30% of the women in the age group of 15–49 years have experienced physical violence and about 6% have experienced sexual violence. In total, 36% have experienced physical or sexual violence (Fig. 29.1).

DOMESTIC VIOLENCE ACT[2]

The Protection of Women from Domestic Violence Act, was introduced in 2005 for effective protection of women from any kind of violence in the family and matters connected therewith.

Domestic violence has been recognized since 1983 as a criminal offence under IPC 498A.

It was not until enactment of the Protection of Women from Domestic Violence Act of 2005, that civil protection was afforded to victims of domestic violence. Protection of Women from Domestic Violence Act provides a definition of domestic violence that is comprehensive and includes all forms of physical, emotional, verbal, sexual and economic violence and harassment in the form of unlawful dowry demands as a form of abuse.

The Act requires appointment of Protection Officers to assist victims and acknowledges the importance of collaboration between government and external organization in protecting women.

OTHER MEASURES TAKEN BY THE GOVERNMENT FOR WOMEN'S SAFETY

The Government has shown a persistent commitment towards improving the law and order and safety for women. India's all-in-one emergency helpline number was launched in February 2019 by Union Home Ministry in 16 states and union territories. The '112' emergency helpline number would provide immediate in assistance to services like police (100), fire (101), health (108), women's safety (1090) and child protection.[6]

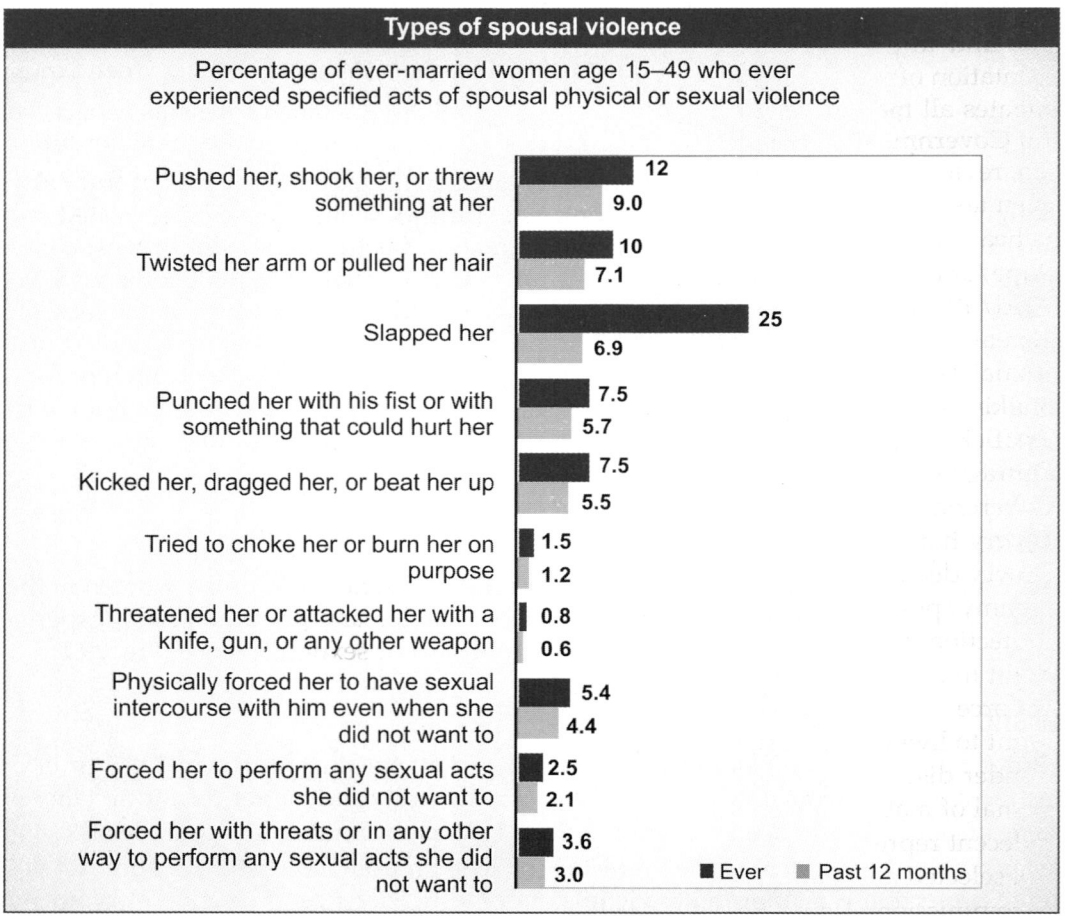

Fig. 29.1: Forms of spousal violence experienced by ever-married women in percentage[1]

Apart from emergency response service, the government also launched the Investigation Tracking System for Sexual Offences (ITSSO) and safe city implementation monitoring portal to improve women's safety.

For smart phones, you need to press the power button three times quickly on your smart phone to activate 112 panic call to the emergency response centre (ERC).

For normal phones you need to press number '5' or '9' to activate a panic call.

A '112 India' mobile app was also launched on Google Playstore and Apple store

THE NATIONAL COMMISSION FOR WOMEN

The National Commission for women is a statutory body of the Government of India generally concerned with advising the government on all policy matters affecting women. It was established in 1992 under the National Commission for Women Act, 1990 (Act No. 20 of 1990 of Government of India).[3]

The objective of the National Commission for Women is to represent the rights of women in India and to provide a voice for their issues and concerns like dowry, politics, equal representation of women in jobs and domestic violence. As per the mandate the Commission investigates all matters relating to safeguards provided for women, presents reports to the Central Government, makes recommendations to the government to safeguard conditions of women, review from time to time and takes up issues of violation of laws relating to women and even takes *suo moto* action.

The heads under which complaints are registered with the commission include:[5]
1. Rape/attempt to rape
2. Acid/attacks
3. Sexual harassment
4. Sexual assault
5. Stalking/voyeurism
6. Trafficking/prostitution
7. Outraging the modesty of women
8. Cybercrimes against women
9. Dowry harassment
10. Dowry death
11. Bigamy/polygamy
12. Protection of women against domestic violence
13. Right to marriage by choice
14. Divorce
15. Right to live with dignity
16. Gender discrimination
17. Denial of maternity benefit
18. Indecent representation of women
19. Sex selected abortion

The commission also participates in planning socioeconomic development of women and work on women's empowerment.

As per the National Family Health Survey-4, it was found that in families approximately 30% of women were employed compared to 97% of men who were employed. Also it was found that amongst working women 50% earn less than the husband. Even where women are working, it was found in 15% households the husband decides how the cash will be spent and in 60% both decide. But regarding the husband's earnings 25–30% husbands will decide how the cash will be spent. Only about 8–10% women are empowered to make decisions about their own health. Also the women are not empowered to fend for themselves as they are not empowered to move out of their homes alone much (only 30–40%) till the age of 25 years. However, amongst older women 45–70% are allowed to fend for themselves.[1]

So as per the survey women are as yet poorly empowered and we have a long way to go. Women's empowerment can help in countering issues of domestic violence.

THE NATIONAL FAMILY HEALTH SURVEY INDIA-4

A survey was conducted by the Ministry of Health and Family Welfare using State modules to get the statistics about existing domestic violence. One eligible woman per household was randomly selected and interviewed in privacy.[1]

NFHS-4 information was obtained from all women by asking the following questions
1. Physical spousal violence—push you, shake you or throw something at you, slap you, twist your arm or pull your hair, punch you with fists or something that can hurt you, kick you, drag you or beat you up, try to choke you or burn you on purpose, or threaten you or attack you with a knife, or any other weapon.
2. Sexual spousal violence—physically force you to have sexual intercourse with him even when you did not want to; physically force you with threats or in any other way to perform sexual acts you did not want to.
3. Emotional spousal violence—say or do something to humiliate you in front of others, threaten to hurt you in front of others, threaten to hurt you or someone close to you, insult you or make you feel bad about yourself.

33% of ever married women have experienced physical violence, sexual or emotional violence. Physical violence is 30%, emotional violence is 14% and 7% have experienced sexual violence.

There has been a decline in spousal sexual and physical violence from 37% in NFHS-3 to 31% in NFHS-4 conducted in 2015-16 over 10 years.

Patterns of Violence

Married women are more likely to experience physical or sexual violence by husbands than by anyone else. Nearly two in five (36%) married women have experienced some form of physical or sexual violence by their husband. For never married women, the most common perpetrators include mothers or step mothers, fathers or step fathers, sisters or brothers and teachers.

Patterns of Background Characteristics of Physical Violence

- Women's experience of physical violence increases with age, from 17% among women of age 15–19 years to 35% among women of age 40–49 years.

- The experience of physical violence is more common among women in rural areas (32%) than among women in urban areas (25%).
- Women's experience of violence declines sharply with women's schooling (from 41% with no schooling to 17% in women with 12 or more years of schooling) and wealth. However, violence still exists in higher socioeconomic strata also, but reporting is less to avoid undue publicity and media coverage.
- Surprisingly women who are employed are more likely (17%) to experience physical violence than women who are not employed (26%).

Patterns of Background Characteristics of Sexual Violence

- Women's experience of sexual violence increases with age from 3% at 15–19 years to 5% at 20–24 years.
- Single, divorced, separated women are far more likely to experience sexual violence (13%).
- Women's experience of violence declines sharply with women's schooling (from 9% with no schooling to 3% in women with 12 or more years of schooling). Women's experience of sexual violence declines similarly with wealth.

Patterns of Background Characteristics for Any Form of Violence

- Ever experience of one or more forms of violence increases sharply with women's number of living children from 24% among women with no children to 43% among women with 5 or more children.
- Women in rural areas are more likely to experience violence (36%) than women in urban areas (28%).
- Women's experience of violence declines sharply with women's schooling and wealth.
- Intergenerational effects of spousal violence are evident in India. Women who report that their fathers beat their mothers are much more likely (58%) to themselves have spousal violence than women who report that their fathers did not beat their mothers.
- Experience of spousal physical or sexual violence varies greatly with the husband's level of alcohol consumption. 71% of women whose husbands often get drunk have experienced spousal violence compared with 22% of the women whose husbands do not drink alcohol.
- 40% of the women who agree with 3–7 reasons for wife beating have experienced spousal violence compared with 23% of women who agree with no reason for wife beating.

Marital Control by Husbands

Women whose current husband demonstrates at least one of the following controlling behaviors is more likely to experience violence: Is jealous or angry if she talks to other men; frequently accuses her of being unfaithful; does not permit her to meet female friends; tries to limit her contact with her family; insists on knowing where she is at all times; and does not trust her with any money.

Attempts by husbands to closely control and monitor their wives' behavior are important early warning signs and correlates of violence in a relationship. Because the concentration of behaviors is more significant than display of a single behavior, the proportion of women whose husbands display at least three of the specific behaviors is also discussed in this section.

Twelve percent of married women with 12 or more years of education have experienced spousal violence, compared with 21% of married women whose husbands have 12 or more years of education. This suggests that women's own education reduces their likelihood of experiencing spousal violence more than their husband's education.

Spousal violence is lower among couples in which husbands and wives have both been to school and are equally educated (24%) than among couples where the husband has more education than the wife or if neither husband nor wife is educated (46%).

Spousal violence varies greatly by state. The prevalence of physical or sexual violence ranges from 4% in Sikkim, 7% in Himachal Pradesh and 45% in Telangana, Bihar, Andhra Pradesh, Tamil Nadu to 55% in Manipur.

One in six (16%) married women have experienced emotional violence by their husband. Acts of emotional violence by the husband against the wife include: Saying or doing something to humiliate her in front of others, threatening to hurt or harm her or someone close to her, or insulting her or making her feel bad about herself.

Only one percent of married women have ever initiated violence against their husband.

Most Women Do Not Seek Help When They are Abused

Only one in four abused women have ever sought help to try to end the violence they have experienced. Two out of three women have only never sought help, but have also never told anyone about the violence. Abused women most often seek help from their own families (65%). The second most common source of help is the husband's family (29%). 15% sought help from a friend. Only 3% sought help from the police. 2% sought help from religious leaders. About 1% seeks help from doctors or medical personnel.

Majority of Women and Men Say that a Husband Is Justified in Beating His Wife

More than half of women (54%) and men (51%) agree that it is justifiable for a husband to beat his wife under some circumstances. Women and men most often agree that wife beating is justified when the wife disrespects her in-laws. Neglect of the house or children is the second most commonly agreed to justification for wife beating for both women and men.

DOMESTIC VIOLENCE ACT AND ITS IMPLEMENTATION

Domestic Violence Act, 2005, hereinafter referred at Protection for Women against Domestic Violence (PWDVA),[2] has been passed with a view to improve the position of women in the domestic front. The Protection of Women from Domestic Violence Act (DVA), 2005, came into force 26.10.2006. It is widely expected that DVA will go a long way to provide relief to women from domestic violence and enforce their 'right to live'. Primarily DVA is meant to provide protection to the wife or female live-in partner from violence at the hands of husband or male live-in partner or relatives. DVA also extends its protection to women who are sisters, widows or mothers. The Act is an extremely progressive one not only because it recognizes women who are in a live-in relationship but also extends protection to other women in the household, including sisters and mothers, thus the Act includes relations of consanguinity, marriage, or through relationships in the nature of marriage, adoption, or joint family, thus 'domestic relationships' are not restricted to the marital context alone. In fact the Act has given a new dimension to the word abuse because unlike the primitive notion abuse includes actual abuse or threat of abuse, whether physical, sexual, verbal, economic and harassment by way of dowry demands.

The primary cause of perpetration of violence on women is still dowry harassment followed by alcoholism, extramarital affairs and birth of a female child or the aggrieved woman's inability to bear children.

According to the National Crime Records Bureau the total number of cases registered under Protection of Women Against Domestic Violence Act from 2012 to 2014 as per the Ministry of Women and Child Development has declined dramatically.

Year	Domestic Violence cases registered
2012	16351 cases
2013	4204 cases
2014	531 cases

The National Commission analyses complaints received:[5]
- This shows the trend of crimes against women and suggests system changes needed for reduction of crimes.
- The complaints are analysed to understand gaps in the routine functioning of the government in tackling violence against women and suggests corrective measures
- The complaints are also used as case studies for sensitization programmes for police, judiciary, prosecutors, forensic scientists, lawyers and administrative functionaries.

The Commission helps in processing complaints on Acts related to justice for women. The complaints are processed in the following manner:[5]
- Investigations by police are expedited and monitored
- Family disputes are resolved through counselling or hearing before the commission. For serious crimes, the commission constitutes an Inquiry Committee which makes spot enquiries, examines witnesses, collects evidences and submits the report with recommendations. Such investigations provide immediate relief and justice to the victims of violence and atrocities. The implementation of the report is monitored by the National Commission for Women. There is a provision for having experts/lawyers on these committees.
- A few complaints are also forwarded to the respective State Commission for Women and other forums like National Human Rights Commission, National Commission for Scheduled Caste and Scheduled Tribes for disposal of complaints.

As per the mandate the commission also undertakes special studies, organizes seminars, conferences and workshops in collaboration with NGOs, voluntary organisations and colleges. It also organizes programmes like Violence Free Homes—a joint Programme held by National Commission for Women, Delhi Police and TISS Mumbai.

CONCLUSION

The question raised in this article is how far the Domestic Violence Act, 2005 has succeeded in fulfilling the requirements of adequately defining all forms of domestic violence and providing redressal and protection to its victims. The issue has been tackled on conceptual and practical grounds, while the aforesaid enactment is an important first step in terms of the concepts it introduces into the Indian legal system, the viability of its implementation may be contested on certain grounds.

In terms of concepts, the aim of the legislation, in addressing the problem of domestic violence on a woman by a man in a domestic relationship, has to a great extent been served. It may be concluded that the range and detail in which various definitions and forms of relief have been drafted, show a clear effort on the part of the legislators to provide adequate redressal and protection. It is only in some cases that implementation has not been adequately provided for example, in the system whereby a breach in a protection orders is addressed. More specifically the case of protection officers is an instance where the Act might have considered using existing administrative machinery instead of creating the necessity for further expenditure.

Low rates of participation in education, lack of economic independence, value biases operating against them, etc. directly and indirectly resulted in the women been given the status of being the secondary gender in Indian society.

It is the Mission of the National Commission for Women to strive towards enabling women to achieve equality and equal participation in all spheres of life by securing her due rights and entitlements through suitable policy formulation, legislative measures, effective enforcement of laws, implementation of schemes/policies and devising strategies for solution of specific problems/situations arising out of discrimination and atrocities against women.[4]

REFERENCES

1. National Family Healthy Survey-4 (NFHS-4) -2015-2016–International Institute for Population Sciences, Deonar, Mumbai 400008, Ministry of Health and Family Welfare
2. Protection of Women from Domestic Violence Act 2005 published by Ministry of Law and Justice
3. National Commission for Women http://ncw.nic.in/mission-and-vision/mission
4. National Commission for Women http://ncw.nic.in/commission/about-us
5. National Commission for Women http://ncw.nic.in/ncw-cells/complaint-investigation-cell
6. 112 is India's all-in-one-emergency helpline number. http://www.indiatoday.in/information/story/112-india-s-all-in-one-emergency-helpline-number-know-all-about-it-1461757-2019-02-21

Chapter 30

Policy Decisions for Women's Health

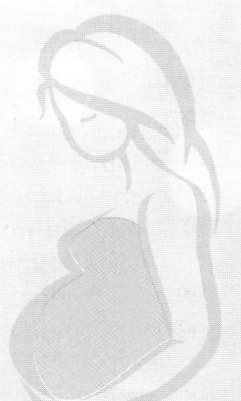

○ Rajesh Darade   ○ Sachin Mumbare

INTRODUCTION

Indian constitution has mentioned the principle of equality of status and opportunity in its preamble. Right to equality and prohibition of discrimination on grounds of gender is one of the six fundamental rights granted by the constitution to the people. Empowerment of women has been recognized as the central point in the development of a nation. So within the framework of Indian democratic system, our Laws, Plans and Programmes have aimed at women's empowerment in every respect. Health policymakers have also recognized the importance of women's health in the national development.

Health of the women is not only important for the overall health status of the country, but also it determines the health status of the children, the future citizens of the country. So, investing in maintaining the health status of the women should not be looked upon as non-productive but it should be envisioned as the fruitful investment required for the healthy future of our country. These principles are kept in mind while making the health policy and decisions, though the quantum and centre of the focus always remained debatable.

Historical Milestones in Policy Decisions Related to Women's Health

1880	Establishment of training centers for dais in Amritsar
1902	First Midwifery Act promulgated to promote safe delivery.
1930	The Child Marriage Restraint Act (Sarda Act) came into effect, fixing the minimum age at marriage at 14 for girls.
1930	Advisory Committee on maternal mortality was set up.
1931	Maternity and Child Welfare Bureau established under Indian Red Cross Society.
1948	India joined World Health Organization as a member state.

1953	National Family Planning Programme launched.
1955	Hindu Marriage Act prescribed the minimum age at marriage—18 for boys and 15 for girls.
1961	Department of Family Planning created.
1970	All India Hospital Postpartum Programme started.
1972	The MTP Act came into force on 1st April 1972.
1974	Family planning services incorporated in MCH care.
1975	ICDS Scheme launched.
1977	National Family Planning Programme renamed as National Family Welfare Programme.
1983	India launched its first National Health Policy.
1992	Child Survival and Safe Motherhood (CSSM) Programme launched on 20th August 1992.
1992-93	First National Family Health Survey conducted.
1994	PCPNDT Act enacted
1995	National Maternity Benefit Scheme came into effect in August 1995 as one of the component of National Social Assistance Programme (NSAP).
1996	National Family Welfare Programme was made target free.
1997	Reproductive and Child Health Programme-1 (RCH-1) launched.
1998-99	National Family Health Survey-2 (NFHS-2) undertaken. National policy for older persons announced.
2000	National Population Policy, 2000 announced.
2001	National Policy for Empowerment of Women launched on 20th March 2001.
2002	National Health Policy, 2002 announced.
2003	PCPNDT Act amended
2004	National Guidelines on Infant and Young Child Feeding were formulated in 2004.
2005	National Rural Health Mission launched.
	Reproductive and Child Health Programme-2 (RCH-2) launched.
	Janani Suraksha Yojana launched
	Indian Public Health Standards for Community Health Centers formulated.
2005-06	National Family Health Survey-3 (NFHS-3) conducted.
2006	Integrated Management of Neonatal and Childhood Illnesses (IMNCI) launched in 16 States, Ministry of Women and Child Development carved out of Ministry of Human Resource and Development.

Review of Policy Decisions Affecting Women's Health

India was the first country to launch National Family Planning Programme in 1952.[1] During the first decade of its existence, family planning was considered more a mechanism to improve the health of mothers and children than a method of population control.[2] Nevertheless, it started offering some health services to the women.

In 1970, All India Hospital Postpartum Programme was started.[3] Though it was intended to offer family planning education and services to women who are in the hospitals for maternity care, it was the first programme to offer something to restore postpartum health of the women.

The MTP Act, which came into force on 1st April 1972, was mainly intended to legalize the abortions. It also helped in reducing maternal morbidity and mortality by allowing the abortions in life-threatening conditions.[4]

Integrated child development services (ICDS): Scheme was launched on 2nd October 1975 with main objectives to improve health status of children in the age group of 0–6 years.[5] One of the objectives of the scheme was to enhance the capability of women to look after the normal and nutritional needs of the child through proper nutrition and health education.

In 1983, India launched its first National Health Policy as a response to commitment to the Alma Declaration of Health for All by 2000 AD.[6,7] It declared maternal health as one of the integral components of the primary healthcare. The identified unacceptable level of maternal health was one of the major problems requiring urgent attention. It clearly stated the need of
1. Launching special programmes for the improvement of maternal and child health with a special focus on under privileged sections of the society.
2. Decentralization of such programmes to the maximum possible extent.
3. Implementation of such programmes through primary level, nearest to the doorsteps of the beneficiaries.
4. Continued efforts for providing training and orientation to the traditional birth attendants.
5. Schemes and programmes to ensure that progressively all the deliveries are conducted by competently trained persons, so that complicated cases receive timely and expert attention.
6. Services within comprehensive programme to provide antenatal, intranatal and postnatal care.

National Health Policy, 1983 set some national goals to be achieved by 1985, 1990 and 2000. All these goals related to women's health were concentrated on maternal health[5] (Table 30.1).

It was very obvious that the National Health Policy towards women's health was centered towards maternal health and family planning. Other aspects of the women's health did not receive much focus and were ignored.

Child survival and safe motherhood (CSSM) programme: An Integrated Maternal and Child Health Programme was launched on 20th August 1992.[8] Few of the aims of CSSM Programme were to reduce maternal mortality to 200 per 100,000 live births, ANC services to 100% pregnant women, 100% deliveries by trained personnel. All these aims were analogous to the goals set by National Health Policy, 1983. So Child Survival and Safe Motherhood Programme was launched to improve the maternal and child health and achieve the goals to be achieved by 2000, set by first National Health Policy.

National Family Health Survey-1, a nationwide health survey, was undertaken in 1992-93 with main objective of providing estimates of fertility, family planning, maternal and child healthcare and utilization rates for services provided to mothers and children. The survey came out with some key findings related to the women's health status.[9] These findings are summarized in Table 30.2.

Table 30.1: Goals related to women's health set by National Health Policy, 1983

S. no.	Indicator	Then current level	Goals set by National Health Policy		
			1983	1990	2000
1.	Maternal mortality rate*	4–5 (1976)	2–4	2–3	<2
2.	Crude birth rate	Around 35	31	27	21
3.	Effective couple protection rate	23.6 (March 1982)	37	42	60
4.	Net reproduction rate	1.48 (1981)	1.34	1.17	1.00
5.	Family size	4.4 (1975)	3.8	—	2.3
6.	Pregnant mothers receiving ANC (%)	40–50	50–60	60–75	100
7.	Deliveries by trained birth attendants (%)	30–35	50	80	100
8.	TT for pregnant women	20	60	100	100

*Per 1000 live births.

Table 30.2: National Family Health Survey-1 findings related to women's health and its comparison with goals set by NHP, 1983

S. no.	Indicator	Finding	Target as per National Health Policy, 1983 (year by which it was to be achieved)
1.	Percent illiterate females (6 + age)	56.7	—
2.	Mothers receiving ANC (%)	62.3	60–75 (1990), 100 (2000)
3.	Mothers receiving TT injection (%)	53.8 (two doses), 7.1 (one dose)	100 (1990).
4.	Deliveries by trained birth attendants/persons (%)	69.4	80 (1990), 100 (2000)
5.	Place of delivery (%)	Health facility—25.5 and home—73.5, Other/do not know—1	—
6.	Maternal mortality rate*	4.37	2–3 (1990)
7.	Crude birth rate	28.7	27 (1990)
8.	Effective couple protection rate (%)	41	42 (1990), 60 (2000)
9.	Family size	3.4	2.3 (2000)

*Per 1000 live births.

The survey clearly showed that many of the targets and goals set for the year 1990 were still not achieved in 1992-93. This stressed the need for widespread changes in policy related to the maternal health.

Reproductive and Child Health Programme-1 was launched in 1997 incorporating four main components, viz. family planning, child survival and safe motherhood, sexually transmitted diseases and reproductive tract infection.[10] Following were the main features of RCH-1:[11]

1. The program integrated all interventions of fertility regulation, MCH and reproductive health.

2. The services provided were made client oriented, demand driven through decentralized participatory planning and target free approach.
3. First Referral Units (FRUs) were decided to be set up at sub-district level to provide comprehensive emergency obstetric care.
4. Facilities of obstetric care, MTP and IUD insertion at PHCs were improved. IUD insertion facilities were made available at sub-center level.
5. Specialist facilities for STD and RTI were made available in all district hospitals and many sub-district level hospitals.
6. Special programme was taken up for urban slums, tribal population and adolescents. Non-Governmental Organizations and Voluntary Health Organizations were involved for the same.

Following were the major policy decisions taken for interventions under RCH-1:[11]

- Additional ANMs provided to many districts (category C in 8 states) and remaining six North Eastern states.
- Public health/staff nurses were provided to 25% PHCs in category C districts.
- Laboratory technicians were provided First Referral Units.
- Private Anesthetists were allowed to conduct emergency obstetric procedures.
- Safe motherhood consultants (specialist doctors) allowed to visit once a week/fortnight to conduct MTPs and ANC checkups.
- 24-hour delivery services at PHC/CHCs with additional honorarium to the staff.
- Transport facility for referral transport for emergency obstetrics care.
- During 2000-01, RCH out-reach scheme was introduced to strength the delivery of maternal and child health services in remote and comparatively weaker districts and urban slums in UP, MP, Rajasthan, Bihar, Assam, Orissa, Gujarat and West Bengal. Border District Cluster Strategy (BDCS), an UNICEF assisted scheme was introduced in 49 districts spread over 17 states to provide focused intervention for reducing infant and maternal mortality rates by half over next two to three years.
- A scheme for training of dais was initiated in 2001-02 in 156 districts, where safe delivery rates were less than 30%. The scheme was extended to all districts of Empowered Action Group States.

National Family Health Survey-2 was conducted in 1998-99. The survey collected most of the type of information collected during NFHS-1. In addition, NFHS-2 covered a lot of new topics related to women's health aspect with important policy implications such as reproductive health, women's autonomy, domestic violence, women's nutrition, anemia and salt iodization. So this survey was the first real attempt to expand the vision beyond maternal and family planning aspects of women's health. The survey came out with some key findings related to the women's health status.[12] These findings are summarized in Table 30.3.

This survey also clearly showed that many of the targets and goals set for the year 1990 were still not achieved in 1998-99.

In 2000 National Population Policy was announced.[13] The policy thought beyond the fertility and mortality rates and dealt with other aspects affecting women's health such as women

Table 30.3: National Family Health Survey-2 findings related to women's health and its comparison with goals set by NHP-1983

S.no.	Indicator	Finding	Target as per National Health Policy, 1983 (year by which it was to be achieved)
1.	Percent illiterate females (6 + age)	49%	—
2.	Female addictions	Alcohol—2% Smoking—3% Chewing pan masala—10% (high rates in North Eastern States)	—
3.	Mothers receiving ANC (%)	65	60–75 (1990), 100 (2000)
4.	Mothers receiving TT injection (%)	67 (two doses)	100 (1990)
5.	Maternal mortality rate*	5.4	2–3 (1990), <2 (2000)
6.	Crude birth rate	25	27 (1990), 21 (2000)
7.	Effective couple protection rate (%)	48	42 (1990), 60 (2000)

*Per 1000 live births.

education, women empowerment, adolescent health and education. The policy set socio-demographic goals to be achieved by 2010. Some of the goals related to women's health are:
- Address the unmet needs for basic RCH services.
- Reduce maternal mortality to less than 100 per 100,000 live births.
- Promote delayed marriage for girls, above 18 (preferably above 20)
- Hundred percent deliveries attended by trained persons. Eighty percent institutional deliveries.
- Universal access to information/counseling and services for fertility regulation and contraception.
- Integrate Indian system of medicine in RCH services.
- Small family norm to achieve replacement level of fertility.

India announced its National Health Policy in 2002.[14] It clearly stated that "Social, cultural and economic factors continue to inhibit from gaining adequate access to even the existing public health facilities. The handicap does not merely affect women as individuals; it also has an adverse impact on the health, general well-being and development of the entire family, particularly children. This policy recognizes the catalytic role of empowered women in improving the overall health standards of the community."

Thus, the National Health Policy, 2002 also thought beyond fertility and maternal aspects of women health. The policy set some goals to be achieved by 2015. Surprisingly the goals were not dominated by fertility rates. Only goal related to maternal care is to reduce MMR to 100 per 100,000 live births by 2010.

Table 30.4: National Family Health Survey-3 findings related to women's health and its comparison with goals set by NHP, 1983

S.no.	Indicator	Finding	Target as per National Health Policy, 1983 (year by which it was to be achieved)
1.	Mothers receiving ANC (%)	50.7 (at least 3 ANC visits)	60–75 (1990), 100 (2000)
2.	Effective couple protection rate (%)	56.3	42 (1990), 60 (2000)
3.	Family size	2.7	2.3 (2000)
4.	Women with BMI less than normal (%)	33	—
5.	Anemia in pregnancy (%)	57.9	—
6.	Anemia in married women (%)	56.2	—

National Family Health Survey-3 was undertaken in 2005-06.[15] This was the first large scale nationwide survey in the new millennium. The survey provided a lot of information related to women's health and provided an opportunity to compare the achievements with set targets or goals and evaluate the health policy. Table 30.4 summarizes the findings of the NFHS-3.

Some important current programmes related to women's health:

Integrated Child Development Services (ICDS)[5] Scheme

Integrated Child Development Services Scheme was launched with objectives to improve the nutritional and health status of children in the age group of 0–6 years. The scheme offers services to the children in that age group as well as pregnant and lactating mothers. A package of services is offered to the beneficiaries in an integrated manner. This policy decision of offering many services under one umbrella of ICDS was taken with a view to increase the overall impact of the services. Following are the services offered through ICDS, with their target group and service providing person (Table 30.5).

ICDS is mainly a centrally funded scheme, with funding ratio of 90:10 (Centre: State) for all components of ICDS for North Eastern States. For other states and UTs ratio is the same, except for supplementary nutrition with funding ratio of 50:50.

The decision of revising norms of setting up of Anganwadi centres and Mini-AWC have also resulted in accelerated improvement in the overall health status of children and women. The revised norms are as follows (Table 30.6).

Central allocation of funds for ICDS increased from 529.3 millions in 2007-08 to 670.5 millions in 2009-10. Other decisions related to ICDS are setting up of countrywide infrastructure for training of ICDS functionaries, monitoring and evaluation of ICDS schemes, revision of the honorarium paid to the AWW, helper, etc.

Reproductive and Child Health Programme-2[16]

RCH-2 was launched on 1st April 2005 with the principal aim of reducing maternal and child morbidity and mortality with special emphasis on rural health. The major strategies are:

Table 30.5: Services provided to women through ICDS

S. no.	Services	Target group	Services provided by	Remarks
1.	Supplementary nutrition	Pregnant and lactating mother	AWW	Supplementary nutrition containing 600 Kcal and 18–20 g per day per beneficiary
2.	Immunization	Pregnant women	ANM/MO	Immunization against TT to reduce maternal and neonatal mortality.
3.	Health check up*	Pregnant and lactating mother	ANM/MO/ AWW	ANC and PNC
4.	Referral services	Pregnant and lactating mother	AWW/ANM/ MO	Referral of high-risk pregnancy and postnatal complications
5.	Nutrition and health education	Women (15–45 years)	AWW/ANM/ MO	As a part of behavior change communication (BCC) strategy, with a long-term goal of capacity building of women, especially in the age group of 15–45 years

ANM: Auxiliary Nurse Midwife, AWW: Anganwadi worker, MO: Medical Officer *AWW helps to identify pregnant women

Table 30.6: Revised policy decision for setting up of Anganwadi for rural/urban projects

S. no.	Population	Norms	Remark
1.	150–400	Mini anganwadi	For tribal/river line/desert/hilly/other difficult areas, one mini-AW for 150–300 population and one AWC for 300–800 population
2.	400–800	One AWC	
3.	800–1600	Two AWCs	
4.	1600–2400	Three AWCs	
5.	Thereafter every multiple of 800	One extra AWC	

- Essential obstetrics care by promoting institutional delivery and skilled attendance at delivery.
- Emergency obstetrics care through first referral units and 24-hour delivery services at PHCs and CHCs.
- Strengthening the referral system.

RCH-2 is a centrally funded programme with more flexibility allowed to the states for planning to achieve the goals.

New initiatives undertaken under RCH-2 are training of MBBS doctors in life-saving anaesthetic skills for emergency obstetric care, setting up of blood storage centres at FRUs, Janani Suraksha Yojana, Vande Mataram scheme, and safe abortion services. Federation of Obstetrics and Gynecology Society of India is helping to train MBBS doctors for emergency obstetrics care.

Janani Suraksha Yojana under NRHM[17]

Janani Suraksha Yojana was launched on 12th April 2005 by modifying National Maternity Benefit Scheme (NMBS), under National Rural Health Mission with aim of reducing maternal and infant mortality through encouraging institutional deliveries. This 100% centrally funded scheme under NRHM combines the benefits of institutional care during ANC, INC and PNC with cash benefit offered to the beneficiaries. The expected end result of the scheme is increased number of institutional deliveries among the poor families, who otherwise cannot afford the institutional care.

For the implementation of the scheme, Indian states have been divided into low performing states (LPS) and high performing states (HPS). The LPS are UP, Uttaranchal, Bihar, Jharkhand, MP, Chhattisgarh, Assam, Rajasthan, Orissa and JK. Remaining states are HPS. The benefit is offered to all women in LPS and below poverty line women above 19 years of age in HPS. ASHA (Accredited Social Health Activist) is responsible for arranging the ANC, INC, PNC and neonatal care. Following is scale of cash assistance provided under the scheme (Table 30.7).

Janani Shishu Suraksha Karyakram under NRHM[18]

Janani Suraksha Yojana did not provide cash assistance for drugs, diagnostic tests, diet, caesarean section, etc. in case of institutional deliveries. So these high out-of-pocket expenses made it difficult for the poor sections to avail the maternal and child health services at institutions. So Janani Shishu Suraksha Karyakram (JSSK) was launched on 1st June 2011 with following services free of cost at government institutions, viz. free and cashless delivery, C-section, drugs, consumables, diagnostics, diet up to 3 days after normal delivery and 7 days after C-section, provision of blood, transport from home to health institutions and back and transport to health facility for referral. Neonatal care up to 30 days after delivery is also provided free of cost. Thus, the scheme has eliminated the out of pocket expenses incurred by pregnant women and sick newborns while accessing the services at government health institutions.

ADOLESCENT HEALTH

Menstrual Hygiene Scheme[19]

The scheme, launched as part of the Adolescent Reproductive and Sexual Health (ARSH) component under RCH II, aims to ensure that adolescent girls in the target group have adequate knowledge about menstrual hygiene and the use of sanitary napkins. The high quality, safe products are made available to them, and environmentally safe disposal mechanisms are readily

Table 30.7: Scale of cash assistance provided under JSY

S. no.	Rural area Mother's package	ASHA's package	Total	Urban area Mother's package	ASHA's package	Total
LPS	1400	600	2000	1000	400	1400
HPS	700	600	1300	600	400	1000

accessible. The sanitary napkins, supplied by central government or Self Help Group (SHG), are provided under NHM's brand, 'Freedays'. These napkins are being sold to adolescents girls at the rate of 6/- per pack of six napkins by Accredited Social Health Activists (ASHAs).

Weekly Iron and Folic Acid Supplementation[20]

MOHFW has launched the Weekly Iron and Folic Acid Supplementation (WIFS) Programme for all adolescent girls and school going adolescent boys. To decrease incidence and prevalence of anemia in adolescent, weekly supervised IFA tablets (100 mg of elemental iron and 500 mcg of folic acid) and biannual de-worming tablets are provided to the beneficiaries.

Rashtriya Kishor Swasthya Karyakram

It includes sexual and reproductive health, nutrition, injuries and violence (including gender-based violence), non-communicable diseases, mental health and substance misuse aspects of adolescent health. Key drivers of the program are community-based interventions like peer educators, outreach by counselors, involvement of parents and the community through a dedicated adolescent health day; communication for information and behavior change, i.e. Social and Behavior Change Communication; and Adolescent Friendly Health Clinics across levels of care.

Other Programmes Related to Adolescent Health under Different Ministries

- Women and Child Development: Kishori Shakti Yojana, Balika Samridhi Yojana, Rajiv Gandhi Scheme for Empowerment of Adolescent Girls (SABLA)
- Human Resource Development: Sarva Shiksha Abhiyan; National Population Education Project (NPEP); Adolescence Education Program (AEP)
- Youth Affairs and Sports: Adolescent Empowerment Scheme; National Service Scheme; Nehru Yuva Kendra Sangathan (NYKS) Programs, National Program for Youth and Adolescent Development (NPYAD)
- Others like: Narcotic Drugs and Psychotropic Substances Act, 1985; AH Strategy

RMNCH+A[21]

RMNCH+A includes Reproductive, Maternal, Neonatal, Child plus Adolescent health encompassing all interventions aimed at reproductive, maternal, newborn, child, and adolescent health under a broad umbrella, and focusing on the strategic lifecycle approach. The RMNCH+A strategy approaches include:

1. Health systems strengthening (HSS) focusing on infrastructure, human resources, supply chain management, and referral transport measures.
2. Prioritization of high-impact interventions for various life cycle stages.
3. Increasing effectiveness of investments by prioritizing geographical areas based on evidence.
4. Integrated monitoring and accountability through good governance, use of available data sets, community involvement, and steps to address grievance.
5. Broad-based collaboration and partnerships with ministries, departments, development partners, civil society, and other stakeholders.

Policy Decisions for Women's Health: Critics

It is very obvious that India's policy on maintaining women's health has centered towards maternal health and family planning. Rest of the physical dimensions of health is not focused and other dimensions are ignored by the policymakers, though National Health Policy, 2002 has mentioned the importance of social and cultural factors in the overall health status of women. Focus on other areas of women's health is needed in the policy on women's health.

IMPORTANT ACTS RELATED TO WOMEN

Medical Termination of Pregnancy Act, 1971[22-26] (Refer Chapters 1 and 2 for Details)

The MTP Act 1971 (Act 34 of 1971) provides provisions for medical termination of pregnancy. The Act was amended in 2002 and 2005. The Act along with MTP rules 2003 specify who, where, when and under what conditions a pregnancy can be terminated. The main features of the MTP Act are as follows:

1. Who can terminate a pregnancy?

A registered Medical Practitioner (RMP), who possesses any recognised medical qualification as defined in Section 2 (h) of the Indian Medical Council Act, 1956 can terminate a pregnancy if that registered medical practitioner fulfills any one of the following four criteria.

a. A RMP, who is registered in a State Medical Register before 1st April 1972 and having experience of not less than three years in the practice of gynaecology and obstetrics;

b. A medical practitioner, who is registered in a State Medical Register after 1st April 1972, and
   i. He has completed six months of house surgery in gynaecology and obstetrics; or
   ii. He has experience of not less than one year in any hospital (where required facilities for MTP are provided), in the practice of gynaecology and obstetrics

c. He has assisted a RMP in the performance of twenty-five cases of MTP, of which at least five have been performed independently, in a hospital established or maintained or a training institute approved for this purpose by the government. With this type training/experience, the RMP can perform only 1st trimester (up to 12 weeks) abortions, and he is not empowered to do 2nd trimester MTP.

d. Medical Practitioner registered in State Medical Register and holding postgraduate degree or diploma in obstetrics and gynaecology.

However, if MTP is being performed in early pregnancy up to 7 weeks and using RU-486 with Misoprostol, the same may be prescribed by a RMP, at his unapproved clinic, provided such a Registered Medical Practitioner has access to a place approved for MTP. For the purpose of access, the RMP should display a Certificate to this effect from the owner of the approved place.

2. Where MTP can be performed?

a. A hospital established or maintained by Government, or

b. A place approved for the purpose of this Act by Government or a District Level Committee constituted by that Government.

The application for approval of a hospital is to be sent to the chief medical officer or civil surgeon in Form A. CMO/civil surgeon can inspect the facilities and give recommendations to the District Level Committee, who after considering the same may grant the approval in Form B. The inspection should take place within 2 months of application and approval must be issued in next 2 months after inspection or rectification of deficiencies, if any. The certificate of approval in form B must be displayed by the owner for the display of the visitors.

As per the National Comprehensive Abortion Care Guidelines, pregnancy may be terminated at Government facilities up to:

a. Eight weeks of gestation at primary health centre (PHC);
b. 12 weeks of gestation at community health centre (CHC) or 24×7 PHC;
c. 20 weeks of gestation at district hospital and above facilities.

3. *Under which conditions MTP can be performed?*

The MTP Act specifies following conditions for termination of pregnancy

a. The continuance of the pregnancy would involve a risk to the life of the pregnant woman or of grave injury to her physical or mental health; or
b. There is a substantial risk that if the child were born, it would suffer from such physical or mental abnormalities as to be seriously handicapped.
c. Any pregnancy alleged by the pregnant woman as a result of rape (presumed to constitute a grave injury to the mental health of the pregnant woman)
d. Pregnancy due to failure of any contraceptive used by wife or husband for the purpose of limiting the number of children (presumed to constitute a grave injury to the mental health of the pregnant woman)

4. *At which gestational week MTP can be performed?*

When length of pregnancy is not more than 12 weeks—one RMP and when the length is more than 12 weeks up to 20 weeks—minimum two RMPs are of the opinion, formed in good faith, that the continuance of the pregnancy would involve a risk to the life of the pregnant woman or of grave injury to her physical or mental health or there is a substantial risk that if the child were born, it would suffer from such physical or mental abnormalities as to be seriously handicapped, then MTP can be performed. The opinion of the RMP/RMPs should be recorded in writing using Form I.

The provisions related to the length of the pregnancy and the opinion of not less than two registered medical practitioners in case of 2nd trimester pregnancy, shall not be applicable to the MTP performed by a RMP in a case where s/he is of opinion, formed in good faith, that the termination of such pregnancy is immediately necessary to save the life of the pregnant woman.

5. *What documentation needs to be kept by the approved institution?*

a. *Form I—Opinion form:* For each MTP done, opinion of form must be duly filled along with the reason of termination of pregnancy. The reason must be written at the specified place and it should never be left blank. The opinion form should be completed within three hours of termination of the pregnancy. Opinion of the second RMP in case of second trimester abortions must also be recorded either at the time of admission or within three hours of termination of pregnancy.

Obstetric conditions/complications like incomplete abortion, inevitable abortion, missed abortion, blighted ovum do not come under the purview of the MTP Act. The records/documentation for these conditions need not to be maintained as per the MTP Act provisions. However, the case records for these conditions must be kept for other legal/academic purposes, as per the existing provisions of general case records.

b. *Form II—Monthly reporting format:* A record of all MTPs done must be sent to CMO using this format. This should include all MTPs including both surgical and medical methods of abortions.

c. *Form III—14 Column Admission Register:* All MTPs conducted at the facility must be recorded in the (confidential) admission register maintained at the facility for each calendar year. The confidentiality of the register must be maintained and it should never be accessible to any unauthorized person, other than authorized by the act.

d. Form A—a copy of the application for approval can also be kept at the centre.

e. Form B—approval letter should be displayed for the public viewing.

f. Form C—consent form: For all MTPs, written consent of the pregnant woman must be recorded using Form C. If the pregnant woman is a mentally ill or minor, then consent of guardian is must. All duly filled and signed consent forms must be kept confidentially.

6. Can MTP be performed at unapproved place under special circumstances?

In case of an emergency, to save life of the pregnant woman, any pregnancy may be terminated by an RMP at an unapproved place. However, the detailed information of the same must be communicated to CMO/CS on the same day or latest by the next day.

7. Can MTP be performed after 20 weeks of gestation?

As per the provisions of the section 5(1) of the MTP Act, in a case where s/he is of opinion, formed in good faith, that the termination of such pregnancy is immediately necessary to save the life of the pregnant woman, the provisions related to the length of the pregnancy (up to 20 weeks) and the opinion of not less than two registered medical practitioners in case of 2nd trimester pregnancy, shall not be applicable to the MTP. MTP can be performed after 20 weeks to save life of the pregnant woman.

8. If a genetic abnormality is detected after 20 weeks of gestation, can a MTP be performed in such case

No. If there is no danger to the life of the pregnant woman, MTP cannot be performed after 20 weeks.

9. What are the proposed amendments in MTP Act (Amendment) 2018?

a. Replacing the twenty weeks criteria by twenty-four weeks and for rape survivors by twenty-seven weeks.

b. Provisions for central supervisory board
c. If in the majority opinion of the Central Supervisory Board, continuance of pregnancy may involve a substantial risk in case the child is born with the following abnormalities:
   i. Chromosomal abnormalities;
   ii. Genetic metabolic diseases;
   iii. Haemoglobinopathies;
   iv. Sex-linked genetic diseases;
   v. Congenital abnormalities; or
   vi. Another abnormalities or diseases as may be specified by the Central Supervisory Board.
   In such cases, the pregnancy, irrespective of the length of pregnancy, shall be terminated in accordance with the provisions of Section 4.
   (Please note that, above provisions are presently not in force, and shall be included only when the act is amended.)

The Surrogacy (Regulation) Bill, 2019[27] (Refer Chapter 25 for Details)

The Surrogacy (Regulation) Bill, 2019 was passed in August 2019 by Lok Sabha and yet to be passed by Rajya Sabha (as on October 2019), before it is converted into an act. The main features of the bill are detailed below.
1. The bill defines "surrogacy" as a practice whereby one woman bears and gives birth to a child for an intending couple with the intention of handing over such child to the intending couple after the birth.
2. It also defines "surrogacy clinic" as surrogacy clinic, centre or laboratory, conducting assisted reproductive technology services, *in vitro* fertilisation services, genetic counselling centre, genetic laboratory, Assisted Reproductive Technology Banks conducting surrogacy procedure or any clinical establishment, by whatsoever name called, conducting surrogacy procedures in any form.
3. Any surrogacy clinic should be registered with appropriate authority constituted under the proposed act. Only registered surrogacy centres can conduct or associate with, or help in any manner, in conducting activities relating to surrogacy and surrogacy procedures.
4. Surrogacy is allowed ONLY in infertile couples, for altruistic purpose, for any condition or disease specified through regulations. It is NOT permitted for commercial purpose, and for producing children for sale, prostitution or any other form of exploitation. Altruistic surrogacy means the surrogacy in which no charges, expenses, fees, remuneration or monetary incentive of whatever nature, except the medical expenses incurred on surrogate mother and the insurance coverage for the surrogate mother, are given to the surrogate mother or her dependents or her representative.
5. A woman acting as a surrogate mother should be:
   a. Holding a certificate of medical and psychological fitness for surrogacy and surrogacy procedures from a registered medical practitioner
   b. Possessing eligibility certificate issued by the appropriate authority.
   c. A married woman having a child of her own and between the age of 25 and 35 years on the day of implantation, and
   d. A close relative of the intending couple.

6. A woman acting as a surrogate mother should not be
   a. Donor of her own gametes,
   b. Acting as a surrogate mother for more than once in her lifetime, provided that the number of attempts for surrogacy procedures on the surrogate mother shall be such as may be prescribed (not yet prescribed).
7. Surrogacy or surrogacy procedures shall not be conducted, undertaken, performed or initiated, unless both, the Director or in-charge of the surrogacy clinic and the person qualified to do so, are satisfied about the fulfillment of the following conditions and the reasons for the same are recorded in writing.
   a. The intending couple is in possession of the essentiality certificate issued by the appropriate authority
   b. A certificate of proven infertility in favour of either or both members of the intending couple from a District Medical Board (a medical board under the Chairpersonship of Chief Medical Officer or Chief Civil Surgeon or Joint Director of Health Services of the district and comprising of at least two other specialists, namely, the chief gynaecologist or obstetrician and chief paediatrician of the district)
   c. An order concerning the parentage and custody of the child to be born through surrogacy, has been passed by a court of the Magistrate of the first class or above, on an application made by the intending couple and the surrogate mother;
   d. An insurance coverage of such amount as may be prescribed in favour of the surrogate mother for a period of sixteen months covering postpartum delivery complications from an insurance company or an agent recognised by the Insurance Regulatory and Development Authority established under the Insurance Regulatory and Development Authority Act, 1999;
8. A separate eligibility certificate for intending couple is required. Appropriate authority can issue the separate eligible certificate to the intending couple, on fulfillment of the following conditions,
   a. The age of the intending couple is between 23 and 50 years in case of female and between 26 and 55 years in case of male on the day of certification;
   b. The intending couple are married for at least five years and are Indian citizens;
   c. The intending couple does not have any surviving child biologically or through adoption or through surrogacy earlier, except couple who has a mentally or physically challenged child.
   d. Any such other conditions as may be specified by the regulations
9. The bill also specifies the offences for advertising commercial surrogacy, exploitation of the surrogate mother, disowning a surrogate child, and selling or importing human embryo or gametes for surrogacy. The penalty specified for such offences can be imprisonment up to 10 years and a fine up to 10 lakh rupees plus cancellation of registration.

After clearance by the Upper House and after the Presidential approval, the bill will be converted into an act. It will be interesting for all the stakeholders to follow the changes, if any, in the proposed bill, before it is converted into the act. The bill does not have any provisions for the centres providing services related to assisted reproduction without surrogacy procedures.

REFERENCES

1. Kohli S. Family Planning in India. Indian Institute of Public Administration, New Delhi 1977; p. 6.
2. Visaria, P. and V. Chari. "India's population policy and family planning programme: Yesterday, today and tomorrow," in Do Population Policies Matter? Fertility and Politics in Egypt, India, Kenya and Mexico, ed. A. Jain. New York: Population Council 1998;53–112.
3. Government of India. Ministry of Health and Family Planning. Department of Family Planning, New Delhi. Family Welfare Planning in India, Yearbook 1972–73; p.90.
4. Family Planning Programme in India- A Brief account. Government of India; Ministry of Health and Family Welfare; Department of Family Planning. New Delhi. 1976. P.9.
5. Government of India; Ministry of Women and Child Development, New Delhi (Internet) www.wcd.nic.in. Available from: http://www.wcd.nic.in/icds.htm . [Retrieved on 23/7/2014]
6. Government of India; Department of Health and Family Welfare, New Delhi. National Health Policy, 1983.
7. Indian Council of Medical Research. ICMR Bulletin 2004; 35:49–58.
8. Child Health Programmes in India. Government of India; Ministry of Health and Family Welfare, New Delhi. (Internet) http://mohfw.nic.in. Available from: http://mohfw.nic.in/WriteReadData/ l892s/ 6342515027file14.pdf. [Retrieved on 23/7/2014]
9. International Institute of Population Sciences (IIPS). 1995. National Family Health Survey (MCH and Family Planning), India 1992-93. Bombay : IIPS.
10. Planning Commission. Government of India. Evolution Of The Family Welfare Programme. (Internet) www. http://planningcommission.nic.in. Available on http://planningcommission.nic.in/ aboutus/ committee/strgrp/stgp_fmlywel/sgfw_ch3.pdf. Retrieved on 20/07/2014.
11. Child Programmes in India. Government of India. Ministry of Health and Family Welfare. Available on https://www.nhp.gov.in/reproductive-maternal-newborn-child-and-adolescent-health_pg. Retrieved on [27/10/2019]
12. International Institute of Population Sciences (IIPS). National Family Health Survey (NFHS-2)-Key Findings. 1998-99. Bombay: IIPS.
13. National Population Policy 2000. Government of India. Ministry of Health and Family Welfare (MOHFW). Available on http://india.unfpa.org/drive/NationalPopulation-Policy2000.pdf. [Retrieved on 22/7/2014.
14. National Health Policy 2002. Government of India. Ministry of Health and Family Welfare (MOHFW). Available on http://mohfw.nic.in/WriteReadData/l892s/18048892912105179110 National %20Health %20 policy-2002.pdf.[Retrieved on 23/7/2014]
15. International Institute for Population Sciences (IIPS) and Macro International. 2007. National Family Health Survey (NFHS-3), 2005-06: India: Volume I.
16. Annual Report 2005-06. Government of India. Ministry of Health and Family Welfare, New Delhi. (2006)
17. National Health Mission. Janani Suraksha Yojana-. Ministry of Health and Family Welfare, New Delhi. Available on https://nhm.gov.in/index1.php? lang=1&level=3&sublinkid=841&lid=309. [Retrieved on 25/10/2019]
18. National Rural Health mission. Guidelines for Janani-Shishu Suraksha Yojana (JSSY). Government of India. Ministry of Health and Family Welfare, New Delhi. Available on http://nrhm.gov.in/ images/ pdf/programmes/jssk/guidelines/guidelines_for_jssk.pdf. [Retrieved on 15/7/2014]
19. National Rural Health mission. Scheme for Promotion of Menstrual Hygiene among adolescent girls in rural India. Available on http://nrhm.gov.in/nrhm-components/rmnch-a/adolescent-health/ menstrual-hygiene-scheme-mhs/schemes.html. [Retrieved on 15/7/2014]
20. National Rural Health mission. Weekly Iron Folic acid supplementation.-Background. Available on http://nrhm.gov.in/nrhm-components/rmnch-a/adolescent-health/weekly-iron-folic-acid-supplementation-wifs/background.html. [Retrieved on 15/7/2014]

21. Government of India; Ministry of Women and Child Development, New Delhi. (Internet). Available from: http:// https://nhm.gov.in [Retrieved on 23/10/2019]
22. Central government Acts. The Medical Termination of Pregnancy Act, 1971. Available on https://indiankanoon.org/doc/634810/ [Retrieved on 23/10/2019]
23. Ministry of Health and Family Welfare. Government of India. 2015. Guidance for implementation of the MTP Act and the PC&PNDT Act. GUIDANCE: Ensuring Access to safe Abortion and Addressing Gender Biased Sex Selection.
24. Government of India; Ministry of Women and Child Development, New Delhi. (Internet). Available from https://mohfw.gov.in/acts-rules-and-standards-health-sector/acts/mtp-act-1971 [Retrieved on 23/10/2019]
25. Government of India; Ministry of Women and Child Development, New Delhi. (Internet). Available from https://mohfw.gov.in/acts-rules-and-standards-health-sector/acts/mtp-act-amendment-2002 [Retrieved on 23/10/2019]
26. Government of India; Ministry of Women and Child Development, New Delhi. (Internet). Available fromhttps://mohfw.gov.in/acts-rules-and-standards-health-sector/acts/mtp-rules [Retrieved on 23/10/2019]
27. The Surrogacy (Regulation) bill, 2019. Available on http://164.100.47.4/BillsTexts/LSBillTexts/PassedLoksabha/156-C_2019_LS_Eng.pdf. Retrieved on [25/10/2019]

Chapter 31

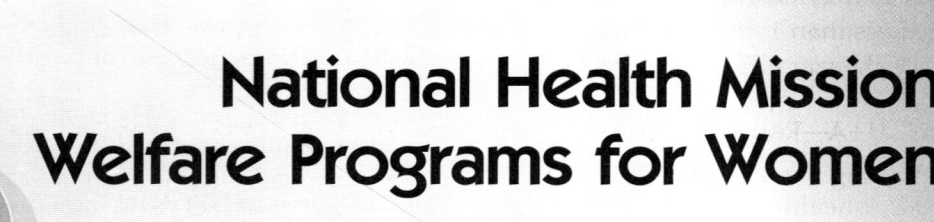

National Health Mission Welfare Programs for Women

○ Suchitra Pandit ○ Rakhee Sahu

The National Health Mission (NHM) encompasses its two sub-missions, the National Rural Health Mission (NRHM) and the National Urban Health Mission (NUHM). The main programmatic components include Health System Strengthening, Reproductive, Maternal, Neonatal, Child, and Adolescent Health (RMNCH+A), and communicable and non-communicable diseases.

NHM Framework for Implementation

Continuation of the National Health Mission, with effect from 1st April 2017 to 31st March 2020, has been approved by Cabinet in its meeting dated 21.03.2018.

GOALS

Outcomes for NHM in the 12th Plan are synonymous with those of the 12th Plan, and are part of the overall vision. Specific goals for the states will be based on existing levels, capacity and context. State-specific innovations would be encouraged. Process and outcome indicators will be developed to reflect equity, quality, efficiency and responsiveness. Targets for communicable and non-communicable disease will be set at state-level based on local epidemiological patterns and taking into account the financing available for each of these conditions.

The endeavor would be to ensure achievement of those indicators are as below:
1. Reduce MMR to 1/1000 live births
2. Reduce IMR to 25/1000 live births
3. Reduce TFR to 2.1
4. Prevention and reduction of anemia in women aged 15–49 years

5. Prevent and reduce mortality and morbidity from communicable, non-communicable injuries and emerging diseases
6. Reduce household out-of-pocket expenditure on total healthcare expenditure
7. Reduce annual incidence and mortality from Tuberculosis by half
8. Reduce prevalence of leprosy to <1/10000 population and incidence to zero in all districts
9. Annual malaria incidence to be <1/1000
10. Less than 1 per cent microfilaria prevalence in all districts
11. Kala-azar elimination by 2015, <1 case per 10000 population in all blocks

RMNCH+A—Reproductive, Maternal, Newborn, Child and Adolescent Health

Improving the maternal and child health and their survival are central to the achievement of national health goals under the National Health Mission (NHM). SDG Goal 3 also includes the focus on reducing maternal, newborn and child mortality. Following the Government of India's "Call to Action (CAT) Summit" in February, 2013, the Ministry of Health and Family Welfare launched Reproductive, Maternal, Newborn, Child plus Adolescent Health (RMNCH+A) to influence the key interventions for reducing maternal and child morbidity and mortality.

The RMNCH+A strategy is built upon the continuum of care concept and is holistic in design, encompassing all interventions aimed at reproductive, maternal, newborn, child and adolescent health under a broad umbrella, and focusing on the strategic lifecycle approach.

The RMNCH+A strategy promotes links between various interventions across thematic areas to enhance coverage throughout the lifecycle to improve child survival in India. The "plus" within the strategy focuses on:
- Inclusion of adolescence as a distinct life stage within the overall strategy.
- Linking maternal and child health to reproductive health and other components like family planning, adolescent health, HIV, gender, and preconception and prenatal diagnostic techniques.
- Linking home and community-based services to facility-based services.
- Ensuring linkages, referrals, and counter-referrals between and among various levels of healthcare system to create a continuous care pathway, and to bring an additive/synergistic effect in terms of overall outcomes and impact.

Key Features of RMNCH+A Strategy

The RMNCH+A strategy approaches include:
- Health systems strengthening (HSS) focusing on infrastructure, human resources, supply chain management, and referral transport measures.
- Prioritization of high-impact interventions for various lifecycle stages.
- Increasing effectiveness of investments by prioritizing geographical areas based on evidence.
- Integrated monitoring and accountability through good governance, use of available data sets, community involvement, and steps to address grievance.
- Broad-based collaboration and partnerships with ministries, departments, development partners, civil society, and other stakeholders.

The RMNCH+A strategy provides a strong platform for delivery of services across the entire continuum of care, ranging from community to various level of healthcare system.

Current Status of key RMNCH+A/RCH Indicators

Indicator	Current status	National Health Policy Target	SDG 2030 Target
Maternal Mortality Ratio (SRS 2014–2016)	130	100 by 2020	<70
Neonatal Mortality rate*	23	16 by 2025	<12
Infant Mortality Rate*	33	28 by 2019	—
Under 5 Mortality Rate*	37	23 by 2025	≤25
Total Fertility Rate*	2.2	Replacement level fertility	—

*SRS 2017

ADOLESCENT HEALTH

There are 253 million adolescents in the age group 10–19 years in India. This age group comprises individuals in a transient phase of life requiring nutrition, education, counseling and guidance to ensure their development into healthy adults. They are susceptible to several preventable and treatable health problems, like early and unintended pregnancy, unsafe sex leading to STI/HIV/AIDS, nutritional disorders like malnutrition, anemia and overweight, alcohol, tobacco and drug abuse, mental health concerns, injuries and violence.

Government of India has recognized the importance of influencing health-seeking behavior of adolescents. The health situation of this age group is a key determinant of India's overall health, mortality, morbidity and population growth scenario. Therefore, investments in adolescent reproductive and sexual health will yield dividends in terms of delaying age at marriage, reducing incidence of teenage pregnancy, meeting unmet contraception need, reducing the maternal mortality, reducing STI incidence and reducing HIV prevalence. It will also help India realize its demographic dividends, as healthy adolescents are an important resource for the economy.

Rashtriya Kishor Swasthya Karyakram (RKSK)

In order to ensure holistic development of adolescent population, the Ministry of Health and Family Welfare launched Rashtriya Kishor Swasthya Karyakram (RKSK) on 7th January 2014 to reach out to 253 million adolescents—male and female, rural and urban, married and unmarried, in and out-of-school adolescents with special focus on marginalized and undeserved groups. The programme expands the scope of adolescent health programming in India—from being limited to sexual and reproductive health, it now includes in its ambit nutrition, injuries and violence (including gender-based violence), non-communicable-diseases, mental health and substance misuse. Key drivers of the program are community-based interventions like outreach by counselors; facility-based counselling; social and behavior change communication; and strengthening of Adolescent Friendly Health Clinics across levels of care.

MATERNAL HEALTH

Government of India adopted the Reproductive, Maternal, Newborn, Child and Adolescent Health (RMNCH+A) framework in 2013. It essentially aims to address the major causes of mortality and morbidity among women and children. This framework also helps to understand the delays in accessing and utilizing healthcare services.

MMR: India's MMR at 130 (SRS 2014-16) has improved significantly from 167 (SRS 2011–13)						
Goal indicator	All India status (Source of data)					NHM Goal (2017)
Maternal Mortality Ratio (MMR)	254 (SRS 2004–06)	212 (SRS 2007–09)	178 (SRS 2010–12)	167 (SRS 2011–13)	130 (SRS 2014–16)	100

According to the latest figure released by Registrar General of India—Sample Registration System (RGI-SRS) Maternal Mortality Ratio (MMR) for the period 2014–16 is 130 maternal deaths per 100,000 live births. With this, India has achieved the Millennium Development Goal (MDG) 5, i.e. India has achieved a reduction in MMR by three quarters between 1990 and 2015. The target was to achieve 139 maternal deaths per 100,000 live births. The table displays the trend in MMR over the years. The average decline in MMR between 2007–09 and 2011–13 had been 11.3 points per year, i.e. compound rate of annual decline was 5.8%, whereas average compound rate of decline is 8% between 2011–13 and 2014–16.

Maternal Health Indicators (NFHS3, NFHS4)

S. no.	Indicator	NFHS 3	NFHS 4
1	Mothers who had antenatal check-up in the first trimester (%)	43.9	58.6
2	Mothers who had at least 4 antenatal care visits (%)	37.0	51.2
3	Mothers who had full antenatal care (%)	11.6	21
4	Mothers who received postnatal care from a doctor/nurse/LHV/ANM/midwife/other health personnel within 2 days of delivery (%)	34.6	62.4
5	Institutional births (%)	38.7	78.9

AREAS OF WORK

Quality Service Provision

Quality antenatal care: Quality and comprehensive ANC incorporates minimum of at least four ANCs including early registration and first ANC in first trimester. The ANC package includes physical and abdominal examinations, Hb estimation, screening for gestational diabetes mellitus, thyroid disorders, HIV/syphilis and urine investigation, TT/Td, immunization, distribution of IFA tablets and calcium (6 months during antenatal period and 6 months during postnatal period) and counselling for nutrition, etc. Early detection of high-risk pregnancies, follow-up and management are important component of antenatal care.

Essential obstetric care during delivery: Government of India provide free institutional delivery at its network of health facilities including sub-centre, primary health centres, community health centres, sub-district hospital, districts hospital, etc. to reduce maternal and neonatal morbidity and mortality. In order to provide essential obstetric care services, Government of India is operationalizing the 24 × 7 PHCs services and providing training to SNs/LHVs/ANMs under skilled attendance at birth.

Postnatal care for mother and newborn: Ensuring postnatal care within first 24 hours of delivery and subsequent home visits on 3rd, 7th, 14th and 42nd day is the important components for identification and management of emergencies occurring during postnatal period. The ANMs, LHVs, and staff nurses are being oriented and trained for tackling emergencies identified during these visits.

Provision of emergency obstetric and neonatal care at FRUs: Provision of emergency obstetric and neonatal care at FRUs is been done by operationalizing all FRUs in the country. While operationalizing, the thrust is on the critical components such as manpower, blood storage units and referral linkages, etc. Availability of trained manpower (Skill Based Training for healthcare providers) is linked with operationalization of FRUs. The initiatives being undertaken in this regard are:

Augmentation of skilled human resources for maternal health:
- To overcome the shortage of skilled manpower particularly Anaesthetists and Gynaecologists, the following key skill-based training programs are being implemented.
- 18 Weeks Training Programme of MBBS Doctors in Life Saving Anaesthesia Skills (LSAS) for Emergency Obstetric Care.
- 16 weeks Training programme of MBBS Doctors in Obstetric Management Skills including C-Section, in collaboration with Federation of Obstetric and Gynaecological Society of India.
- 10 days Training Programme in Basic Emergency Obstetric Care for Medical Officers (BEmOC)
- 3 weeks Training Programme for ANMs/SNs/LHVs as Skilled Birth Attendants (SBA) Referral
- Skills Labs (Daksh training): For improving the skills of healthcare providers and to enhance their capacity for providing quality RMNCH +A services, Government of India established National and State Skills Lab.

Referral Services at both Community and Institutional Level

Government of India has a thrust to establish a network for basic patient care transportation through ambulances with an aim to reach to the beneficiary in rural area for quick service delivery.

Technical Guidelines and Service Delivery Guidelines

Training

Capacity building programme for various categories of health, works through various training programme is as follows:

Skilled attendance at birth: Government of India has a commitment to provide skilled attendance at every birth both at community and institution levels. To manage and handle some common obstetric emergencies at the time of birth, staff nurses (SNs) and ANMs have been permitted to give certain injections and also perform certain interventions under specific emergency situations to save the life of the mother.

Dakshata: Maternal mortality and morbidity and perinatal mortality are major public health problems. Majority have an intrapartum origin and are a consequence of interventions carried out around the time of delivery. In light of this, the Government of India, in 2015, developed 'Dakshata' for rapidly improving the quality of care during intrapartum and immediate postpartum period across delivery points in the country. Currently, Dakshata is being implemented in more than 1500 facilities in seven states of the country.

The package provides the complete set of resources to assist the states in planning and implementing the Dakshata programmes. For the realization of this, operational guidelines, learning resource package, assessment tools, planning and budgeting tools are included in the package.

STRATEGIES AND INTERVENTIONS

Flagship Programmes

Janani Suraksha Yojana (JSY): Janani Suraksha Yojana (JSY), a demand promotion and conditional cash transfer scheme, was launched in April 2005 with the objective of reducing maternal and infant mortality. It is being implemented with the objective of reducing maternal and neonatal mortality by promoting institutional delivery among poor pregnant women.

Janani Shishu Suraksha Karyakram (JSSK): Government of India has launched JSSK on 1st June, 2011, which entitles all pregnant women delivering in public health institutions to absolutely free and no expense delivery including cesarean section. The initiative stipulates free drugs, diagnostics, blood and diet, besides free transport from home to institution, between facilities in case of a referral and drop back home. Similar entitlements have been put in place for all sick newborn accessing public health institutions for treatment till 30 days after birth. In 2013, this has been expanded to sick infants and antenatal and postnatal complications.

Pradhanmantri Surakshit Matritva Abhiyan (PMSMA): Carrying forward the vision of our Hon'ble Prime Minister, the PMSMA was launched in 2016 to ensure quality antenatal care and high risk pregnancy detection in pregnant women on 9th of every month.

LaQshya: In order to further accelerate decline in MMR in the coming years, MoFHW has recently launched 'LaQshya—labour room quality improvement initiative. LaQshya program is a focused and targeted approach to strengthen key processes related to the labor rooms and maternity operation theatres which aim at improving quality of care around birth and ensuring respectful maternity care.

Comprehensive abortion care services: Comprehensive and safe abortion services are provided at public health facilities including 24 × 7 PHCs/FRUs (DHs/SDHs/CHCs) including the delivery points. Supply of Nischay Pregnancy detection kits to sub centres for early detection of pregnancy is undertaken.

Provision of RTI/STI services: Under NHM, provision of STI/RTI care services is an important strategy to prevent HIV transmission and to promote sexual and reproductive health services in all the FRUs, CHCs and at 24 × 7 PHCs.

Village health and nutrition day: Village health and nutrition day (VHND) are being organized at Anganwadi center at least once every month. It is a platform to provide antenatal/post-partum care for pregnant women, promote institutional delivery, immunization, family planning and nutritional counseling.

Newer interventions: Midwifery: Government of India has initiated midwifery services throughout the country in 2018, with an objective to provide access to quality maternal and neonatal health services, to promote natural birthing, to ensure respectful care and to reduce over medicalization. The midwifery services initiatives aim to create a cadre for Nurse Practitioners in Midwifery who are skilled in accordance to ICM competencies, knowledge and capable of providing compassionate women-centric pregnancy care.

Information Systems for Maternal Health

Maternal death surveillance and response (MDSR): The process of maternal death review (MDSR) has been implemented and institutionalized by all the states since 2017. Guidelines and tools for conducting community-based MDSR and facility-based MDSR have been provided to the states. The states are reporting deaths along with its analysis for causes of death. Maternal near-miss review is also being conducted at premier institutions.

RCH portal/MCTS portal: Name-based tracking of pregnant women and children has been initiated by Government of India as a policy decision to track every pregnant woman, infant and child up to 5 years of age by name for provision of timely ANC, institutional delivery, and PNC along with immunization and other related services.

MCP card: Ministry of Health and Family Welfare and Ministry of Women and Child Development (MOWCD) has been launched as a tool for documenting and monitoring services for antenatal, intranatal and postnatal care to pregnant women, immunization and growth monitoring of infants.

JANANI SHISHU SURAKSHA KARYAKRAM

The New Initiative of Ministry of Health and Family Welfare

Institutional deliveries in India increased substantially after launched of Janani Suraksha Yojana (JSY). However, 25% women still hesitate to access health facilities for delivery due to out-of-pocket expenditure during stay at health facilities on drugs, diet, and diagnosis and arrangement blood, etc.

Building on the progress of this safe motherhood scheme. In 2014, the programme was extended to all antenatal and postnatal complications of pregnancy and similar entitlements have been put in place for all sick newborns and infants (up to one year of age) accessing public health institutions for treatment.

Entitlements

- JSSK launched on 1st June, 2011 entitles all pregnant women delivering in public health institutions to absolutely free and no expense delivery, including cesarean section.
- The initiative entitles all pregnant women delivering in public health institutions to absolutely free and no expense delivery, including cesarean section. The entitlements include free drugs and consumables, free diagnostics, free blood wherever required, and free diet for 3 days during normal delivery and 7 days for C-section. This initiative also provides for free transport from home to institution, between facilities in case of a referral and drop back home.

JANANI SURAKSHA YOJANA

The Yojana has identified Accredited Social Health Activist (ASHA) as an effective link between the government and pregnant women.

Important Features of JSY

The scheme focuses on poor pregnant woman with a special dispensation for states that have low institutional delivery rates, namely the states of Uttar Pradesh, Uttarakhand, Bihar, Jharkhand, Madhya Pradesh, Chhattisgarh, Assam, Rajasthan, Orissa, and Jammu and Kashmir. While these states have been named Low Performing States (LPS), the remaining states have been named High Performing states (HPS).

Eligibility for Cash Assistance

The eligibility for cash assistance under the JSY is as shown below:

LPS	All pregnant women delivering in government health centres, such as subcenters (SCs)/primary health centers (PHCs)/community health centers (CHCs)/first referral units (FRUs)/general wards of district or state hospitals
HPS	All BPL/scheduled caste/scheduled tribe (SC/ST) women delivering in a government health centre, such as SC/PHC/CHC/FRU/general wards of district or state hospital
LPS and HPS	BPL/SC/ST women in accredited private institutions

Cash Assistance for Institutional Delivery (in Rs)

The cash entitlement for different categories of mothers is as follows:

Category	Rural area Mother's package	ASHA's package*	Total	Urban area Mother's package	ASHA's package**	Total (Amount in Rs.)
LPS	1400	600	2000	1000	400	1400
HPS	700	600	1300	600	400	1000

*ASHA package of ₹600 in rural areas includes ₹300 for ANC component and Rs. 300 for facilitating institutional delivery.
**ASHA package of ₹400 in urban areas includes ₹200 for ANC component and Rs. 200 for facilitating institutional delivery.

DAKSHATA

Empowering providers for improved MNH care during institutional deliveries April 2015.

A strategic initiative to strengthen quality of intrapartum and immediate postpartum care.

Goal of the initiative: To improve the quality of maternal and newborn care during the intra- and immediate postpartum period, through providers who are competent and confident (Dakshata).

Objectives

The major objectives of the initiative are:

Objective 1: To strengthen the competency of providers of the labour room, including medical officers, staff nurses, and ANMs to perform evidence-based practices as per the established labour room protocols and standards.

Objective 2: To implement enabling strategies to ensure transfer of learning towards improved adherence to evidence-based clinical practices.

Objective 3: To improve the availability of essential supplies and commodities in the labour room and the postpartum wards.

Objective 4: To improve accountability of service providers through improved recording, reporting and utilization of data.

Objective 5: (intermediate term objective): Implementation of the MNH tool kit at the delivery points, in a phased manner.

Key Activities under Dakshata

- Sensitization workshop for district and facility level officials on Dakshata program
- Identification and mapping of target facilities with resource availability
- Hiring of quality improvement mentor
- Rapid assessment of resource availability and practices status
- Ensuring availability of essential supplies and other resources
- Preparation of training micro-plan for each facility
- 3 days on-site training of labour room staff at district hospitals
- Post-training follow-up and support to district hospital
- 3 days training of staff from subdistrict level facilities at DH
- Post-training follow-up and support to SDL facilities by trainers and mentors
- Implementation of data recording tools and dashboard indicators

PRADHAN MANTRI SURAKSHIT MATRITVA ABHIYAN

Objective

PMSMA was launched to provide fixed-day assured, comprehensive and quality antenatal care universally to all pregnant women (in 2nd and 3rd trimester) on the 9th of every month.

Introduction

- While antenatal care is routinely provided to pregnant women, special ANC services are provided by OBGY specialists/radiologist/physicians at government health facilities under PMSMA.
- As part of the campaign, a minimum package of antenatal care services are provided to pregnant women in their 2nd/3rd trimesters at Government health facilities (PHCs/CHCs, DHs/urban health facilities, etc.) in both urban and rural areas.
- Using the principles of a single window system, it is envisaged that a minimum package of investigations and medicines such as IFA and calcium supplements, etc. would be provided to all pregnant women attending the PMSMA clinics.
- One of the critical components of the Abhiyan is identification and follow-up of high risk pregnancies and red stickers are added on to the mother and child protection cards of women with high risk pregnancies.

Engagement with Private/Voluntary Sector

- Hon'ble Prime Minister of India highlighted the aim and purpose of introduction of the Pradhan Mantri Surakshit Matritva Abhiyan in the July 31, 2016 episode of Mann Ki Baat and asked doctors to dedicate 12 days in a year to this initiative.
- A National Portal for PMSMA and a mobile application have been developed to facilitate the engagement of doctors from private/voluntary sector.
- OBGY specialists/Radiologist/Physicians working in the private sector are encouraged to volunteer for the campaign and can register for the campaign through any of the following mechanisms:
- Toll Free Number—Doctors can call 18001801104 to register
- SMS—Doctors can SMS 'PMSMA <Name> to 5616115
- PMSMA Portal—Register atpmsma.nhp.gov.in
- Register using the 'Volunteer Registration' Section of the Mobile Application

PMSMA 'Nearest Facility' Search

As a step towards Hon'ble Prime Minister's dream of 'Digital India', a mobile/web-based application has been designed to help pregnant women find their nearest PMSMA facility. In order to access this service, pregnant women can visit https://pmsma.nhp.gov.in/or download the 'PMSMA' mobile application.

PMSMA 'I Pledge for 9' Achievers Awards

- PMSMA 'I Pledge for 9'Achievers Awards have been devised to celebrate individual and team achievements, identify and recognize excellence in performance in PMSMA at various levels and focus on awarding government teams and private sector doctors who have volunteered for the programme.
- The National PMSMA 'I Pledge for 9' Achievers Awards ceremony was held in June 2018. Contributions of states/UTs were recognized through a physical award ceremony as well

as through a virtual a 'Hall of Fame' for wide public and social recognition of their contributions. (https://pmsma.nhp.gov.in/hall-of-fame-2/).
For further information please visit: www.pmsma.nhp.gov.in

LABOUR ROOM AND QUALITY IMPROVEMENT INITIATIVE

Overview of LaQshya

Ministry of Health and Family Welfare, Government of India, launched an ambitious program LaQshya on 11th December 2017.

Following facilities are being taken under LaQshya initiative on priority:
- All government medical college hospitals.
- All district hospitals and equivalent health facilities.
- All designated FRUs and high case load CHCs with over 100 deliveries/60 (per month) in hills and desert areas.

Key Features

- LaQshya program envisages to improve quality of care in labour room and maternity OT.
- Under the initiative, multi-pronged strategy has been adopted such as improving infrastructure upgradation, ensuring availability of essential equipment, providing adequate human resources, capacity building of healthcare workers and improving quality processes in labour room.
- Implementation of 'fast-track' interventions (NQAS assessment, trainings, mentoring, reviews, etc.)
- Capacity-building of healthcare workers by skill-based training like Dakshta and improving quality processes in the labour room.
- To strengthen critical care in Obstetrics, dedicated obstetric ICUs at medical college hospital level and obstetric HDUs at district hospital are operationalized under LaQshya program.

Strategies

- Reorganizing/aligning labour room and maternity operation theatre layout as per standard guidelines issued by the Ministry of Health and Family Welfare, Government of India.
- Ensuring all government medical college hospitals, district hospitals have dedicated obstetric HDUs and obstetric ICU as per GoI MOHFW Guidelines, for managing complicated pregnancies that require life-saving critical care.
- Ensuring strict adherence to clinical protocols for management and stabilization of the complications before referral to higher centers.
- Continued mentoring and hand holding support to improvise skills.
- Regular MDSR, C-section audit and referral audits and linkage among lower level facilities.
- Collating best quality practices across states which can be replicated by other states.

Quality Improvement Cycles

- 6 focused quality improvement cycles (Documentation, RMC, timely management of complications in pregnancy, judicious use of oxytocin, essential and emergency newborn care, infection prevention and biomedical waste management) each for two months.
- First month for improvement followed by second month for sustaining improvement.
- Improvement using PDCA approach and quality tools.
- Each cycle supported by onsite coaching team visits.
- Support resource package for each cycle.
- Onsite training and monitoring by coaches.
- Documentation of improvement activities.

Digital Innovation

- LaQshya web portal—all LaQshya related data will be uploaded on the portal for prompt report generation as well as visualization of dashboard to monitor progress in key maternal newborn indicators at various levels (facility, district, state and national)
- Safe delivery App—job aid as well as training tool for health workers.

Certification, Incentives and Branding

- Quality improvement in labour room and maternity OT will be assessed through NQAS (National Quality Assurance Standards). Every facility achieving 70% score on NQAS will be certified as LaQshya certified facility.
- Furthermore, branding of LaQshya certified facilities will be done as per the NQAS score. Facilities scoring more than 90%, 80% and 70% will be given Platinum, Gold and Silver badge accordingly.
- Facilities achieving NQAS certification, defined quality indicators and 80% satisfied beneficiaries will be provided incentive of Rs. 6 lakhs, Rs. 3 lakhs and Rs. 2 lakhs for Medical College Hospital, District Hospital and FRUs respectively.

Way Forward

- New innovations for escalating quality of healthcare services for mothers and newborn.
- Increased satisfaction of beneficiaries and positive birthing experience.
- Increased demand of services from beneficiaries of public health facilities.
- LaQshya certification of all health facilities.
- Sustained efforts to achieve SDG targets and goals related to maternal newborn health.
- Maintain and accelerate unprecedented progress—end all preventable maternal, newborn and child deaths.

FAMILY PLANNING

Factors that influence population growth. *Factors influencing population growth can be grouped into the following 3 categories:*

Unmet need of family planning: This includes the currently married women, who wish to stop child bearing or wait for next two or more years for the next childbirth, but not using any contraceptive method. Total unmet need of Family Planning is 12.9 (NFHS-IV) in our country.

Age at Marriage and first childbirth: In India 26.8% (NFHS-IV) of the girls get married below the age of 18 years and out of the total deliveries 6.1% are among teenagers, i.e. 15–19 years. The situation regarding age of girls at marriage is more alarming in few states like, Bihar (39.1%), Rajasthan (35.4%), Jharkhand (38%), UP (21.2%), and MP (30%). Delaying the age at marriage and first child birth could reduce the impact of Population Momentum on population growth.

Spacing between births: Healthy spacing of 3 years improves the chances of survival of infants and also helps in reducing the impact of population momentum on population growth. SRS 2016 data shows that in India, spacing between two childbirths is less than the recommended period of 3 years in 48.1% of births.

Some Positives
Total fertility rate (TFR)
Total fertility rate (TFR) in the country has recorded a steady decline to the current levels of 2.2 (SRS 2017)

2005	2006	2007	2008	2009	2010	2011	2012	2013	2014	2015	2016	2017
2.9	2.8	2.7	2.6	2.6	2.5	2.4	2.4	2.3	2.3	2.3	2.3	2.2

Survey Data (NFHS)
Nationwide, the small family norm is widely accepted (the wanted fertility rate for India as a whole is 1.9: NFHS-3) and the general awareness of contraception is almost universal (98% among women and 98.6% among men: NFHS-3).

As per NFHS-4 TFR for India is 2.2. The NFHS-4 survey shows 53.5% use of contraceptives among married women (aged 15–49 years) and prevalence of modern method 47.8%. Strategies under family planning programme in the country:

Policy level	*Service level*
Target free approach	More emphasis on spacing methods
Voluntary adoption of family planning methods	Assuring quality of services
Based on felt need of the community	Expanding contraceptive choices
Children by choice and not chance	

Current Family Planning Programme under Public Sector
The public sector provides the following contraceptive methods at various levels of health system:

National Health Mission Welfare Programs for Women

Spacing methods	Limiting methods
IUCD 380 A and Cu IUCD 375	**Female sterilization:**
Injectable Contraceptive MPA (Antara Programme)	Laparoscopic
Combined Oral Contraceptive (Mala-N)	Minilap
Centchroman (Chhaya)	**Male sterilization:**
Progesterone-Only Pill (POP)	No scalpel vasectomy
Condoms (Nirodh)	Conventional vasectomy
Emergency contraception	
Emergency Contraceptive pills (Ezy pills)	

Above services are provided at various levels of public sector facilities; following table provides details of the same:

Family planning method	Service provider	Service location
Spacing Methods		
IUCD 380 A, IUCD 375	Trained and certified ANMs, LHVs, SNs and doctors	Subcentre and higher levels
Injectable contraceptive MPA (Antara Programme)	Trained ANMs, SNs and doctors	Subcentre and higher levels
Oral contraceptive pills (OCPs)	Trained ASHAs, ANMs, LHVs, SNs and doctors	Village level subcentre and higher levels
Condoms	Trained ASHAs, ANMs, LHVs, SNs and doctors	Village level subcentre and higher levels
Emergency Contraception		
Emergency contraceptive Pills (ECPs)	Trained ASHAs, ANMs, LHVs, SNs and doctors	Village level subcentre and higher levels
Limiting Methods		
Minilap	Trained and certified MBBS doctors and specialist doctors	PHC and higher levels
Laparoscopic sterilization	Trained and certified MBBS doctors and specialist doctors	Usually CHC and higher levels
NSV: No scalpel vasectomy	Trained and certified MBBS doctors and specialist doctors	PHC and higher levels

Note: Contraceptives like OCPs, condoms are also provided through Social Marketing Organizations.
National Health Mission (NHM)
Ministry of Health and Family Welfare
Key people: Dr. Anbumani Ramadoss
Launched—April 2005
Edited—24th September 2019

Chapter 32

Janani Suraksha Yojana (JSY)

○ Balaji Jadhav ○ Shweta Khade

INTRODUCTION

Janani Suraksha Yojana (JSY) under the overall umbrella of National Rural Health Mission (NRHM) is being proposed by way of modifying the existing National Maternity Benefit Scheme (NMBS). The Yojana, launched on 12th April 2005, by the Hon'ble Prime Minister, is being implemented in all states and UTs with special focus on low performing states. JSY integrates the financial assistance with antenatal care during the pregnancy period, institutional care during delivery and immediate postpartum period in a health centre by establishing a system of coordinated care by field level health worker called ASHA (Accredited Social Health Activist). The JSY would be a 100% centrally sponsored scheme. The success of the scheme would be determined by the increase in institutional delivery among the poor families.

In India, 301 maternal deaths per 100,000 live births during 2001–03 have reduced to 167 during 2011–13. Infant Mortality Rate (IMR) has declined from 58 deaths per 1000 live births in 2005 to 37 in 2015 (SRS Bulletin 2015). In 2005–06, only 39 per cent of Indian women delivered in a health facility. JSY helped raise institutional delivery to 74 per cent in the first eight years since its implementation. (Sidney et al., 2017).

Vision
- To reduce overall maternal mortality ratio and infant mortality rate
- To increase institutional deliveries in BPL families.

Target Group
All pregnant women belonging to the below poverty line (BPL) households and
- Age of 19 years or above
- Up to two live births.

Strategy

It is to link the financial assistance under JSY to institutional delivery.

This would, however, entail carrying out following:
- Early registration of the beneficiaries with the help of ASHA
- Early identification of complicated cases;
- Providing at least three antenatal care, and post-delivery visits;
- Organizing appropriate referral and provide referral transport
- Convergence with Integrated Child Development Services (ICDS) worker
- Ensuring transparent and timely disbursement of the financial assistance to the mother and the incentive to ASHA

The strategy also involves the following:
- Operationalization of 24/7 delivery services at PHC and first referral units (FRUs) to provide the obstetric care,
- Accreditation of private sector specially in the rural areas to provide obstetric services to the JSY beneficiaries.

IMPORTANT FEATURES OF JSY

1. Tracking Each Pregnancy

Each beneficiary registered should have a JSY card along with a MCH card (Figs 32.1 and 32.2). **ASHA/AWW/any other identified link worker** under the overall supervision of the ANM and the MO PHC should mandatorily prepare a **micro-birth plan.** This will effectively help in monitor in antenatal check-up, and the post-delivery care.

Role of Registered Accredited Worker/ASHA

- Identify pregnant woman from BPL families as a beneficiary of the scheme,
- Report to the ANM and bring the women to registration,
- Assist to obtain BPL certification if BPL card is not available,
- Provide and/or help the women to receive at least three ANC visits,
- Counsel for institutional delivery and fix before 7th month of pregnancy the place of delivery
- Assist in receiving two tetanus toxoid injection, supplement iron folic acid tablets
- When the pregnant woman is in labour or faces complication, escort the women to the pre-determined health centre and stay with her till the delivery is complete and woman is discharged,
- Arrange to immunize the newborn till the age of 10 weeks,
- Register birth or death of the child or mother,
- Post-natal visits within 7 days of pregnancy and track mother's health,
- Counsel for initiation of breastfeeding within one-hour of delivery and its continuance till 3–6 months.

Fig. 32.1: JSY card

2. Eligibility for Financial Assistance (Table 32.1)

Table 32.1

Low performing states (LPS): Total 10, namely 8 Empowered Action Group (EAG) states (Uttar Pradesh, Uttaranchal, Madhya Pradesh, Chhattisgarh, Rajasthan, Bihar, Jharkhand and Orissa) and the states of Assam and J&K even after the third live birth	**All pregnant women** delivering in Government health centers like sub-centre, PHC, community health Centre (CHC)/first referral unit (FRU)/General wards of sub-divisional, district and state hospital
High performing states (HPS)	BPL/Scheduled caste (SC)/scheduled tribe (ST) women delivering in govt. health centre: PHC/CHC/FRU/General wards of district/state hospital
LPS and HPS	All BPL/SC/ST delivering in accredited private institutions

3. Cash assistance at Institutional Delivery (Table 32.2)

Table 32.2

Category	Rural area		Total	Urban area		Total
	Mother package	ASHA package	₹	Mother package	ASHA package	₹
LPS	1400	600	2000	1000	400	1400
HPS	700	600	1300	600	400	1000

ASHA package:
In rural area is ₹600, divided in 2 components (ANC and institutional delivery) ₹300 each.
In urban area is ₹400, divided in 2 components (ANC and institutional delivery) ₹200 each.

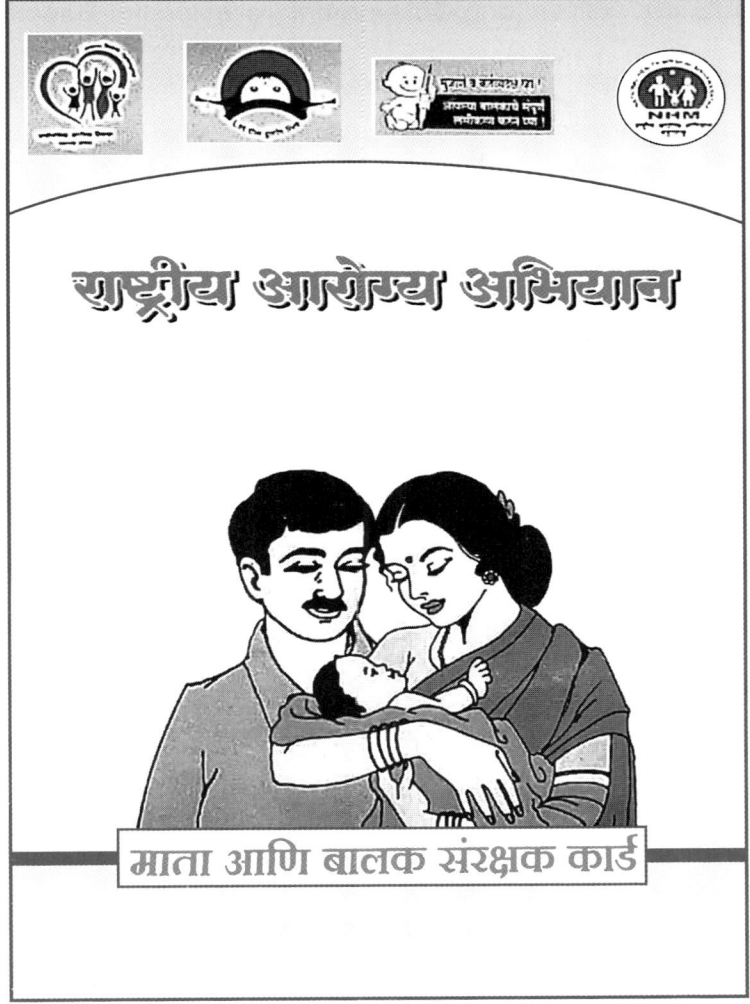

Fig. 32.2: MCH Card

4. **Disbursement of Financial assistance to Beneficiary for Institutional Delivery**
a. It should be disbursed *effectively at the institution itself.*
b. In order to streamline payment separate bank account has to be opened to manage the JSY funds in the nearest nationalized bank for JSY under the concerned Rogi Kalyan Samiti.
c. At the time of institutional delivery payment of Rs. 1000/- and above financial assistance is given which would be jointly approved by the Medical Officer and a paramedic staff like Staff Nurse or Health Worker (female), preferably the senior most in the hospital.

5. Financial Assistance: Delivery at a Government Institution (for Rural Beneficiaries)
(Table 32.3)

Table 32.3

	Delivery place	Payment made by
A	Sub-Centre, PHC	Auxiliary Nurse Midwife (ANM)/ASHA
B	CHC	Medical Officer (MO)
C	Tertiary centre	MO/Chief Medical Officer (CMO)/Superintendent

6. Financial assistance: Delivery at Government Institutions (for Urban beneficiaries)

Area/Municipal/Sub-Divisional/District Headquarter/State Headquarter/Government Medical hospital: Will be given by MO incharge/College Superintendent or their authorized representatives at the time of delivery.

For the purpose of JSY benefit, the mother has to bring along identity card, JSY, MCH card and a referral slip issued by the medical staff of the government institution/accredited private institution who have conducted 3 ANC visits.

7. Delivery at an Accredited Private Institution

- Produce a **genuine BPL** or **SC/ST certificate,** referral slip from ASHA/ANM/MO and MCH-JSY card for accessing benefits under JSY.
- Disbursement of financial assistance available under JSY should be **given to the beneficiary only** and not to any other person or relative.
- Such accredited private institution would also be responsible for any post-natal complication arising out of the cases handled by them.
- The accredited private institution should not deny their services to any referred targeted expectant mother.

8. Financial Assistance for Home Delivery

BPL pregnant women aged 19 years and above preferring to deliver at home by a trained traditional birth attendant or skilled birth attendant is entitled to financial assistance of ₹500 per delivery.

Note:
1. **Require age proof like** birth certificates, voter ID card, school leaving certificate
2. If BPL card not available, then Antodaya Anna Yojana cards can be substituted
3. Limited only for *2 live births* and not for stillbirths
4. Home delivery will be treated as an institutional delivery provided the mother and the child are subsequently admitted to the hospital for post-delivery care.

9. Compensatory Financial Assistance

If the mother or her husband, of their own will, undergoes sterilization, immediately after the delivery of the child, compensatory financial assistance available under the existing family welfare scheme should also be disbursed to the mother at the hospital itself.

ASHA PACKAGE

In rural areas, it includes the following components:
a. Financial assistance for **Referral transport:** Not be less than ₹250/- per delivery.
b. The **transactional cost:** Not more than ₹150/-
c. **Financial incentive to ASHA:** Not be less than ₹200/- per institutional delivery.
d. ASHA should get this money **after her postnatal visit** to the beneficiary and that the child has been immunized for BCG.
e. Expectant mother reaching any institution for delivery of her own **(without the help of ASHA)** should get transport cost (limited to ₹250/-) out of ASHA package immediately after reaching the institution on registration for delivery.
f. In case ASHA has provided ANC but could not accompany the pregnant mother due to some exigencies (to be recorded), but has **arranged one escort to accompany** and stay till delivery and discharge to mother is done, payment to ASHA should be done **within 7 days** of the delivery.
g. No payment to ASHA package in case of delivery at home/accredited private institution.
h. All payments to ASHA should be done by **ANM only**.

SUBSIDIZING COST OF CESAREAN SECTION OR MANAGEMENT OF OBSTETRIC COMPLICATIONS

- Generally, PHCs/FRUs/CHCs, etc. would provide emergency obstetric services free of cost.
- To manage complications or for cesarean section financial assistance up to ₹1500 per delivery could be utilized for hiring services of specialists from the private sector.

Accreditation of Private Health Institution

In order to increase choice of delivery care institution, a number of private health institutions can be accredited to provide delivery service.

Fund Arrangement under JSY

a. For Government Medical College/Capital Hospital, fund will be placed directly from Mission Directorate to the head of the institution in a separate account under the supervision of governing body of the college/hospital. Superintendent, CMOs of the institution would make assessment of the number of delivery taking place and the requirement of funds and communicate the same to the Mission Directorate. The utilization certificate has to be submitted to the NRHM Directorate from time to time for the release of further funds.
b. For block PHC/CHC/municipal/sub-division/district headquarter hospital. The district should allocate sufficient amount of money **in a separate account** under the supervision of the Rogi Kalyan Samiti.

Flow of Fund

a. District authorities would advance ₹10,000/- to each ANM as a recoupable impress money in account for JSY fund.

b. This money would be kept in a joint account of ANM and Sarpanch/Naib Sarpanch, whichever is a lady.
c. ANM will advance fund, as per the requirement to each ASHA/AWW and get the expenditure statement reconciled in the monthly meeting.
d. ANM will be solely responsible for recoupment of all the advances given to ASHA/AWW.

Establish a Grievance Redressal Cell

A grievance redressal cell is to be established in the district, **under the Chief District Medical Officer,** supported by the District Programme Management Unit mainly to facilitate meeting people's genuine grievances on:
- Eligibility for the scheme.
- Quantum of financial assistance.
- Delays in disbursement of the financial assistance.

Display of Names of JSY Beneficiaries

The list of JSY beneficiaries along with the date of disbursement of financial assistance to her should **mandatorily be displayed** on the display board and be updated on a month-to-month basis.

MONITORING

For assessing the effectiveness of the implementation of JSY, monthly meeting of all ASHAs/AWWs related health link workers working under an ANM should be held by the ANM, and at sector level under supervision of medical officer possibly on a fixed day (**may be on the third Friday**) of every month, if Friday is a holiday, meeting could be held on the following working day.

Operational Guideline for Implementation of JSY

In the monthly meeting, the ANM, should prepare a Monthly Work Schedule for each ASHA/village level health worker on the following aspects of the coming month:
- **Feedback on previous month's schedule:**
  a. Number of pregnant women missing ANCs.
  b. Number of cases for which the ASHA/Link worker did not accompany the pregnant women for delivery.
  c. Number of home deliveries out of the identified beneficiaries.
  d. Number of postnatal visits missed by ASHA.
  e. Cases referred to first referral unit (FRU) and review of their current health status.
  f. Number of children missing immunization.
- **Fixing Next Month's Work Schedule (NMWS): To include**
  i. Names of the identified pregnant women to be registered and to be taken to the health centre/Anganwadi for ANC.
  ii. Names of the pregnant women to be taken to the health centre for delivery (wherever applicable).

iii. Names of the pregnant women with possible complications to be taken to the health centre for check-up and/or delivery.
iv. Names of women to be visited (within 7 days) after their delivery.
v. List of infants/newborn children for routine immunization.
vi. To ensure availability of fund in account.
vii. Check whether referral transport has been organized.

Reporting

For the purpose of monthly reporting the ANM is to report both physical and financial progress in a particular format.

Result

- JSY has clearly increased the number of institutional deliveries,
- Over 50% of women who previously had a home delivery had opted for an institutional delivery.
- Equity in access for women (SC/ST/BPL) to institutional deliveries

Shortfalls

Despite this increase, there is persistence of home deliveries, with a wide range—from 7.7% to almost 63%. Women who deliver at home had higher proportions of SC/ST and non-literate or primary school dropouts. Causes are listed below:

1. The JSY excludes a significant proportion of women by virtue of the criteria, and these women who are excluded are those under 19 years, multiparous, poor women, often with no access to a BPL card, all of whom are at higher risk of maternal and perinatal outcomes.
2. Non-affordability of transport costs.
3. Poor service quality and high costs in institutions
4. Cultural preference for the home delivery and a lack of awareness about how quality care could reduce risks
5. Messages on JSY (financial assistance) have not reached
6. Nonpayment and delayed payments of financial assistance
7. Out-of-pocket payments are high in instructional delivery on drugs, investigations, blood and blood products.
8. Lack of 24 × 7 operationalization of PHC and referral services
9. Lack of skilled human resources and basic emergency obstetric services
10. Lack of cleanliness, toilet facility, water and electricity supply

Recommendations

1. Removal of the exclusionary criteria for home and institutional deliveries which limit this entitlement for the most vulnerable women.

2. Streamlining payments and addressing issues of leakage.
3. Out-of-pocket expenses to women are stopped.
4. Expanding the base of institutions to provide services, skill building for existing staff, use of printed protocols, recording and reporting complications, and clarifying the role of the ASHA in the JSY.
5. Development of additional facilities so that unmet need for emergency obstetric care and cesarean sections is increased, training of skilled birth attendants, enabling facility based newborn care across facilities, developing optimal HR (human resource) policies, and establishing a pattern of differential financing across facilities.

CONCLUSION

JSY has unarguably resulted in an increase in institutional deliveries, and has enabled poor women to access public health facilities. It has also perhaps for the first time, challenged the public health system, forcing the providers and the system to deliver services for safe childbirth. This has been made possible by the commensurate increases in infrastructure and human resource provided through other NRHM inputs. Notwithstanding these successes, much more needs to be done.

With the JSY, a beginning to address maternal mortality has been made, but is far from sufficient. The pressure built up on the system has to be sustained, and accelerated. Urgent and focused action is needed and if not forthcoming, our goals for reduction of maternal mortality are likely to elude us for a long time.

BIBLIOGRAPHY

1. Ministry of Health & Family Welfare, Government of India; Operational Guidelines for Maternal and Newborn Health; 2010.
2. Ministry of Health & Family Welfare, Government of India; Operational Guidelines for implementation Janani suraksha yojana; 2010.
3. Ministry of Health & Family Welfare, Government of India; program evaluation of Janani suraksha yojana; 2011.
4. Sidney, Kristi, Rachel Tolhurst, Kate Jehan, et al. (2016) 'The money is important but all women anyway go to hospital for childbirth nowadays'—a qualitative exploration of why women participate in a conditional cash transfer program to promote institutional deliveries in Madhya Pradesh, India, *BMC Pregnancy and Childbirth*. Accessed on 4/7/2017. https://doi.org/10.1186/s12884- 016-0834-y
5. The Impact of India's Janani Suraksha Yojana Conditional Cash Transfer Programme: A Replication Study NATALIE CARVALHO The Journal of Development Studies, 2019 Vol. 55, No. 5, 989–1006, https://doi.org/10.1080/00220388.2018.1506578

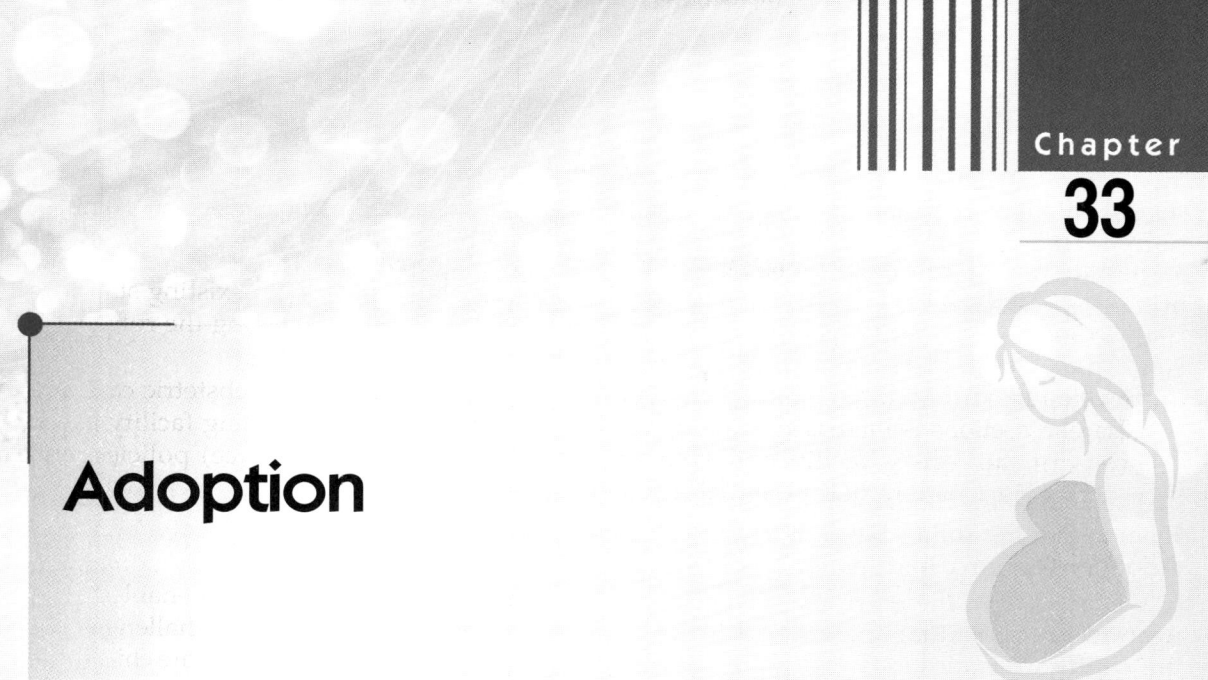

Chapter 33

Adoption

○ Namrata Rajput ○ Amit Upadhyay

Adoption has been recognised for centuries, but being a part of personal laws, there is no uniformity among the different communities. Unitar Whinnie said "It legally establishes a parent–child relationship between persons not so related. The child is absorbed in the family of adopter and is treated as if it were their own Natural Child. By adoption, an artificial but a permanent family relationship is created between the child and the adopter".[1] "Adoption" means the process through which the adopted child is permanently separated from his biological parents and becomes the legitimate child of his adoptive parents with all the rights, privileges and responsibilities that are attached to the relationship. Ministry of Women and Child development, Government of India has established an independent body called "Central Adoption Resource Authority" (CARA). It is responsible to regulate all in-country and inter-country adoptions. In this process, a couple gets an opportunity to fill a void in their lives simultaneously giving security, shelter and future to the child.

Most common reasons for couple to decide for adoption are:[2]
1. Long standing infertility
2. *Medical conditions:* Sometimes people suffer from serious diseases and they don't want to pass it on their kids. Women who are facing serious medical conditions and problem to carry pregnancy also pursue adoption.
3. Single parents
4. Need for a second child
5. As part of an altruistic gesture
6. Need for a child of the other sex when one already has a biological child to complete the family.

Children who are orphan, abandoned or surrendered and who have no family of any sort as decided by the courts of India are available for adoption. Orphan is a child who is without a legal parent or guardian while abandoned child is who is deserted by parents or guardian. A surrendered child is one whose rights are relinquished by parents or guardians in view of multiple emotional, physical and/or social factors. Cradle points may be set up by Specialized Adoption Agencies (SSA) with the help of hospitals or nursing homes for safe abandonment and rehabilitation. All efforts are to be made to restore the child to its biological parents and only after a stipulated period of time and efforts, the Child Welfare Committee declares the child to be legally free for adoption. In case of a surrendered child, the SAA follows the procedure laid down for the same including adequate counselling of the biological parents and only after signing a deed of surrender, 60 days later the child is legally free for adoption.

There are a few fundamental principles that govern adoptions of children from India which include that the child's best interests are kept in mind. All adoptions are registered on Child Adoption Resource Information and Guidance System and confidentiality shall be maintained.

Under CARA, there are many specialized adoption agencies (SAA). These specialized agencies are under the supervision of SARA (State Adoption Resource Agency). These agencies are child care institutions which are recognized and registered by the State Government as specialized adoption agencies. These are primarily a non-profit organization who have been looking after the child welfare activities for at least a period of 3 years and meets all the requirements laid down by the Indian Government.

Every Specialised Adoption Agency shall:[2]
a. Be responsible for the care, protection and well-being of every child in its charge
b. Protect the child from any kind of abuse, neglect and exploitation
c. Prepare the Child Study Report of all orphan, abandoned and surrendered children, through its social worker, and upload them in Child Adoption Resource Information and Guidance System, within seven days from the date such children are declared legally free for adoption by the Child Welfare Committee;
d. Arrange medical tests
e. Try to restore to the biological family or legal guardian;
f. Create a memory album, which shall include a photo album of the child, history and details of the child's life (details of surrendering parents not to be mentioned), and interests of the child, which shall be handed over to the adoptive family along with the medical history of the child at the time of handing over the child to the prospective adoptive parents in pre-adoption foster care;
g. Make efforts to place each child in adoption, who has been declared legally free for adoption by Child Welfare Committee;
h. Be responsible to complete referral process of a child to prospective adoptive parents and the legal procedure related to adoption as provided in these regulations;
i. Prepare every adoptable child psychologically for his assimilation with the adoptive family, wherever required;
j. Facilitate interaction of the child with prospective adoptive parents, wherever required;
k. Ensure that siblings and twins are placed in the same family, as far as possible;
l. Preserve adoption records in a manner, that such record is accessible to authorised persons only;

Eligibility Criteria for Prospective Adoptive Parents[2]

1. The prospective adoptive parents (PAPs) shall be physically, mentally and emotionally stable, financially capable and shall not have any life-threatening medical condition.
2. The age of prospective adoptive parents, as on the date of registration, shall be counted for deciding the eligibility and the eligibility of prospective adoptive parents to apply for children of different age groups shall be as under:

Age of the child	Maximum composite age of prospective adoptive parents (couple)	Maximum age of single prospective adoptive parent
Up to 4 years	90 years	45 years
Above 4 and up to 8 years	100 years	50 years
Above 8 and up to 18 years	110 years	55 years

3. A couple who have at least 2 years of stable marital relationship.
4. Couples in a live-in relationship are not eligible.
5. PAP should have adequate financial resources to provide a good upbringing and be in good physical and mental health.
6. An unmarried or a single male person is not permitted to adopt a girl child.
7. The minimum age difference between the child and either of the prospective adoptive parents shall not be less than twenty-five years.
8. The age criteria for prospective adoptive parents shall not be applicable in case of relative adoptions and adoption by step-parent.
9. Couples with three or more children shall not be considered for adoption except in case of special need children as defined.

For the process of adoption, prospective adoptive parents have to register. PAP's can approach the SAA close to their residence with requisite documents and registration fee. They can, however, register at any SAA or can transfer registration to another SAA but only one. The next step is counselling. The PAPs are then given pre-adoption counselling to prepare them for the process. A social worker makes a visit to the home for home study. This is an assessment of the environment, family, motivational and emotional need of the prospective parents. The home study report is prepared within 2 months of registration which is valid for 3 years. A medical examination report is also done which is valid for one year. The SAA makes best possible efforts to offer child to the PAPs as per their preference. A child study report and medical examination report is shown to the PAPs. If they want, they can get an independent medical examination done by their physician. In case the PAP does not like the child offered to them, a maximum of two more are shown. If they still do not select, then the PAP shall be eligible for reconsideration only after 3 months have lapsed. Once the child is accepted by PAP, the SAA files a petition in the competent court in whose jurisdiction SAA is located. There will be a court hearing following which the court gives the order for adoption. The court has to dispose of the case within 2 months of filing. The local registrar notified under the Registration of Births and Death Act, 1969 (18 of 1969) shall issue birth certificate within five working days in favour of an adopted child on an application filed by the Specialised Adoption Agency or adoptive parents, incorporating the names of the adoptive parents as parents and the date of birth of the child as mentioned in the adoption order of the court, in accordance with circulars issued from time to time by the Registrar General of India.

The Specialized Adoption Agency, which has prepared the home study report shall prepare the postadoption follow-up report on 6 monthly bases for 2 years from the date of pre-adaptation foster placement with the prospective adoptive parents in the format as provided in Schedule 12 and upload the same in CARA guidance system with photos of the child.

Various Acts related to adoption in India are as follows:
1. **Hindu Adoptions and Maintenance Act, 1956**
2. **Guardians and Wards Act, 1890**
3. **Juvenile Justice (Care and Protection of Children) Act, 2000**

Hindu Adoptions and Maintenance Act, apply to Hindus and all those considered under the umbrella term of Hindus as described below. As per the provision of this Act, the following person can adopt a child in India.
- A person who is a Hindu by religion in any of its forms or development, including the Virashaiva, a Lingayat or a follower of the Brahmo, Prarthana or Arya Samaj
- A person belongs to a Buddhist, Jain or Sikh can adopt a child
- A person who has been converted to the Hindu, Buddhist, Jain or Sikh religion

Juvenile Justice (Care and Protection of Children) Act, the right to adopt a child was restricted to Hindus, Buddhists, and Jains. Now it has been extended to Muslims, Christians, Jews, Parsis and all other communities.

A landmark Judgement of the Supreme Court in 2014 ruled that any person can adopt a child irrespective of the religion he or she follows and *even if the personal laws of that particular religion do not permit it.*[3]

The JJ Act 2000 is a secular law enabling any person irrespective of the religion to adopt a child. Prior to this, Muslims, Christians, Jews, Parsis only had the power of guardianship in which one possesses legal rights on the child only till he/she turns adult.

The bill amending the Juvenile Justice (care and protection of children) Act, 2015 allows orphaned, abandoned or surrendered children to be adopted for rehabilitation. Such children may be given for adoption by a court in keeping with guidelines of the Government and CARA once declared free for adoption by Child Welfare Committee (CWC).[4]

This Act also allows person living abroad to accept a child after filing an application in civil court.[5]

Guardians and Wards Act, 1890. The Guardians and Wards Act, 1890 establishes the rights and duties of the guardian of a ward. The responsibility of being a guardian under the Act has been vested to the husband or the father of a minor. The wife or the mother of a minor also holds the capability to be the guardian of the minor. This statute only makes a child a ward, not an adoptive child. According to this statute, once the child turns to the age of 21, he is no longer consider as a ward and treated as an individual identity. It is under this act that Muslims, Christians, Parsis and Jews were allowed to take a child under their care.

In today's world, in developing countries like India, adoption serves a very important social purpose. There are a large number of orphans, abandoned, handicapped and destitute children in our society. Adoption provides an option for such children who are in need of homes and parents. On the other sides, there are a large number of the people in India and abroad who do not have children. Adoption serves the object of providing homes for homeless children and for providing richer family life to those persons who have no children or who have only one child and wants to adopt another child. In today's world, institutions involved in adoption are gaining a lot of importance. There is urgent need to grant liberal finance help to such institutions, so that they may be able to provide better facilities to those children who are living under their care and protection.

REFERENCES

1. Adopted Children - How they grew up, 1967, P. 36.
2. http://cara.nic.in/
3. https://www.indiatoday.in/india/story/supreme-court-gives-adoption-rights-to-muslims-181849-2014-02-20
4. http://www.legalserviceindia.com/article/l327-Adoption-under-Juvenile-Justice-Act.html
5. https://www.prsindia.org/billtrack/juvenile-justice-care-and-protection-children-amendment-bill-2018

Contact details of CARA
Central Adoption Resource Authority,
Ministry of Women and Child Development
West Block 8, Wing 2
1st Floor, RK Puram
New Delhi-110066 (India)
Telephone Numbers:+91-11-26180194
e-mail: carahdesk.wcd@nic.in

For adoption queries:
Toll-Free No: 1800 11 1311 /011-26760471/011-26760472/011-26760473
Available between 9:00 am to 5:30 pm in all working days (Mon-Fri)

Chapter 34

Government Policies Regarding Adolescent Reproductive Health

○ Ashwini Bhalerao Gandhi ○ Sampath Kumari

INTRODUCTION

According to 2011 census data, India has the largest population of adolescents in the world being 253 million individuals aged 10 to 19 years. The UNICEF's flagship the state of the world's children report states that the country's adolescent constitute 20% of world's 1.2 billion adolescent population. This age group comprises individuals in their transient phase of life requiring nutrition, education, counselling and guidance to ensure their development into healthy adults. However, data on adolescent from national surveys including National Family Health Survey III (NFHS III), District level household survey III (DLHS III), and Sample Registration Survey (SRS) call for focussed attention with respect to health for this age group.

Given the above scenario, government of India has recognized the importance of influencing health seeking behaviour of adolescents. The health situation of this age group is a key determinant of India's overall health, mortality, morbidity, and population growth scenario.

In keeping with the spirit of convergence under National Rural Health Mission (NRHM), the Reproductive and Child Health phase II (RCH II), and Adolescent Reproductive and Sexual Health Programme (ARSH) strategy emphasizes the need for intersectoral linkage with other departments at the policy and programme levels to create a supportive environment for adolescent interventions and to improve awareness level among adolescents.

HEALTH PROGRAMMES FOR ADOLESCENTS

1. Rashtriya Kishor Swasthya Karyakram (RKSK)

The beneficiaries are adolescent age group, the benefits are to
- Improve nutrition
- Improve sexual and reproductive health

- Enhance mental health
- Prevent injuries and violence
- Prevent substance misuse

2. Kishori Shakthi Yojana (KSY)

The beneficiaries are adolescent girls, the benefits of this programme are:
- Educational activities through non-formal and functioned literacy pattern
- Immunization
- A general health check up every six months
- Treatment for minor ailments
- Deworming
- Prophylaxis measures against anaemia, goiter, vitamin deficiencies, etc.
- Referral to primary healthcare (PHC) or district hospitals in case of acute need
- Convergence with Reproductive Child health scheme, reproductive and child health phase (RCH)

3. Balika Samridhi Yojana (BSY)

Girl children belonging to families below the poverty line are given benefits, who are born on or after 15th August, 1997. The benefits are restricted to two girl children in a household. The goals are to change the negative attitude of the family and community towards the girl child at birth and towards her mother.

The programme aims to:
- To improve enrolment and retention of girl children in school
- To increase age of marriage of girls and
- To assist the girls to undertake income generation activity.

4. Reproductive and Child Health (RCH) and Adolescent Reproductive Sexual Health [ARSH] Programme

The beneficiaries are adolescent married and unmarried girls and boys. The goals are

Promotive services
- Focussed care during antenatal period
- Counselling and provision of emergency contraceptives
- Counselling and provision of reversible contraceptives
- Information/advice on sexual and reproductive health (SRH) services

Preventive services
- Services for TT and prophylaxis against nutritional anaemia
- Nutritional counselling
- Services for early and safe pregnancy and management of postabortion complications

Curative services
- Treatment for common RTI/ STI
- Treatment and counselling for menstrual disorders
- Treatment and counselling for sexual concerns of male and female adolescents
- Management of sexual abuse among girls

Referral services
- The primary facilities must be in a position to make appropriate referrals for care and support, especially for HIV/AIDS
- Voluntary counselling and testing centre (VCTC)
- Prevention of parent to child transmission

Outreach services
- Periodic health check-ups and community camps
- Periodic health education activities
- Co-curricular activities

5. Adolescent Friendly Health Services

- Monitoring growth and development
- Monitoring of behaviour problems
- Offer information and counselling on developmental changes, personal care and ways of seeking help
- Reproductive health including contraception and STI treatment, pregnancy care and post-abortion management
- Integrated counselling and testing for HIV
- Management of sexual violence
- Mental health services including management of substance abuse

6. The Adolescent Education Programme (AEP) under NACP for AIDS Control

The adolescent education programme (AEP) under National AIDS Control Programme (NACP) for AIDS control. The beneficiaries are adolescents—the aim is to promote
- Co-curricular adolescent education in classes IX–XI
- Life skills education in classes I–VIII

7. Rashtriya Bal Swasthya Karyakram (RBSK)

The beneficiaries are children's from birth to 18 years of age. The aim is screening and early referral of all congenital and other conditions.

8. Weekly Iron and Folic acid Supplement (WIFS) *Under National Health Mission (NHM)*

The beneficiaries are school going adolescent girls and boys in 6th to 12th class enrolled in government/government aided municipal schools and out of school adolescent girls.

The aim is to:
- Reduce the prevalence and severity of anaemia in adolescent population (10 to 19 years).
- Administration of supervised weekly iron folic acid supplements (100 mg elemental iron 500 micro gm folic acid) using a fixed day approach.
- Screening of target groups for moderate/severe anaemia and referring these cases to an appropriate health facility.
- Biannual deworming (Albendazole 400 mg), six months apart for control of helminthic infestation.
- Information and counselling for improving dietary intake

ORGANIZING EFFECTIVE SERVICES

For ensuring effective services, the following components are crucial:

Service Providers
- Adequate and appropriate (identified) service providers in place.
- At all health facilities, defining the staff profile is needed and it has to be ensured that the identified staff is present in all clinic sessions.
- Service providers are clearly aware of their role and responsibilities in relation to the functioning of the health facility.
- Service providers have the competencies required to provide the specific health services effectively.

Location, Ambiance and Supplies
- The medical officer in charge must be able to take a decision to locate/setup clinic in the existing infrastructure. The decision should be guided based on the availability of a separate room for the clinic, timing, frequency of organizing the clinic, and the expected level of utilization of services by the adolescent. If there is no clash of timings, the same room that is used for OPD in the morning may be used for adolescent clinic in the afternoon.
- The waiting area is to be identified with appropriate seating arrangement, provision of drinking water, and clean functional toilets. Also reasonable cleanliness must be ensured. The specified supplies, equipment and basic amenities should be available in each type of health facility.

Guidelines and Procedures
Clinical management guidelines and standard operational procedures are in place for the provision of the specified health services. The existing guidelines in the RCH programme would be followed.

Information, Education and Communication (IEC) and Resource Materials
- An adequate number of information booklets should be made available as take away material in these clinics.

- Communication aids in local language are to be used. Partnerships with local NGOs may be explored specifically for this purpose.

Conducive Environment at Health Facilities

Attention should be given to the following factors:

Staff

- On all clinics days it must be ensured that the designated staff is present.
- Punctuality and regularity must be enforced.
- Staff attending to the adolescents must have the qualities that put the adolescents at ease for them to avail services they need and are being offered.
- Follow-up action may be taken up by them to enhance their credibility with the adolescents.

Registration Procedure

By registration and retrieval of records of adolescent clients will be made simpler. If the client does not wish to reveal personal details, address, etc., the staff should not insist on it.

Privacy and Confidentiality

- Arrangements of visual and audio privacy.
- Clinic rooms must have window curtains and a bed screen surrounding the examination table.
- It is advisable to give clear instruction to the staff about not allowing anyone into the clinic when a client is already there in order to ensure privacy.
- The confidentiality policy of the clinic may be displayed and clearly expressed to the client in the first session itself.
- Client records to be kept out of reach of unauthorised persons.

Clinic Timings

It is advisable to have clinic timings that suit the needs of the adolescents. Due attention is to be given to school timings and work timings of adolescents who are engaged in employment in that area.

Appropriate Signboard

The clinic is to have an appropriate signage reflecting the location of the clinic and its operational timings. Display board of the PHC may indicate availability of services for adolescents. State and district programme managers can decide on the appropriate branding of the clinics giving them a distinct identity. Suggestion such as 'Yuva', 'Saathi', and 'Mitr' may be considered. The name may be identified in consultation with young people.

Information, Education and Communication (IEC)

In case a dedicated spaces available for running a clinic for adolescents, relevant posters and communication materials may be displayed. Reading material should be available on relevant issues, especially the handouts the adolescents can take without having to request for them. Resource material are to cover topic related to growth and development, puberty, sexuality concerns, myths, misconceptions, pregnancy, safe sex, contraception, unsafe abortions, menstrual disorders, anaemia, sexual abuse, RTI/STI, etc.

Capacity Building of Providers
- Selection of providers: Subcentres/primary healthcare (PHCs)
- Medical officer in charge
- Lady health visitor (LHV), auxiliary nurse midwife (ANM), multi-purpose health worker—male (MPW-M) (posted at headquarters)
- ANMs/MPW-M (posted at subcentre attached to PHC)
- Community health centre (CHCs) and district hospitals
- Medical officers (preferably a lady medical officer)

Environment Building Standard
- At the district level, a one day ARSH orientation is to be organised by the district health officer (DHO), reproductive and child health (RCHO) for the district level officers of different departments including civil society representative and district level Zillah Panchayat members.
- At block level, one day meeting of Panchayati raj institution (PRIs), women and child development (WCD)/education/youth departments is to be organised by the medical officers.
- At the PHC level, a half day meeting is to be organized by the LHV/ANM for self-help groups, office bearers and village health communities (VHC) members.
- At the village level, the ANMs while participating in the meeting of women's groups or self-help groups or VHCs must generate support for adolescents for information and services. They can take help of ASHA/AWW and other community-based functionaries in organising such group activities.
- Folk media and mass media as applicable for the setting must be engaged for the purpose of environment building in the community.

Communication with Adolescents
Communication activities are to be conducted at the level of village outreach, Anganwadi centre or youth group. The target group would include unmarried and married females and males. Such group communication activities are to be conducted once a month by ANM, ASHA, AWW, youth coordinators and/or link workers.

Monitoring and Supervision
Management systems should be in place to improve/sustain the quality of health services. Mechanisms are to be in place to monitor the performance of the health facilities and needs for corrective/ameliorative actions. Monitoring as a function comprises supervision, analysing

data and reporting on progress. Effective supervision is necessary to ensure that activities and subactivities are carried out in the desired manner. It is needless to say that supervision is not to be perceived as a control function. It is a tool to observe activities, detect problems, and explore solutions and implement appropriate solutions to ensure that the same problems do not occur in the future.

Flow of Data

The monthly reports submitted by the MOs are to be compiled by the DHO on a monthly basis and submitted to the state RCH society/State Programme Management Unit (SPMU). At the state level the state RCH society/state programme management unit is expected to review RCH II programme implementation on a periodic basis. During these periodic reviews, the ARSH monthly reports from the districts are to be discussed. Appropriate review and feedback mechanism at the national, state and district levels are to be in place to ensure that timely corrective actions are initiated. Quality of outreach activities may be further assessed during supervisory visits. Depending on the maturity of the health system, the mechanism for quality assurance and improvement may be instituted. Further, community monitoring mechanism may also provide inputs on client satisfaction with special reference to adolescents.

India as a country has matured enough to understand the adolescents are the future of the nation. We need to nurture this age group. The various government policies if well implemented will give far reaching results.

BIBLIOGRAPHY

1. A profile of adolescents and youth in India 2011, Census of India, United Nations Population Fund (UNFPA), India.
2. .http://aepatc.org
3. http://nhm.gov.in/index1.php?long= 1 & level =1 & sublinkid=969&lid=49
4. http://rchiips.org/NFHS/nfhs3.shtml
5. http://wed.nic.in/kishori-shakti-yojana.(under ministry of women and child development)
6. http://www.Censusindia.gov.in/vital_statistics/SRS_Statstical _report.html
7. http://www.nhm.gov.in/rashtriya-kishore-swasthys-karyakram-rksk-pg
8. http://www.nthmhp.hov.in/content/adolescent-reproductive-sexual-health-programme.
9. http://www.unicef.org/reports/state-of-worlds-children-2019.

Chapter 35

Lifestyle Modifications for Empowering Women

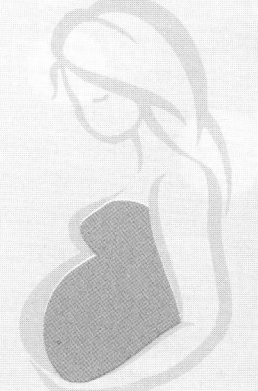

○ Charmila Ayyavoo ○ CN Aditi

"Girls are one of the most powerful forces for change in the world. When their rights are recognized, their needs are met, and their voices are heard, they drive positive changes in their families, their communities and the world"

—Kathy Calvin, United Nations Foundation, President and CEO

Positive changes can be brought about in society if girls and women are empowered. For empowerment, they need options which have no restraints. If these options are provided without any curbs particularly in their lifestyle, they will be more benefited. Having the capacity to make one's own resolutions will lead to empowerment.[1]

The factors in lifestyle which can lead to a positive change for woman are health parameters, education of women, human rights and gender equality. In the Hunger Report released by Bread for the World in 2015, it has been reported that stunting of younger children is reduced in countries where women are empowered. Women's empowerment will serve to address the issue of undernourishment of young children.[2]

Women's Health

Changes in lifestyle are needed for women for better health. Young girls should be motivated to follow a healthy lifestyle from the beginning so that these changes are a part of their routine. The changes advocated by the American Psychological Association to help girls and women to have an enduring positive lifestyle are:[3]

1. Plan the change which can be followed without trouble. It should have realistic goals which can be achieved.
2. Big plans which will have difficulty in following should be avoided. The changes to be followed should be of small scale.

3. Change in all types of activity at the same time should be avoided. One type of behaviour at a particular point in time should be changed.
4. To help in achieving the goal, a friend or a motivator's help should be sought.
5. A support group for boosting the morale should be available.

Women should be encouraged to eat nutritious food, reduce the intake of caffeine and exercise correctly. Women and girls in low income families tend to eat lesser than their male counterparts. According to the World Health Organisation (WHO), girls are facing hurdles in achieving good health because of sociocultural practices.[4] It points out that

- Men and women are in disparate relationships where women are perceived as weaker.
- Society has discouraged education chances for girls.
- Earning jobs are less for women.
- A girl's capacity to procreate is given prime importance.
- There are more occasions for women to face domestic violence than men.

WHO further points out that undernutrition because of poverty may lead to poor health in both boys and girls but girls face more discrimination. In consequence the health of the girl is poorer than a boy. This has also contributed to an increase in exposure to HIV/AIDS.

MENSTRUAL HYGIENE

Menstruation is a normal event in a girl's life. It is subjected to so many social and cultural taboos. Girls face discrimination because of menstruation. On behalf of the Menstrual Hygiene Management Consortium, Tamil Nadu many awareness programs on science behind menstruation, safe and eco-friendly methods of disposal of sanitary napkins and socio-cultural taboos regarding menstruation are being conducted in many schools and colleges. It is seen that unhealthy practices in usage of clothes, ash, cow dung during menstruation is still followed in many rural areas. In urban areas, young girls do not change sanitary napkins correctly. They tend to use it for long periods and napkins which are wet can lead to irritation of the genital tract and infection. Use of dirty pads is also prevalent which can also lead to infections. Girls should be taught about the reproductive system, the menstrual cycle, the scientific facts about reproduction so that they are empowered to make the right choices. During the conduct of awareness programs, the girls informed that they

1. Are not allowed to attend school during menstruation.
2. Are asked to sleep separately from the family.
3. Are not allowed to eat certain foods.
4. Are not allowed to take a shower or bathe.
5. Are not allowed to play sports.
6. Are not allowed to visit temples or religious functions.

Menstruation is considered to be "dirty" by society. Girls are discriminated against because of menstruation. It is imperative that girls acquire knowledge and make empowered choices.

NUTRITIONAL PARAMETERS

Anaemia

There is impairment in an individual's well-being if there is iron deficiency and anaemia. It will lead to reduction in work capacity, well-being and increase weariness and apathy. The loss to an individual's productivity will be high. Anaemia can lead to poor quality of life and the future generation's health is also spoiled as anaemic women are prone to have children with impediments to learning skills and impaired growth profiles. Anaemia in the mother will increase the chance of abortions, stillbirths, preterm deliveries, hypertension in pregnancy and eclampsia.[5] Anaemia needs to be prevented and treated at younger ages in girls. This is of particular importance if they belong to a society which tends to get its girls married in the adolescent period. Anaemia is prevented if WASH is followed which is access to clean water, sanitation and hygiene. This will lead to a reduction in anaemia due to reduction in nutritional losses due to infection and inflammation. Girls should be encouraged to consume a diet rich in green leafy vegetables and fruits. The intake of fast foods and snacks should be discouraged to prevent nutritional anaemia. Women of reproductive age should be encouraged to take iron and folic acid supplementation when anaemia is prevalent in the community.

The main reasons for inequality in health parameters between genders are poverty and access to healthcare. Girls are more prone for nutritional problems when the society that they live in is less privileged.

Weight

a. Underweight

Women of ideal weight will give birth to healthy children of high intelligence. Even though women are in charge of meals in most households, they are the last to eat. They tend to eat less too. This will perpetuate a vicious cycle of undernourished women giving birth to sick children. The key to breaking this cycle is access to nutritious food for women. This will serve to be of utmost importance for the survival of future generations. The interventions to improve women's health should begin from young ages in girls. The effect of correction of nutritional deficiencies on status of health parameters in women, stunting rates in young children and the outcome at birth are proved without doubt now. In India, the Government is promoting long standing Poshan Abhiyaan since 2018 with the aim to reduce malnutrition.[6] The Government has planned an improvement in collection of data, monitoring the implementation and appraisal systems on nutritional status in the country. There are other programs to change the health parameters of women in the country. The Nutritional Rural Livelihoods Mission (NRLM) started in 2011 has motivated the marginalised women in rural areas to work together as self help groups (SHG). These groups are encouraged to have an increased say in the resources of their families and the women are encouraged to change their attitude towards health and nutrition.[7] Many states are encouraging programs like Jeevika (Bihar), Kudumashree (Kerala) and Swabhimaan in Bihar, Odisha and Chhattisgarh which encourage nutritional changes through the SHGs. They have been successful in empowering women. These types of interventions need to be increased and details should be provided to women who need them and should help to cause a constant change in their nutritional habits.

b. Overweight

The other end of the spectrum is the issue of increasing weight of women especially in the urban areas. The increase in weight during the growing ages is increasing the chances of obesity in the reproductive years which can lead to metabolic diseases and problems during pregnancy. During the period of adolescence, there is propensity to overeating, reduced physical activity and changes in body contour, insulin sensitivity, emotional behaviours, etc.[8] Adolescence is a period of developmental plasticity and behaviours in this age tend to be maintained during adulthood. A girl who tends to have unhealthy eating habits will continue to do so as a woman and this will lead to many complications as an adult. Girls in their young age should be encouraged to change their lifestyle behaviour by getting involved in sports and physical activities and eating right.[9] Treatment of obesity issues are very costly and may involve surgical options in adulthood. Adolescence should be utilised as a window of opportunity for changing the lifestyle so that body fat accumulation does not occur.

Healthy Bones

The incidence of osteoporosis is increasing in Indian women. In 2015, about 20%, i.e. 46 million women above the age of 50 years suffered from osteoporosis. It is a major health problem in women.[10]

Genetic factors account for the height of an individual as well as the strength of the skeleton. But for bones to be healthy, lifestyle characteristics like food and exercise are important.

EXERCISE

Exercising daily is a must. Moderate intensity aerobic exercises like cycling and fast walking for at least 2–3 hours is essential from the age of 19–64 years. Exercises which utilise weight bearing and resistance exercises are beneficial in increasing bone density. This will serve to prevent osteoporosis in older ages. Exercises to strengthen the muscles should also be a part of the daily activities.

A diet rich in calcium will help in sustaining bone strength. If leafy green vegetables, milk products, dried fruit are taken, they help in strengthening bones. Vitamin D is also needed for absorption of calcium and bone strength. It is obtained from food and sunlight. The sources in food are fish, meat, eggs and dietary supplements. Sunlight is also a source of vitamin D. Girls should be encouraged to play in the sun for strong bones throughout life.

EDUCATION

A woman is a human with talent, passion, dreams, strength, courage and another million different things beyond her biological destiny. She doesn't necessarily have to like Barbie dolls. She doesn't necessarily have to wear pink. She doesn't necessarily need all the gold given to her as 'gifts'.

What she needs is an education to be empowered, freedom to explore, courage to stand for herself and some moral support from her family.

Girls need to be educated so that the family flourishes. They can grow up frustrated and discontented which may propagate a toxic environment in their future. Instead they need a voice in their younger ages and should not compromise with their ambitions. Fuelling a stigma that is having far-reaching adverse effects on millions of girls around the world should be avoided.

GENDER EQUALITY

If a man in his forties is asked why his mother was so important to him, his answer would be somewhere along the lines of ," she sacrificed her entire life for me", "she lived for the family's happiness", "she missed out on everything good in life".

This word 'sacrifice' holds a lot of emotions, power and the most often ignored 'stereotype'. Why is drinking a necessary evil for men? When did compromise start being glorified as a maternal trait?

There is no denying that being amicable, selfless, and tolerant are admirable qualities in a woman but that is not definitely everything that she is.

Renunciation and immolation are two sides of the same coin "sacrifice".

Compromising on education, independence, esteem and constitutional rights is immolating oneself but definitely it is not for the greater good. It will propagate a domino effect of bigotry, oppression, discrimination and more oppression.

No one likes that next door aunty with gossip juicier than the paparazzi can give and a network wider than the All India radio. Have anyone ever wondered why she comments on girls going to school? Why she has to say something when someone comes home late? Why is she bothered?

May be she is jealous, vexed or simply bored. Hers is a voice fighting to be heard. Her resentment is the backlash of her snuffed out passion. Her judgement is based on the prejudice she faced. Her tales are an echo of a half done education. She envies the self respect, confidence, financial stability and freedom that other women seem to have.

While appearances seem to be deceptive, deluded are those who say not to make an appearance at all. "Your physical appearance is a plus but not your whole package" is a very true statement. But a plus is a plus. A healthy, well-groomed, hygienic appearance is basic. Women should seize the freedom to dress, to style themselves so that they can be comfortable and confident. It is not a crime to look and feel good. They should be the person they want to be. Giving up these little joys of life at a young age for those unknown voices is just taking another step toward the vortex that the graduate woman of today is striving to avoid.

Freedom comes with responsibilities. Women are accountable to their families, the society, and the government. The difference is that they should do it out of their own volition and interest. A woman cannot be defined. She comes in all shapes and forms. Every woman is strong in her own way. Envisioning the modern woman as a jean clad biker with cropped hair is just redefining stereotypes and not breaking it.

Women should be allowed to ask for "what they want". They should be given space for different opinions and ideas. They should be taught to be flexible but yet solid. Men are not the enemies. All are in this together battling against a norm that evolved with mankind in a desperate need to establish balance in the tumultuous road of life.

CONCLUSION

WHO Regional Director for South-East Asia, Dr. Poonam Khetrapal Singh has stated that Women's empowerment is a public health imperative. In the past few years, there is a strong conviction which is evidence based among society, policymakers and the Government that empowerment of the girl child is very important both locally and globally. If priority is given to implementing changes in the lifestyle of a young girl in health, education, hygiene and nutrition and providing an opportunity for her to thrive in an environment which is gender neutral, it will help in the formation of a world which is healthier and happier.

REFERENCES

1. Bayeh, Endalcachew. "The role of empowering women and achieving gender equality to the sustainable development of Ethiopia". *Pacific Science Review B: Humanities and Social Sciences*. January 2016:2(1);38.
2. Lateef A. Speaking Up for Nutrition: The Role of Civil Society. InThe Road to Good Nutrition 2013 (pp. 158–168). Karger Publishers.
3. American Psychological Association. *Making lifestyle changes that last.* http://www.apa.org/helpcenter/lifestyle-changes (2010).
4. Health topics; Women's Health; World Health Organisation;2019.
5. Comprehensive implementation plan on maternal, infant and young child nutrition. In: Sixty-fifth World Health Assembly Geneva, 21–26 May 2012. Resolutions and decisions, annexes. Geneva: World Health Organization; 2012:12–13
6. Press Information Bureau; Government of India; Ministry of Women and Child Development; 26-July-2019; National Nutrition Mission
7. The National Rural Livelihoods Project; July 5, 2011.
8. Alberga AS, Sigal RJ, Goldfield G, Prud'homme D, Kenny GP. Overweight and obese teenagers: Why is adolescence a critical period? Pediatr.Obes. 2012;7:261–273.
9. Hills AP, Andersen LB, Byrne NM. Physical activity and obesity in children. Brit J Sport Med 2011;45:866–870.
10. Anuradha V Khadilkar; Epidemiology and treatment of osteoporosis in women; an Indian Perspective; Int J Womens Health, 2015;7:841–850.

Medical Councils and Doctors: Medical Ethics Training—the Need of the Hour

○ Shivkumar S Utture

It is indeed disheartening and frustrating to read about the increasing incidents of assaults by patient's relatives on medical practitioners and establishments. In spite of the passing of the Law on Assault on Clinical Establishment and Personnel (which was passed due to the decisive role played by IMA members all over Maharashtra), there does not seem to be any paradigm shift in tendency of patient's relatives expressing their anguish in the form of violence and rioting, thus causing physical and psychological trauma to medical practitioners. Hence I believe that along with protection of Law, practitioners of modern medicine require educating themselves on the hitherto neglected subject of Medical Ethics.

The unremitting progress of medical science and the unforeseen changes in medical practice make it impossible to predict future development in medicine. It is said that in modern medicine fifty percent of current knowledge undergoes radical changes every five years. Hence both medical students and practitioners must face the arduous problem of recycling their knowledge and get ready for their continuing medical education.

Only the fundamental traits of medical ethics will withstand the powerful pressure coming from future innovations in medicine. Basic principles of medicine and human nature form the essential foundation of doctor–patient relationship and will remain unchanged no matter how deep the changes fostered by scientific progress and socioeconomic evolution. Medicine is one of the few professions that sets a code of behavior for its practitioners. The Medical Council of India vide its notification in 2002 has laid some basic regulations relating Professional Conduct, Etiquette and Ethics for registered medical practitioners. The Code of Medical Ethics details the duties and responsibilities of the physicians in general, duties of physicians to their patient, duties of physicians in consultation, responsibilities of physicians to each other, duties of physicians to the public and paramedical staff, unethical acts, misconduct and disciplinary action and punishment thereof. Unfortunately 90% of medical practitioners are unaware of existence of such a Code of Medical Ethics. Could this be the reason behind increasing distrust and decreasing faith of patients towards their training doctors culminating into a spurt of cases of assault on Medical Practitioners and Establishments in the recent past? The patient's trust in his doctor depends on the doctors respect for patients rights and his full technical and practical knowledge to deliver the proper and adequate treatment.

The essential component of continued medical training and Professional Ethics was clearly defined by Hippocrates 2500 years ago and still remains intact in modern practice of medicine. So what needs to be done to fill this vacuum in study of Medical Ethics? I feel we require to tackle this problem in a two pronged fashion.
1. Introduction of Medical Ethics as a separate subject during undergraduate and postgraduate medical training.
2. Imparting thorough knowledge of medical ethics by prestigious organizations like IMA as an integrated continuing medical education (CME)

Luckily better sense has prevailed and MCI is all set to introduce training of medical students on ethics guidelines with special emphasis on doctor–patient relationship. Medical schools must deliver ethically informed training programs that develop doctor's skills and promote patient's autonomy. Trust and respect, the essentials of doctor–patient relationship are missing from student experience of bedside medicine training given in the terribly competitive and stressed environment in medical institutions these days. Unfortunately the number of role models in medical colleges is diminishing as unethical practices flourish and this adds to the frustration amongst students. The students see divergence in the way that they are exposed to this important subject throughout their medical training period. The course on medical ethics must be made compulsory with requisite attendance for award of medical degree.

Recognizing the need for medical ethics to evolve with changing social circumstances, the Medical Council keeps the Code under continuous review. The Code embodies two cardinal values of the medical profession. It is committed to maintaining high standards of proper conduct and good practice to fulfill doctors' moral duty of care. Importantly also, the Code upholds a robust professional culture to support self-governing through identifying role-specific obligations and virtues of the medical profession. These obligations and virtues define the moral ethos and shape the professional identity of the medical community.

The code marks the profession's commitment to integrity, excellence, responsibility, and responsiveness to the changing needs of both patients and the public. This Code is only a guide and is by no means exhaustive.

Contravention of this Code, as well as any written and unwritten rules of the profession, may render a registered medical practitioner liable to disciplinary proceedings.

THE INDIAN MEDICAL COUNCIL ACT 1956

The Medical Council of India (MCI) has the following roles:
- Inspection/visitation with a view to maintain proper standard of medical education in India.
- Permission to start new medical colleges, new courses including PG or higher courses, increase of seats, etc.
- Recognition/de-recognition of Indian qualifications/foreign qualifications.

- Maintenance of All India Medical Register of persons who hold any of the recognised medical qualification or for the time being registered with any of the State Medical Councils or Medical Council of India.
- Registration of RMPs for those states where State Councils are not in existence
- Issue of Good Standing Certificates for doctors going abroad

Conducting inquiry and hearings of ethical complaints from complainant/RMP who are not satisfied by the verdict given by State Medical Council.

THE MAHARASHTRA MEDICAL COUNCIL ACT 1965

Set up in 1965 as a statutory body the MMC designed its missions to primarily focus on maintaining an updated register of allopathic practitioners, developing a code of ethics for its registered practitioners, attending to the complaints led by users of the medical service and taking necessary disciplinary actions against the doctors found guilty, and inspecting and accrediting medical colleges and institutions across the state for diploma studies.

Let us now look at some of the rules and regulations which affect individual RMPs in their daily practice.

PROFESSIONAL MISCONDUCT (INFAMOUS CONDUCT)

As per Medical Council of Indian Amendment Act No. 24 of 1964, the council has specified a Warning Notice that violation of this code shall constitute "Infamous conduct in a professional sense", i.e. it will be professional misconduct. It is defined as that conduct which is considered as reasonably disgraceful or dishonorable by the professional brethren of good repute and competency.

MCI PROFESSIONAL CONDUCT AND ETHICS AND REGULATIONS, 2002

The Medical Council of India vide its notification in 2002 has laid some basic regulations relating to Professional Conduct, Etiquette and Ethics for registered medical practitioners.

IMC Code 1.2.3—Renewal of Registration

A physician should participate in professional meetings as part of continuing medical education programmes, for at least 30 hours every five years, organized by reputed professional academic bodies or any other authorized organisations. The compliance of this requirement shall be informed regularly to Medical Council of India or the State Medical Councils as the case may be.

It is compulsory for all doctors of modern medicine practising in the state of Maharashtra to renew their registration with MMC every five years. One of the requirements is completion of thirty credit hours of CME every 5 years. Trust is essential to the practice of medicine. The patient's trust imposes upon the doctor a corresponding duty to be trustworthy and accountable. Whereas a patient's trust is fundamental to the process of healing, the ability to heal depends importantly on one's professional knowledge and skills. It is therefore necessary for every doctor to attain continuous professional development through lifelong learning in order to fulfill the duty of care to patients.

MCI Code 6.4.1—Dichotomy or Fee Splitting

A physician shall not give, solicit, or receive nor shall he offer to give solicit or receive, any gift, gratuity, commission or bonus in consideration of or return for the referring, recommending or procuring of any patient for medical, surgical or other treatment. A physician shall not directly or indirectly, participate in or be a party to act of division, transference, assignment, subordination, rebating, splitting or refunding of any fee for medical, surgical or other treatment. Dichotomy or fee splitting is not only unethical but also illegal. Same thing applies to when doctor sends a patient for various investigations like radiological, pathological, etc.

MCI Code 7.4—Adultery or Improper Conduct

Abuse of professional position by committing adultery or improper conduct with a patient or by maintaining an improper association with a patient will render a Physician liable for disciplinary action as provided under the Indian Medical Council Act, 1956 or the concerned State Medical Council Act.

Association with unqualified assistants by the doctor is unethical if:
a. In his day-to-day practice he employing them
b. He/she assists unqualified practitioner or quack in his private practice in any way—giving anesthesia, attending delivery cases, etc.
c. He/she covers up the unqualified practitioner by issuing medical certification of "Ill Heath" to patients not treated by himself.

MCI Code 6.1.1—Advertising

Soliciting of patients directly or indirectly by a physician, by a group of physicians or by institutions or organisations is unethical.

MCI Code 6.1.2—Printing of Self Photograph

MCI Code 6.1.2: Printing of self photograph, or any such material of publicity in the letter head or on signboard of the consulting room or any such clinical establishment shall be regarded as acts of self advertisement and unethical conduct on the part of the physician. However, printing of sketches, diagrams, picture of human system shall not be treated as unethical.

Canvassing and advertising directly or indirectly to promote private practice is unethical.
a. Displaying unusually large signboards depicting anything other than his name, qualification and nature of his specialization (e.g. giving photographs, diagrams of the equipment).
b. Displaying signboards at other than at his residence and clinic, e.g. at chemists shops, religious places.
c. Guaranteeing a cure for certain ailments by notifying in the lay press.
d. By publicly exhibiting his scale of refund if not cured.
e. Advertising his name while notifying his association with social welfare activities. However, writing an article in the lay press or giving a talk on the Radio/TV on subject matters of public health, community welfare, etc. are not acts of professional misconduct.

MCI Code 6.3—Running an open shop (Dispensing of Drugs and Appliances by Physicians)

A physician should not run an open shop for sale of medicine for dispensing prescriptions prescribed by doctors other than himself or for sale of medical or surgical appliances. It is not unethical for a physician to prescribe or supply drugs, remedies or appliances as long as there is no exploitation of the patient. Drugs prescribed by a physician or brought from the market for a patient should explicitly state the proprietary formulae as well as generic name of the drug.

MCI Code 6.8—Relation with Pharmaceutical and Allied Health Sector Industry

Code of conduct for doctors and professional association of doctors in their relationship with pharmaceutical and allied health sector industry. A medical practitioner shall not receive any gift, travel facility, hospitality, cash or monetary grants from any pharmaceutical or allied health sector industry and their sales people or representatives.

MCI Code 7.2—Medical Records

A RMP should maintain the medical records of his/her indoor patients for a period of three years as per regulation 1.3. Refusal to provide the same within 72 hours when the patient or his/her authorised representative makes a request for it as per the regulation 1.3.2 is unethical.

MCI Code 7.7—Medical Certificate

Signing professional certificates, reports and other documents
Medical practitioners who deliberately issue a false, misleading or inaccurate certificate could face disciplinary action under the Indian Medical Council (Professional Conduct, Etiquette and Ethics), Regulations, 2002.

MCI Code 7.17—Publishing Photographs and Case Reports

A registered medical practitioner shall not publish photographs or case reports of his/her patients without their permission, in any medical or other journal in a manner by which their identity could be made out. If the identity is not to be disclosed, the consent is not needed.

MCI Code 7.20—Specialisation/Additional Qualification

A physician shall not claim to be specialist unless he has a special qualification in that branch and registered with the State Medical Council under additional qualification.

It must be clearly understood that instances of professional misconduct as given in the said Gazette Notification are not intended to constitute a complete list of the infamous acts. MCI or State Medical Councils will consider and deal with any other form of professional misconduct. It is emphasized that the code should not be violated in letter or spirit. The concerned council will consider and decide upon the facts brought before them in each case of infamous conduct.

CONCLUSION

As far as practising doctors are concerned the concept of "Learning how to Learn" finds its prevalent application in Ethics Self Education. Ethical responsibility is the heart of the physicians competent professional behavior. We must learn to ethically review our attitudes and to update constantly our ethics knowledge. World over national medical associations have taken the initiative with regards to education in medical ethics and protection of patient rights. But ultimately we require to introspect and ask ourselves "Is virtue (ethics) something that can be taught? Or does it come by practice? Or is it natural aptitude that requires to be nurtured? It is only when we are able to answer these questions and accept that professionalism and professional behavior are closely related and learn to adopt and value patient focused care that we can play a decisive role in shaping a civilized world which respects human life with compassion.

Self regulation is the best regulation.

BIBLIOGRAPHY

1. Indian Medical Council Act, 1956.
2. Indian Medical Council (Professional Conduct, Etiquette and Ethics) Regulations 2002.
3. Maharashtra government gazette, 28 April 2010, Maharashtra Medicare Service persons and Medicare Service Institutions (Prevention of Violence and Damage or loss to property) Act, 2010 (Maharashtra Act No 11 of 2010).
4. Maharashtra Medical Council Act, 1965.

Domestic Violence Act

○ Reena J Wani ○ Preeti Deshpande

INTRODUCTION

Domestic violence has no boundaries. It is prevalent in different counties, cultures and socio-economic stratas. Women have been oppressed all over the world for several generations.

United Nations has organized four world conferences on women over the decades. The 1995 Fourth World Conference on Women in Beijing marked a significant turning point for the global agenda for gender equality. The Beijing Declaration and Platform for Action was adopted unanimously in 189 countries. It has an agenda for women's empowerment and considered the key global document on gender equality. It sets strategic objectives and actions for the advancement of women in critical areas of concern such as women and poverty, training of women, health, violence against women, the girl child, human rights and media issues related to women.

The world has a long way to go still. India certainly has a very long way to go.

Indian culture and mythology is filled with stories of female Goddesses and stories of Swayamwaras. But there is a difference between history, stories and reality. Let's have a reality check—India is a male dominant society. The medieval era saw a downturn in women's status in the society with customs like Sati. Widows were expected to live a life of severe austerity. So the woman's life was doomed if her husband died!

The winds of change began way back in the 19th century in the British era itself. Hindu Widows' Remarriage Act was passed in 1856.

Raja Ram Mohan Roy was the "Father of Indian Renaissance". He was known for his efforts to abolish Sati, child marriage, polygamy and dowry and he demanded inheritance rights for women. In 1828 he set up the "Brahmo Samaj", a reformist movement to fight against social evils.

Though a lot has improved, we still are largely an unfair society in the practical sense. We may feel the urban population is relatively liberal but even in the urban scenario women are not empowered.

From time to time various Acts have been passed for the cause of women in India.
- The Dowry Prohibition Act, 1961
- The Equal Remuneration Act, 1976
- The Child Marriage Restrain Act, 1976
- The Medical Termination of Pregnancy Act, 1971
- The National Commission for Women Act, 1990
- The Protection of Human Rights Act, 1993
- Protection of Women from Domestic Violence Act, 2005
- Protection of Women against Sexual Harassment at Workplace Bill, 2010

Domestic violence is a major issue in all stratas of Indian society till today. Contrary to the belief, actually domestic violence is also seen in higher socioeconomic classes but reporting is poor to avoid undue publicity and media coverage. We need to fight against domestic violence as a society.

Protection of Women Against Domestic Violence Act, 2005[1] (PWDVA)

Main Features of the Act

The definition of an 'aggrieved' person' is wide and covers not just the wife but a woman who is the sexual partner of the male irrespective of whether she is his legal wife or not. The daughter, mother, sister, child (male or female), widowed relative, in fact, any woman residing in the household who is related in some way to the respondent, is also covered by the Act.

The respondent under the definition given in the Act is not only "any male, adult person who is, or has been, in a domestic relationship with the aggrieved person" but so that his mother, sister and other relative. The relatives do not go scot free and the case can also be filed against relatives of the husband or male partner.

The information regarding an act or acts of domestic violence does not necessarily have to be lodged by the aggrieved party but by "any person who has reason to believe that" such an act has been or is being committed. This means that neighbors, social workers, relatives, etc. can all take initiative on behalf of the victim.

This fear of being driven out of the house effectively silenced many women and made them silent sufferers. The court, by this Act, can now order that the women cannot only reside in the same house but that a part of the house can even be allotted to her for her personal use even if she has no legal claim or share in the property.

It allows the magistrate to protect the woman from acts of violence or even "acts that are likely to take place" in the future and can prohibit the respondent from dispossessing the aggrieved person or in any other manner disturbing her possessions, entering the aggrieved person's place of work or, if the aggrieved person is a child, the school.

The respondent can also be restrained from attempting to communicate in any form, whatsoever, with the aggrieved person, including personal, oral, written, electronic or telephonic contact". The respondent can even be prohibited from entering the room/area/house that is allotted to her by the court.

The Act allows magistrates to impose monetary relief and monthly payments of maintenance. The respondent can also be made to meet the expenses incurred and losses suffered by the aggrieved person and any child of the aggrieved person as a result of domestic violence and can also cover loss of earnings, medical expenses, loss or damage to property and can also cover the maintenance of the victim and her children.

It allows the magistrate to make the respondent pay compensation and damages for injuries including mental torture and emotional distress caused by acts of domestic violence. It gives a penalty up to one year imprisonment and/or a fine up to ₹20,000/- for the offence. The offence is also considered cognizable and non-bailable.

It goes even further and says that "under the sole testimony of the aggrieved person, the court may conclude that an offence has been committed by the accused".

The Act also ensures speedy justice as the court has to start proceedings and have the first hearing within 3 days of the complaint being filed in court and every case must be disposed of within a period of sixty days of the first hearing.

It makes provisions for the state to provide for Protection Officers and the whole machinery by which to implement the Act. It is the role of protection officers to assist the Magistrate in the discharge of his functions. They are supposed to make the Domestic Incident Report. They are supposed to ensure that legal aid is provided to the aggrieved person. They are to maintain a list of service providers, shelter homes and medical facilities. Their role is also to ascertain that the aggrieved person gets monetary relief.

The Act also provides for the penalty for not discharging duty of Protection Officer.

The Acts enunciate certain duties of central and state government to make wide publicity and training programs for the Police Officers.

The Act also provides for the assistance of welfare experts if found necessary by the Magistrate.

The Act recommends service providers to facilitate the processes. Any voluntary association registered under the societies Registration Act 1860 or a company registered under the Companies Act, 1956, or any other law in force with the objective of protecting the rights of women shall register itself as a service provider. A service provider can record the Domestic Incidence Report in prescribed form if the aggrieved person desires and forward a copy to the Protection Officer or Magistrate. The service provider can get the aggrieved person medically examined and forward the medical report to the Protection Officer and police station. The service provider can ensure shelter is provided to the aggrieved person if she so desires. No legal suit can lie against the service provider who is deemed to be acting in good faith to prevent domestic violence.

Loopholes in the Present System against Domestic Violence
Un-clarified Responsibility and Insufficient Official Resource

In practice duty of each role, such as the Protection Officers and service providers, still seems ambiguous.

Lack of Training of Police Officers and Magistrates

There is a lack of training of police officers and magistrates regarding the Act's requirements and its purpose, as well as a lack of sensitivity towards the issue of domestic violence. This lack of training has led to the re-victimization of women within the justice system, either through police non-response to calls for help, sending women back home to their abusers by branding their victimization as mere domestic disputes, or magistrates allowing for numerous continuances of cases, prolonging the court process and forcing victims to come to court to face their trauma time and again.

Dual System: Family Court and Criminal Court

There are mainly two legal approaches for women, who have suffered domestic violence, one is filing for divorce through Family Court, and the other is filing application to Magistrate according to Domestic Violence Act which might go through Criminal Legal System. The dual system sometimes makes the legal proceeding more complex even tedious for them. Also, the social impression of each approach puts some stress on them.

Misled as A One-way Affair

The act is deeply controversial due to its insistence that firstly, the person who commits domestic violence is always a male, and secondly, that on being accused, the onus is on the man to prove his innocence. Therefore, there are a lot of chances of the Act being misused by unscrupulous women.

Overweening Ambition and Lack of Proportion

In attempting to anticipate all possible ways to protect all aggrieved women from any sort of harm, the framers of the law have put their faith in all women being essentially honest victims, without worrying about proof of claims.

Disparities in Implementation

There are major disparities in implementation of the law in various states. Not surprisingly, states that invested in implementation of the Act in terms of funds and personnel also reported the highest number of cases filed.

Fading Attempts of NGOs as Service Provider

Very few NGOs have registered themselves as service providers under the Act, the registered service providers as well as protection officers' lack experience with domestic violence work and a few protection officers are assigned in each district to handle the caseload.

Failure to Mandate Criminal Penalties

Advocates and protection officers have noted additional inadequacies of the PWDVA, including the Act's failure to mandate criminal penalties for abuse along with its civil measures, its failure to explicitly provide a maximum duration of appellate hearings which delays women's grant of relief, the residency orders' failure to give women substantive property rights to the shared household (only giving them the right to reside there), and a basic lack of infrastructure linking law enforcement officials, officials under the Act, and service providers together in order to best and most efficiently serve domestic violence victims.

Shaking Responsibilities

The Act has by and large affected those who have access to quality legal aid. Though the Act provides for state legal aid, the quality of services in such cases is really poor. The state has passed on all responsibility to the service providers. They have to provide medical aid to abused women, arrange for short stay homes and arrange for compensation. It becomes a burden on these providers who do not have the wherewithal.

Lack of Follow-up

Needless to say, lack of follow-up can endanger victims' safety as well as allow for corruption and inefficiency within the organizations intended to help them. In addition, a Times of India July 19th, 2009 article reported the PWDVA's lack of retroactivity, citing the Mumbai High Court's decision to set aside an order permitting an abused woman to reside in her husband's flat since his eviction attempt occurred prior to the PWDVA's enactment in 2005.

Victims of domestic violence may hide such incidents. Fear of community reaction and lack of support, fear that no one would believe them, feeling of shame, threat from perpetrators and lack of information about negative health consequences may prevent them from coming forward. Domestic violence is known to cause physical, emotional, social and economic consequences.

A "victim" is a person who is not fully capable of comprehending the situation at hand because of the victimhood faced. The belief is that the person so victimized that she may not be in a frame of mind to make decisions independently. Victims are also in need of compassion, care, validation and support.

Our Role as Medical Professionals

The first and foremost responsibility of medical institutions is that they cannot refuse treatment to the aggrieved woman under any circumstances.

Detection of injuries arising from domestic violence and identification of "domestic violence as a syndrome" is a concept somewhat similar to "battered baby syndrome". If identified the person in charge will be required to counsel the woman in privacy and inform her about the reliefs under this law.

The treatment and documentation should be done with gendered understanding in view. Also referrals to other related services such as counselling and legal aid is a part of the duty of the medical professionals. Hospitals may have to function as temporary shelter homes. Domestic violence is to be recognized as a medical emergency.

Role of Policymakers

The role of policymakers is also coordinating with healthcare professionals, protection officers and crisis intervention services. They must arrange for social support, counselling, temporary shelter in hospitals and shelter homes, police and legal help as well.

Role of Service Providers and Non-government Organisations

Many non-government organisations have taken up issues of gender-based violence. They are involved in providing support, shelter homes, rehabilitation and empowerment of victims of domestic violence. They are also involved in running social and community awareness and sensitization programmes.

One such organization is the Family Planning Association of India established since 1949. It works closely with NGOs and the government. It is the founding member of the International Planned Parenthood Federation. It has taken up issues of gender-based violence, i.e. violence against an individual based on his biological sex or gender identity. Gender-based violence includes physical violence, sexual, verbal, emotional and psychological abuse, also coercion, economic and educational deprivation.

Impact of Domestic Violence is at Multiple Levels (Fig. 37.1)

Domestic violence has an impact on the women's health. As per the WHO these women are twice as likely to experience depression, anorexia or alcohol disorders. They are 16% more likely to have low birth weight babies and 1.5 times more likely to get HIV and sexually transmitted diseases. Domestic violence increases chances of injuries and premature death. Also there is a higher chance of unwanted pregnancies, anaemia and chronic ill health.[2]

Various programmes are run by NGOs, National Women's Commission and Medical Organizations to create awareness and change the outlook of the society. Stree Hinsa Mukt Bharat Abhiyan is one such programme run by the Family Planning Association of India with an objective to catalyze the civil society for preventing and mitigating violence against women.[3] It includes encouraging the society to take a pledge to denounce violence. Doctors involved in this programme have to identify the history of domestic violence and provide treatment, counselling and referrals. Empowering young women with life skills and training. It also entails enabling men and boys to break away from the rigid norms of patriarchy.

Effect of Domestic Violence on Children

UNICEF along with a corporate organization The Body Shop conducted a survey called "Behind Closed Doors" to study the impact of domestic violence on children.[4] There is an increased risk that the children may become victims of abuse themselves. There is a significant risk of harm to the child's physical, emotional and social development. There is a strong social likelihood that this will become a continuing cycle of violence for the next generation (Fig. 37.2).

The survey suggested that policymakers must increase awareness about the impact of domestic violence on children, create public policies and laws to protect children, enhance social services that address impact of violence of children.

There are multiple pathways through which intimate partner violence can lead to adverse health outcomes. This figure highlights three key mechanisms and pathways that can explain many of these outcomes. Mental health problems and substance use might result directly from any of the three mechanisms, which might, in turn, increase health risks. However, mental health problems and substance use are not necessarily a precondition for subsequent health effects, and will not always lie in the pathway to adverse health.

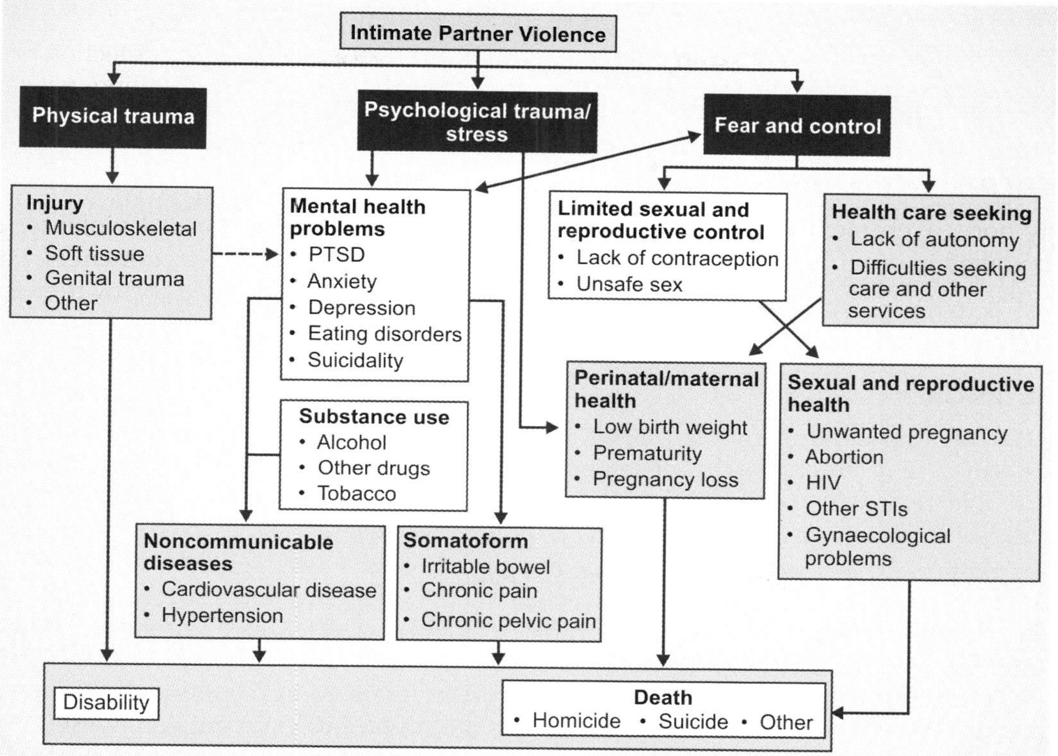

Fig. 37.1: Pathways and health effects on intimate partner violence [2]

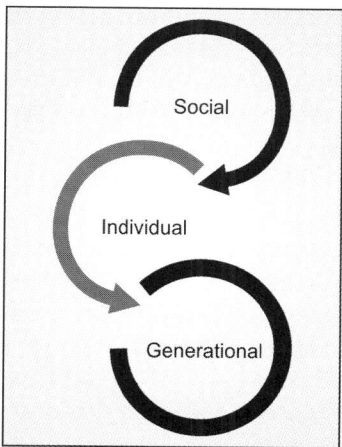

Fig. 37.2: Impact of domestic violence

The Domestic Violence Act currently does not specifically address the issue of the effect of violence on children.

Role of the Private and Corporate Sectors

Corporate social responsibility is a growing priority in the private sector.

The private sector can:
- Finance initiatives that seek to prevent domestic violence and protect victims
- Actively engage in partnerships with NGOs
- Increase awareness through employee education
- Take action to persuade the government to take the issue of domestic violence and its impact on children seriously

CONCLUSION

The enactment of Domestic Violence Act, 2005 is an answer to violation of women's human rights which may be criminally prosecuted. Though this legislation has been thoroughly prepared, lacunas will always be there leading to accused circumventing the law.

Whether or not the Act will be misused only time will tell.

There cannot be any perceptible change in women's status overnight. It will take at least a decade before things change. This Act provides them a safeguard and a sort of sword in their hand so that they will not be seen as an animal or a doormat. One precondition for improving the implementation of the DV Act is to increase women's awareness of it. Also, effective trainings for their respective roles of each department involved in the implementation of the Act are necessary. To complete the system, there should be sufficient budget invested.

In social-cultural level, to bring the idea of gender equality to public is one tough mission for the government. The process of social change is obscure, however, the effects are obvious. Only in a more gender-equal society, women who have suffered violence could get rid of shame/self-blame and such happenings could be de-stigmatized. Family, school, peer groups, and media are all agencies of social change, which all together should join the cultural revolution and mental revolution to construct India into a more female-friendly society. Domestic violence concerns so many elements. Low rates of participation in education, lack of economic independence, value biases operating against them, etc. directly and indirectly resulted in the women been given the status of being the secondary gender in the Indian society.

In conclusion, I would like to quote Yehuda Bauer, the Israeli historian and scholar of the Holocaust, "Thou shalt not be a victim, thou shalt not be a perpetrator, but above all thou shalt not be a bystander." Domestic violence is as heinous a crime as the Holocaust.

As healthcare professionals, we must understand that providing emotional support is as important as taking care of the medicolegal aspects of domestic violence. The physical wounds will heal but unless the survivor is given adequate psychosocial support in the right way from the first contact, the emotional trauma can last lifelong. Mental health professionals like psychologists can be involved in the care. NGOs should be involved to support, rehabilitate and empower women. They can be given vocational training and made self-sufficient.

Changing perceptions of gender education, creating and supporting peer groups can help in bringing about a positive change.

Domestic Violence Act Highlights
a. Applicable if habitually assaults or makes the life of the aggrieved person miserable by cruelty of conduct.
b. Force the aggrieved person to lead an immoral life.
c. Otherwise injuries or harms the aggrieved person.
d. Economic abuses: Deprives of all or any economic or financial resources, household necessities of the aggrieved person and her children's.

Important Features
1. Women's right to secure housing: The Act provides for the women's right to reside in the matrimonial or shared household whether or not she has any title or rights in the household.
2. Power of the court to pass protection orders that prevent the abused from entering the workplace or residence of the victim or any other place frequented by the abused or attempting to communicate with the abused.

Appointment of Protection Officers and NGOs to provide assistance to the women with respect to:
1. Medical examination
2. Legal aid
3. Safe shelter, etc…

Offence under DVA is a cognizable, non-bailable and punishable. Punishment with imprisonment for a term which may extend to 1 year or with a fine which may extend to 20000/- rupees or with both.

REFERENCES
1. The Protection of Women from Domestic Violence Act, 2005, No.43 of 2005.
2. Global and regional estimates of violence against women: prevalence and health effects of intimate partner violence and non-partner sexual violence, World Health Organization 2013.
3. Stree Hinsa Mukta Bharat Abhiyan, FPA India.
4. Behind Closed Doors; The Impact of Domestic Violence on Children, Survey by UNICEF with The Body Shop.

Section VI

Recent Updates

38. Assault on Doctors and Remedies against the Same
39. Anti-ragging Rules and Regulations in the Medical Education System in India
40. Biomedcial Waste Management
41. Clinical Establishment Act in Day to Day Practice

Chapter 38

Assault on Doctors and Remedies against the Same

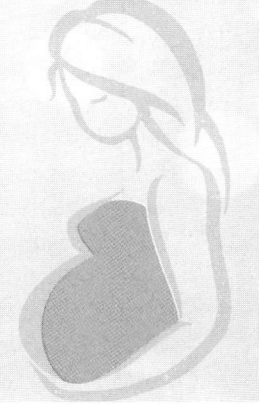

○ Vipin Checker

*Any Behavior Responsible for Physical or Mental Harm
To Healthcare Professional is Violence..!*

Have you read?
1. Dhule doctor may lose vision as dead patient's kin thrash him—May 15, 2017, TOI, Maharashtra
2. 1 in 2 doctors face violence at public hospitals: Study—March 21, 2017 Times Of India
3. Is India at War with its Doctors? December 15, 2017, The New Indian Express

Violence against doctors is unacceptable and needs to be condemned. The medical fraternity is very disturbed and concerned about the rising incidents of physical violence and assaults or attacks on doctors and their staff, clinical establishments, etc.

The Government of India had constituted an Inter-Ministerial Committee, which had promised to soon enact a Central Act for violence against doctors. But, sadly, this has yet to see the light of the day. It is time that the medical profession unites and stand firm till the government brings a Bill for violence against doctors in the coming Parliament session.

If the doctors and other healthcare staff, etc. are always under a constant threat and pressure from the ongoing violence and assault, then they will not be able to do justice to their profession and also they shall not be able to treat and cure their patients who are under emergency and undergoing risk and danger of their life properly and promptly.

It is, therefore, in the interest of public at large that such cases of physical violence against doctors must be condemned and controlled and must not be allowed to happen.

Persons committing such offences and crimes can be punished under the following laws:

Criminal Law

The Act of physical violence, assault, attack on doctors, nurses, their staff, clinical establishments, etc. amounts to following criminal offences, which are punishable under the provisions of Indian Penal Code (IPC), 1860:
- *Criminal conspiracy*: Section 120A and Section 120B of IPC
- Offences against the public tranquility
  - *Unlawful assembly*: Section 141, 143 and 144 IPC.
  - *Rioting*: Section 146 IPC, Section 147 IPC and Section 148 IPC.
  - *Affray*: Section 159 IPC and Section 160 IPC.
- Offences affecting the public health, safety, convenience, decency and morals
  - *Public nuisance*: Section 268 IPC, Section 269 IPC and Section 294 IPC.
- Offences affecting human body
  - *Hurt:* Section 319 IPC, Section 323 IPC and Section 324 IPC.
  - *Grievous hurt:* Section 320 IPC, Section 325 IPC, Section 326 IPC and Section 326A IPC.
  - *Act endangering life or personal safety of others*: Section 336 IPC, Section 337 IPC and Section 338 IPC.
  - *Wrongful restraint:* Section 339 IPC and Section 341 IPC.
  - *Criminal force and assault:* Section 350 IPC, Section 351 IPC, Section 352 IPC and Section 355 IPC.
- Offences against property
  - *Theft*: Section 378 IPC and Section 379 IPC.
  - *Mischief*: Section 425 IPC and Section 426 IPC.
  - *Criminal trespass*: Section 441 IPC and Section 447 IPC.
- *Offence of defamation: Section* 499 IPC and Section 500 IPC.
- *Offences of criminal intimidation, insult and annoyance*: Section 503, Section 504 IPC and Section 506 IPC.
- *Offences of outraging, insulting the modesty of women*: Section 354 IPC, Section 354A IPC, Section 354B IPC, Section 354C IPC and Section 509 IPC.

If any person commits any of the above mentioned offence, then the doctors and their staff can lodge a police complaint under **Section 154 of the Criminal Procedure Code** and get an FIR lodged against the said offender.

Civil Law

Doctors, hospitals, its staff, clinical establishment, etc. can also file civil suits like suit for permanent injunction, suit for damages and suit for defamation against the aforesaid Acts and offences of physical violence, assault, attack, etc.

Besides the above mentioned remedies under IPC or CrPC, around 15 States and Union Territories (UTs) in India have their respective State or UT legislations on the issue of physical violence or assault on doctors, for example, Delhi Medicare Service Personnel and Medicare

Service Institutions Act, 2008; Bihar Medical Service Institution and Person Protection Act, 2011, etc. In all these legislations, punishment is imprisonment which may extend to 3 years or with fine up to Rs. 10,000/- or both and compensation of twice the purchase price of property damaged and loss caused to be recovered as arrears of land revenue on default. However, the said legislations framed by the 15 States or UTs are not effective and also there is no awareness about the same either amongst the doctors or the concerned police authorities.

Then there are **laws relating to sexual harassment at the workplace**. Women can file a complaint against the offence of sexual harassment at workplace as per the provisions of the Sexual Harassment of Women at Workplace (Prevention, Prohibition and Redressal) Act, 2013 (hereinafter referred to as Act, 2013).

As per the provisions of the Act, 2013, the hospitals, clinical establishments, etc. should constitute an Internal Committee for redressing the complaints relating to the sexual harassment at workplace made by any aggrieved women.

Violence is much more common in healthcare than in other industries. Violence in healthcare may take a variety of forms. Violent events can happen with anyone. Doctors are usually unprepared to face the episodes. Violence is one of the most serious problems in worldwide healthcare and needs to be addressed in channelized way. Violence is a serious problem all over the world. In India violence has become an epidemic in recent years.

Over 30–40% of Indian doctors have faced violence once in lifetime. Violence is reported on daily basis across India, some resulting in grievous injuries. Today doctors are facing big challenge of violence in clinics, hospitals and healthcare in general. Violence against doctors is seriously threatening. It is affecting doctors' professional as well as personal lives. It is an effect of an unwell, pathetically backed healthcare system. I, believe the hospitals cannot be allowed to become war zones. Patients need a peaceful environment and the doctors also need a stable and peaceful ambience for delivering 100% quality care. Because of violence doctors have started practicing defensive medicine. Violence is creating an ambience of suspicion amongst doctors as well as patients.

Incidence: 55–60% Resident doctors face violence. 30–40% Private doctors face violence. Small nursing homes are worst sufferers. Solo establishments have no support system.

Frequently Asked Questions (FAQs)

What do you think are the causes of violence?
- Failure of communication.
- Poor public image of the profession.
- Mob mentality—'Aggression will make the hospital work harder,' "gundas" will teach them to respect me and my patient'.
- Government apathy.
- Low health literacy.
- Rising healthcare costs.
- Poor security for hospitals and doctors.
- Psychological stress amongst relatives.
- Lack of funds, human resources with family.

- Ignorance—about disease and prognosis, lack of knowledge regarding medical science.
- Poor conditions at public hospitals, belief that private healthcare is profit driven.
- Rising costs of healthcare.

What are the Patient, Organization Related Provocative Risk Factors?
- Working with staff who have a history of behavioral issues or who do not possess good interpersonal relations.
- Working alone in hospitals.
- Poor unprofessional designs of the hospitals.
- Lack of emergency communication.
- Prevalence of firearms, knives and other weapons among patients and their families and friends.
- Lack of facility, policies and staff training for recognizing and managing escalating hostile and assaultive behaviors from patients and visitors. High worker turnover.
- Long waits for patients and overcrowded, uncomfortable waiting rooms.
- Unrestricted movement of the public in clinics and hospitals.
- Perception that violence is tolerated and victims will not be able to report the incident to police and/or press, charges . . . starts from your reception area.
- Working when understaffed—especially during mealtimes and visiting hours. Overworked, numerous patients, understaffing of doctors.
- Junior doctors mostly get attacked. They are the first responders in critical situation, lack of training in proper communication, not introduced as part of the team.
- Lack of surveillance and security.
- Lack of institutional/organisational policies, action plans to deal with violence.
- Medical jousitng between professionals (unfortunately true).
- Poor image of medical profession.
- Role of media in distorting facts.
- Government and judicial apathy. Lack of organisation and unity among medical professionals. United we stand divided we fall.

What are the types of healthcare violence?
- Verbal abuse
- Mobbing
- Psychological harassment
- Threat
- Physical violence
- Vandalism
- Cyber trolling
- Phone calls
- Messages
- Writing on various social media sites like facebook.

What are the problems with the present acts?
- Nineteen states have Medicare Act.
- No CRPC code for Act.
- Not known to police stations.
- Not executed or applied.
- Not a single conviction till date.
- Culprits are indirectly helped, not arrested or get free within 24 hours
- No use of Acts which are only on paper! It is impossible to work under stress.
- We are left with safe practice only.
- Doctors have lost hope for safety.
- Threat to dignity, self-respect.
- Families of doctors feel threatened.
- The intellectual fraternity is suppressed by goons.
- Doctors scared to rise up to social or political platform; prefer to remain subdued.

As a doctor what do you expect from the government?
- No healthcare violence. Hospitals should be safe zones by Government policy.
- Promote such policies to people.
- Strict execution of the policies.
- Enforce legislation to safeguard healthcare sector: Central Medicare Act.
- Launch awareness programs on consequences of healthcare violence.
- Protective measures for doctors.

So what is the solution my elite reader?
- Central Effective Medicare Act.
- Transparent doctor–patient relationship.
- Government safety measures.
- Reducing healthcare expenses, timely, correct, authentic, professional, documented communication. Counseling sessions for doctors. Ethics, safety, quality and professionalism in clinical practice. Increasing public awareness.
- Involvement of public face in counselling and awareness. Medical curriculum should include—ethics, quality, professionalism, communication skills, interpersonal relationship assessment, patient psychology assessment, documentation in clinical practice.

Integrated Approach—Professional
- Doctors also need to change the mode of practice and attitude towards practice.
- Positive and effective way of communication. Ethics, safety, quality and professionalism in clinical practice.
- Accreditation and certification for channelized approach in practice.
- Patient and relatives' psychology assessment, documentation in clinical practice.
- Satisfactory time for patient examination and relatives counseling.
- Informed consent for all procedures.

- Introduction of all team members.
- Staff can be outnumbered or harmed
- Multi-disciplinary team meetings with families of critical patients.
- Avoid maligning fellow colleagues.
- Report incidents of violence or any perceived threats of violence immediately.

Integrated Approach—Institutional
- Security and surveillance.
- Limitation to number of individuals entering the hospital premises.
- Activating emergency response codes and systems.
- Immediate response teams to violence with clearly designated roles of employees and security personnel.
- Incident reporting.
- Mob management.
- Media management.
- CCTV surveillance at all important risk areas.
- Liasioning with local leaders, RWAs, local district administration.
- Local police.

Integrated Approach—Medical Council Level
- Medical curriculum to include team development—group practice modules, communication skills development.
- Communication and documentation awareness programme.
- Accreditation of healthcare.
- Awareness of medical protective laws.
- Inter-personal relationship protocol awareness.

So what do you think should be the role of community?
- Community should be informed about certain facts by awareness programmes.
- Medicine is a science to deal with illnesses.
- Doctors deal with complex nature of diseases.
- Unforeseen circumstances out of changing nature of diseases.
- Unpredictable patient responses to disease management protocols.
- Medical science has evolved over centuries, achieved many milestones but has not yet conquered death . . . ! Public awareness is must to underline these things to people.

I am a staunch IMAite, and AMCite, so is there a role of association?
Guidelines
- Report: To authorities and medical associations.
- React: Through crisis management groups/defense cell.
- Reach out: To community

- Regulate: Strong central regulation. Self-regulation
- Retaliate by constitutional means.
- Social and national violence registry.
- CCTV installation and maintenance campaign.
- Anti-violence videos, pictures in public places and
- Reception area of hospitals
- Memorandum to civic bodies, police officers.
- Demand letter for Central Medicare Act. Demand letter for declaring hospitals as crisis safe zone.
- Management groups or defense cell.
- Local guidelines/SOP. Broadcast or mobile app. confidentiality.
- Legal support.
- Involve prominent personalities.
- Cyber lynching and cyber trolling.
- Involve local politicians.
- Press meets and press coverage.

SUMMARY

Some remedies

Here are a few suggestions to avoid doctor–patient disputes.

There is an urgent need to legislate a Central Act on prevention of violence against doctors while on work and duty. Any act of violence against doctors should be made a punishable, non-bailable offence with imprisonment of up to 14 years. Also, the State Acts on violence against doctors should be advertised and also acted upon by the state government. Workshops, seminars, etc. should be organized to educate the general public and doctors about the penal provisions in case of violence against doctors. This can be done by the government and professional associations. Patients' rights should be displayed in every hospital and clinic. Associations should educate their doctors about etiquettes, conduct and ethics. Patients should be educated about the significance of informed consent. Patients should be educated about triage in emergency. Patients should be sensitized that error of judgment does not automatically mean negligence. There should be a grievance redressal mechanism for both patients and doctors in every healthcare establishment. Right communication is the key to a strong doctor–patient relationship, based on mutual trust and respect. The charges should be clear and transparent. There should not be a large difference between the estimated cost of treatment and the actual cost of treatment. There should be no hidden charges or kickbacks. It is important to acknowledge the altered dynamics of doctor–patient relationship, which has undergone a paradigm shift from doctor's right to take decision to patient's rights to take decision. The rules should be rational treatment, rational prescription, transparency in investigations and treatment. Hospitals should identify high risk areas and install audio-based CCTV cameras in all sensitive and high risk areas. Bodies of deceased patients cannot be held as hostage for financial disputes. Hospitals should make adequate security arrangements; protection to be given to doctors and nurses working in the night shift in particular. Provide transparent daily billing to avoid future disputes. CPR and first aid to be available everywhere. Briefing to the legal heirs should be timely. Nurses and paramedical staff to be trained about soft communication. Besides the doctors and patients who are direct stakeholders in this, the media and police too have an important role to play in preventing violence against doctors and hospital staff.

Guideline for Media

No media trial. Negative news about the doctors should not be published. Name of the doctor and patient should not be published. No news article should be published without proper verification.

Guideline for Police Officers

To be sensitized about the Violence Against Doctors Act. To be sensitized about the guidelines as laid down by Hon'ble Supreme Court in Jacob Mathew case.

Acknowledgements

Dr Jayesh Lele, Past President IMA MS, Dr KK Agarwal and Dr Vinay Agarwal, Past National Presidents of IMA and IMA Maharashtra State.

SOURCE REFERENCES AND SUGGESTED READINGS

1. http// Times of India india times .com/city/mumbai/dhule-doc-may-lose-vision-as –dead-patients-kin-thrash-him/article show/57639925.cms
2. http// Times of India india times .com/city/delhi/1-in-2-doctors-face-violence-at-public-hospitals-study/srticleshow/57740477.cms
3. http// www.news18.com/news/india/ima-to-go-ahead-with-nationwide-strike-tomorow-in-support-of-protesting-bengal-doctors-2189301.html

Chapter 39

Anti-ragging Rules and Regulations in the Medical Education System in India

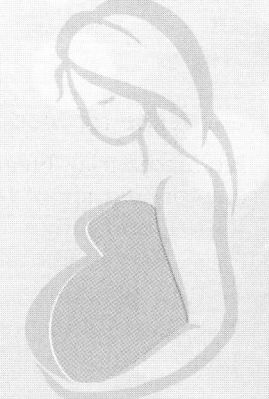

○ Manisha Khare

INTRODUCTION

The unfortunate story of Dr Payal Tadvi, the budding postgraduate student of Mumbai's Nair Hospital who allegedly committed suicide by hanging herself after months of harassment by her seniors, has stunned us all. While the enquiry still goes as it has prompted us to make all medical students and faculty aware about the anti-ragging rules and regulations and its legal implications.

Ragging is a disturbing reality in the higher education system of our country, especially for courses like medicine, engineering, and management. It is very serious problem, where many unethical acts take place under the name of ragging which affects human dignity, sometimes leading to severe depression and even driving the victim to commit suicide.

While discrimination is rampant across our society, it is worth examining the peculiar ecosystem that pervades our medical education, which creates an exceptionally undemocratic and intimidating atmosphere. Medical training in India continues to be extremely hierarchical and regimented. This is especially true during the medical residency period where the maximum work is assigned to the junior most resident doctor. Add to this the enormous workload especially in public institutes.

Despite the fact that over the years ragging has claimed hundreds of innocent lives and has ruined careers of thousands of bright students, the practice is still perceived by many as a way of 'familiarization' and an 'initiation into the real world' for young college going students.

Facts about Ragging

Ragging continues to make news at worryingly regular intervals.
- About 9 teenagers are killed every year

- Hundreds get seriously injured and/or disabled
- Countless of innocent youths suffer extreme forms of physical and sexual abuses for months.

As per data collected by the University Grants Commission (UGC), 5003 cases of ragging of students have been registered across India between April 18, 2012 and September 2019. A total of 52 cases of death have been reported allegedly due to ragging in the last seven years.

In a Study funded by the University Grants Commission (UGC), where about 10,000 students were questioned, it was observed that 40% students were ragged in some form, out of these only 8.6% students reported it. Such poor reporting is out of fear of getting boycotted by the seniors or lack of confidence in the administration that any action would be taken. The study also found language and region to be the basis of more than 25% ragging incidents, while caste was a factor in 8% cases.

It makes one question our understanding of this phenomenon, particularly in the context of the deeper psychological and sociological determinants that eventually manifest as ragging behaviours.

Psychology of the Ragger

It is important to understand the psychology behind ragging, senior students desire to show off their power and superiority, to feel important by helping the juniors, and to avenge their own ragging experience by doing to juniors what they themselves faced.

At times it may act as catharsis and be used to vent anger or unconscious frustration. It may also help to satiate one's sadistic tendencies. Sometimes ragging may be done under the influence of alcohol or peer pressure.

Psychology of the Victim

The juniors are already nervous and apprehensive about the new college and hostel life and their nightmare comes true when their seniors start abusing them. Depending on the upbringing, temperament and personality, each individual reacts to the circumstances differently. While some may forget about the incident and move on with their life, others may go into depression and may discontinue studies or even commit suicide.

Effects on the Victim

It may evoke stress and the victim may suffer from psychological (anxiety, negative self esteem, anger, irritability, nightmares), behavioral (alcohol, substance abuse, aggressive behavior), cognitive (lack of attention, concentration reduced productivity, forgetfulness) and physical problems (sleep disorders, increased blood pressure/ heart rate, etc).

Other Effects

The effects are not only restricted to the victim but the family and friends are also affected. The family is worried about the well-being of their child, they may also face financial trouble due to expenditure on the victim's health. The friends are under constant apprehension that they may be the next victim. This also hampers the reputation of the institute.

Due to all of the above reasons, all sections of the society raised their voice to prohibit ragging and demanded that the Government must take proactive steps to eradicate this menace to the society.

On the 8th May, 2009, the Hon'ble Supreme Court ordered the Union Government to implement a plan for prevention of ragging.

Following this Judgment the UGC and other regulatory authorities like All India Council for Technical Education (AICTE), Medical Council of India (MCI), Dental Council of India (DCI), etc. published a single set of regulations that would cover the entire nation and all educational institutions.

The following regulations of UGC came into effect on June, 2009.

What is Ragging?

"Ragging in essence is a human right abuse . . . in present times shocking incidents of ragging have come to the notice . . . The student is physically tortured or psychologically terrorized…."

Supreme Court of India (Feb. 11 2009)

Ragging constitutes one or more of any of the following acts:

1. Any conduct by any student or students whether by words spoken or written or by an act which has the effect of teasing, treating or handling with rudeness a fresher or any other student;
2. Indulging in rowdy or undisciplined activities by any student or students which causes or is likely to cause annoyance, hardship, physical or psychological harm or to raise fear or apprehension thereof in any fresher or any other student;
3. Asking any student to do any act which such student will not in the ordinary course do and which has the effect of causing or generating a sense of shame, or torment or embarrassment so as to adversely affect the physique or psyche of such fresher or any other student;
4. Any act by a senior student that prevents, disrupts or disturbs the regular academic activity of any other student or a fresher;
5. Exploiting the services of a fresher or any other student for completing the academic tasks assigned to an individual or a group of students;
6. Any act of financial extortion or forceful expenditure burden put on a fresher or any other student by students;
7. Any act of physical abuse including all variants of it: sexual abuse, homosexual assaults, stripping, forcing obscene and lewd acts, gestures, causing bodily harm or any other danger to health or person;
8. Any act or abuse by spoken words, emails, post, public insults which would also include deriving perverted pleasure, vicarious or sadistic thrill from actively or passively participating in the discomfiture to fresher or any other student;
9. Any act that affects the mental health and self-confidence of a fresher or any other student with or without an intent to derive a sadistic pleasure or showing off power, authority or superiority by a student over any fresher or any other student.

10. Any act of physical or mental abuse targeted at another student on grounds of colour, race, religion, caste, ethnicity, gender, sexual orientation, appearance, regional origins, linguistic identity, place of birth /residence, or economic background.

Measures for Prohibition of Ragging

There are a number of such measures at institution level, university level, district level, etc. Some of them that are important for students to know are as follows:
1. No institution shall permit or condone any reported incident of ragging in any form; and all institutions shall take all necessary and required measures, to achieve the objective of eliminating ragging, within the institution or outside.
2. All institutions shall take action in accordance with these regulations against those found guilty of ragging and/or abetting ragging, actively or passively, or being part of a conspiracy to promote ragging.
3. Every public declaration of intent by any institution, in any electronic, audiovisual or print or any other media, for admission of students to any course of study shall expressly provide that ragging is totally prohibited in the institution, and anyone found guilty of ragging and/or abetting ragging, whether actively or passively, or being a part of a conspiracy to promote ragging, is liable to be punished in accordance with these regulations as well as under the provisions of any penal law for the time being in force.
4. The telephone numbers of the anti-ragging helpline and all the important functionaries in the institution, including the head of the institution, faculty members, members of the anti-ragging committees and anti-ragging squads, district and subdivisional authorities, Wardens of hostels, and other functionaries or authorities where relevant, shall be published in the brochure of admission/instruction booklet or the prospectus.
5. The application for admission, enrolment or registration must be accompanied by an anti-ragging affidavit signed by a student in a prescribed format and another anti-ragging affidavit signed by a parent/guardian.
6. Any distress message received at the anti-ragging helpline shall be simultaneously relayed to the head of the institution, the warden of the hostels, the nodal officer of the affiliating university, if the incident reported has taken place in an institution affiliated to a university, the concerned district authorities and if so required, the district magistrate, and the superintendent of police, and shall also be web-enabled so as to be in the public domain simultaneously for the media and citizens to access it.
7. On receipt of the recommendation of the anti-ragging squad or on receipt of any information concerning any reported incident of ragging, the head of institution shall immediately determine if a case under the penal laws is made out and if so, proceed to file a first information report (FIR), within twenty-four hours of receipt of such information or recommendation, with the police and local authorities, under the appropriate penal provisions.
8. The commission shall maintain an appropriate database to be created out of affidavits, affirmed by each student and his/her parents/guardians and stored electronically by the institution, and such database shall also function as a record for ragging complaints received, and the status of the action taken thereon.

9. Any incident of ragging in an institution shall adversely affect its accreditation, ranking or grading by NAAC or by any other authorised accreditation agencies while assessing the institution for accreditation, ranking or grading purposes.
10. The commission may accord priority in financial grants-in-aid to those institutions, otherwise eligible to receive grants, which report a blemish less record in terms of no reported incident of ragging. These grants can be withdrawn to institutes which do not comply with anti-ragging measures.

Punishable Ingredients of Ragging

i. Abetment to ragging
ii. Criminal conspiracy to rag
iii. Unlawful assembly and rioting while ragging
iv. Violation of decency and morals through ragging
v. Injury to body causing hurt or grievous hurt
vi. Wrongful restraint
vii. Wrongful confinement
viii. Use of criminal force
ix. Extortion
x. Assault/sexual offences/unnatural offences
xi. Criminal intimidation
xii. Offences against property
xiii. Attempt to commit any or above of the offences
xiv. Any offence flowing from the definition of ragging

Punishments under Indian Penal Code against Acts of Ragging

Every single incident of ragging or abetting in ragging puts an obligation on the institution to get the FIR registered. There are provisions in the IPC, which can be used by a student to register an FIR in the nearest Police Station. These provisions are:

294	Obscene acts and songs
323	Punishment for voluntarily causing hurt
324	Voluntarily causing hurt by dangerous weapon or means
325	Punishment for voluntarily causing grievous hurt
326	Voluntarily causing grievous hurt by dangerous weapon
339	Wrongful restraint
340	Wrongful confinement
341	Punishment for wrongful restraint
342	Punishment for wrongful confinement
506	Punishment for culpable homicide not amounting to murder

Administrative Action in the Event of Ragging

The institution shall punish a student found guilty of ragging after following the procedure and in the manner prescribed herein under:

The anti-ragging committee of the institution shall take an appropriate decision, in regard to punishment or otherwise, depending on the facts of each incident of ragging and nature and gravity of the incident of ragging established in the recommendations of the anti-ragging squad. To those found guilty, one or more of the following punishments, namely:

a. Suspension from attending classes and academic privileges
b. Withholding/withdrawing scholarship/fellowship and other benefits.
c. Debarring from appearing in any test/examination or other evaluation process.
d. Withholding results.
e. Debarring from representing the institution in any regional, national or international meet, tournament, youth festival, etc.
f. Suspension/expulsion from the hostel.
g. Cancellation of admission.
h. Rustication from the institution for period ranging from one to four semesters.
i. Expulsion from the institution and consequent debarring from admission to any other institution for a specified period.
j. Fine up to Rs. 25,000/-
k. Imprisionment—six months to three years
l. Where the persons committing or abetting the act of ragging are not identified, the institution shall resort to collective punishment.

How to Report Ragging

1. The UGC has installed a National Anti-Ragging Helpline No. 1800-180-5522 (24 × 7 Toll free no.), helpline@antiragging.in where anyone can register complain.
2. It can be notified through contact details of ARC members
3. Any other member of the institute (HOU, colleagues)
4. External source (through family members, friends)

Procedure for Handling Complaints

Informing the Chairperson (within 2 hours of receipt of complaint)
↓
ARC will conduct a preliminary on the spot enquiry and collect the details, submit the preliminary report to the Chairperson (within 24 hours)
↓
ARC will conduct a detailed enquiry gather evidences and submit its report along with the recommendations to the Chairperson in 15 days.
↓
The Chairperson will take action as per the recommendations.
↓
If the victim student/parents are not satisfied with the action taken by the committee, a FIR should be filed with the local police

CONCLUSION

Though the anti-ragging act is in place since over a decade, its implementation is half-hearted. The higher education institutions must provide an environment where the students learn the values of democratic, mutually respectful relationships, non-violent conflict resolution, autonomous and critical thinking, compassion and caring, respect for differences, fairness and so on. There is need for the teachers to instil confidence in their students to report ragging of any form and ensure healthy working atmosphere between the juniors and seniors. The hostel wardens too have to be vigilant and encourage the students to report all sorts of bullying. There is a requirement of active participation of media and civil society as well in controlling ragging.

BIBLIOGRAPHY

1. Dr Ch Venkateswarlu, Effects of ragging on human dignity-a critique, International Journal of Multidisciplinary Educational Research Volume 1, Issue 4, Sept 2012, 229–242.
2. Dr Snjay Nagral, Medicine's own caste system, Mumbai Mirror, July 30, 2019.
3. Garg R, Ragging: A public health problem in India. Indian J Med Sci. 2009 Jun; 63(6):263–271.
4. Prof. Mohan Rao, Psychosocial Study of Ragging in Selected Educational Institutions in India, December, 2015.
5. Ragging: Prohibition, Prevention and Punishment, The University Grants Commission vide its letter no F.1-16/2007 (CPP-II) dated June 17, 2009
7. Shri Adhir Ranjan Chowdhury, MP. The Prohibition And Eradication Of Ragging Bill, 2016, Bill No. 142 of 2016.
8. Summary of the judgment of the Hon. Supreme Court, Delivered on the 8th May 2009.

Chapter 40

Biomedical Waste Management

○ Bipin Pandit ○ Vipin Checker

DEFINITION

It is defined as "any waste, which is generated during the diagnosis, treatment or immunization of human beings or animals or research activities pertaining thereto or in the production or testing of biological material or in health camps, including the categories mentioned in Schedule I appended to BMW rules 2016."

"Any solid and/or liquid waste including its container and any intermediate product, which is generated during the diagnosis, treatment or immunization of human beings or animals."

Who Generates BMW?

Biomedical waste generated by hospitals, nursing homes, clinics, dispensaries, veterinary institutes/animal houses, pathological laboratories, blood banks/blood donation camps, ayush hospitals, clinical establishments, research/educational institutes/research labs, health camps, medical or surgical camps, vaccination camps, blood donation camps, first aid rooms of schools and forensic laboratories.

BMW CHARACTERIZATION (Fig. 40.1)

Classification of BMW

Non-hazardous waste	1. Biodegradable
	2. Non-biodegradable
Potentially infectious waste	Dressings, swabs, laboratory wastes, instruments used in patient care
Potentially toxic waste	Radioactive, chemical, pharmaceutical

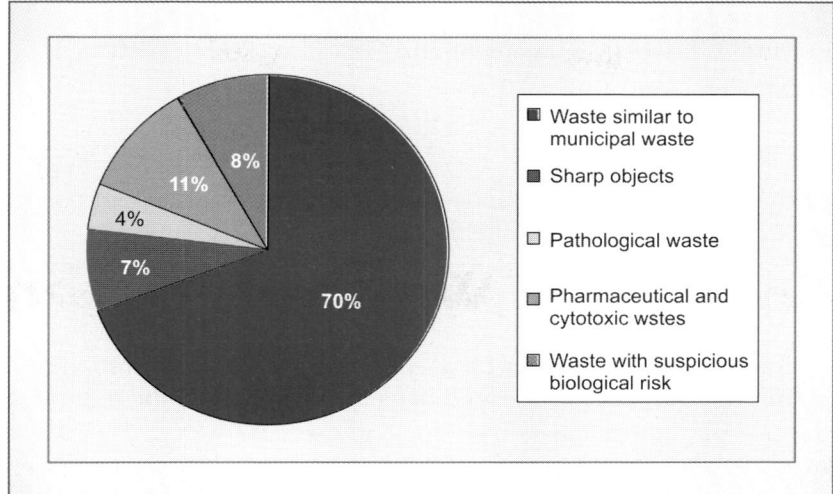

BMW characterisation

Categories of Persons Exposed to Risk of Infection

Sanitation workers and environment, medical paramedical staff, patients and public.

Health Hazards

Risk of HIV and HBV, nosocomial infections, others.

Routes of Transmission

Inhalation, airborne, vector, vehicle, direct and indirect contact, intact/non-intact mucous membranes, uncontaminated stuff.

Precautions

- Medical, paramedical and sanitation staff should be vaccinated against hepatitis B.
- Use of heavy duty gloves especially when dealing with infectious waste.
- Recapping needles should be discouraged.
- All necessary compliances in accordance with BMW (Management) Rules 2016 to avoid unwanted occurrence.

ENVIRONMENT RELATED LEGISLATIONS

- The Air (Prevention and Control of Pollution) Act, 1981
- The Water (Prevention and Control of Pollution) Act, 1974
- The Environment (Protection) Act, 1986
- The Hazardous Waste (Management and Handling) Rules, 2016
- The National Environmental Tribunal Act, 1995

- The Biomedical Waste (Management) Rules, 2016
- The Municipal Solid Waste (Management and Handling) Rules, 2000
- The E-Waste (Management) Rules, 2016

KEY FEATURES OF BMW (M) RULES, 2016

- The ambit of the rules has been expanded to include vaccination camps, blood donation camps, surgical camps or any other healthcare activity.
- Occupier shall take all necessary steps to ensure that biomedical waste is handled without any adverse effect to human health and the environment and in accordance with these rules.
- Make a provision within the premises for a safe, ventilated and secured location for storage of segregated biomedical waste in colored bags or containers in the manner as specified.
- Phase-out the use of chlorinated plastic bags, gloves and blood bags within two years. Pretreatment of the laboratory waste, microbiological waste, blood samples and blood bags through disinfection or sterilization onsite in the manner as prescribed by WHO or NACO.
- Do not give treated bio-medical waste with municipal solid waste. Conduct health check up at the time of induction, provide training to all its healthcare workers and immunize all health workers at the time of induction and thereafter at least once every year.
- Report major accidents.
- The details of training programmes conducted, number of personnel trained and number of personnel not undergone any training shall be provided in the Annual Report.
- Ensure occupational safety of all its healthcare workers and others involved in handling of biomedical waste by providing appropriate and adequate personal protective equipment.
- Establish a Bar Code System for bags or containers containing biomedical waste for disposal. Untreated human anatomical waste, animal anatomical waste, soiled waste and, biotechnology waste shall not be stored beyond a period of forty-eight hours.
- Existing incinerators to achieve the standards for retention time in secondary chamber and Dioxin and Furans within two years.
- Ensure segregation of liquid chemical waste at source and ensure pre-treatment or neutralization prior to mixing with other effluent generated from health care facilities (HCFs).
- Biomedical waste has been classified into four categories instead ten to improve the segregation of waste at source.
- Procedure to get authorization simplified.
- Automatic authorization for bedded hospitals.
- The validity of authorization synchronized with validity of consent orders for bedded HCFs.
- One-time authorization for non-bedded HCFs.
- Operator of a common biomedical waste treatment and disposal facility to ensure the timely collection of biomedical waste from the HCFs and assist the HCFs in conduct of training.
- Maintain and update on day-to-day basis the biomedical waste management register and display the monthly record on its website according to the biomedical waste generated in terms of category and color coding as specified.

- Establish a system to review and monitor the activities related to biomedical waste management by forming a committee and maintain their record.
- Every occupier or operator of common biomedical waste treatment facility shall submit an annual report to the prescribed authority in Form-IV, on or before the 30th June of every year.
- Occupier shall make available the annual report on its website and all the healthcare facilities shall make own website within two years.

CATEGORIES OF BMW AND SEGREGATION CHART (Fig. 40.2)

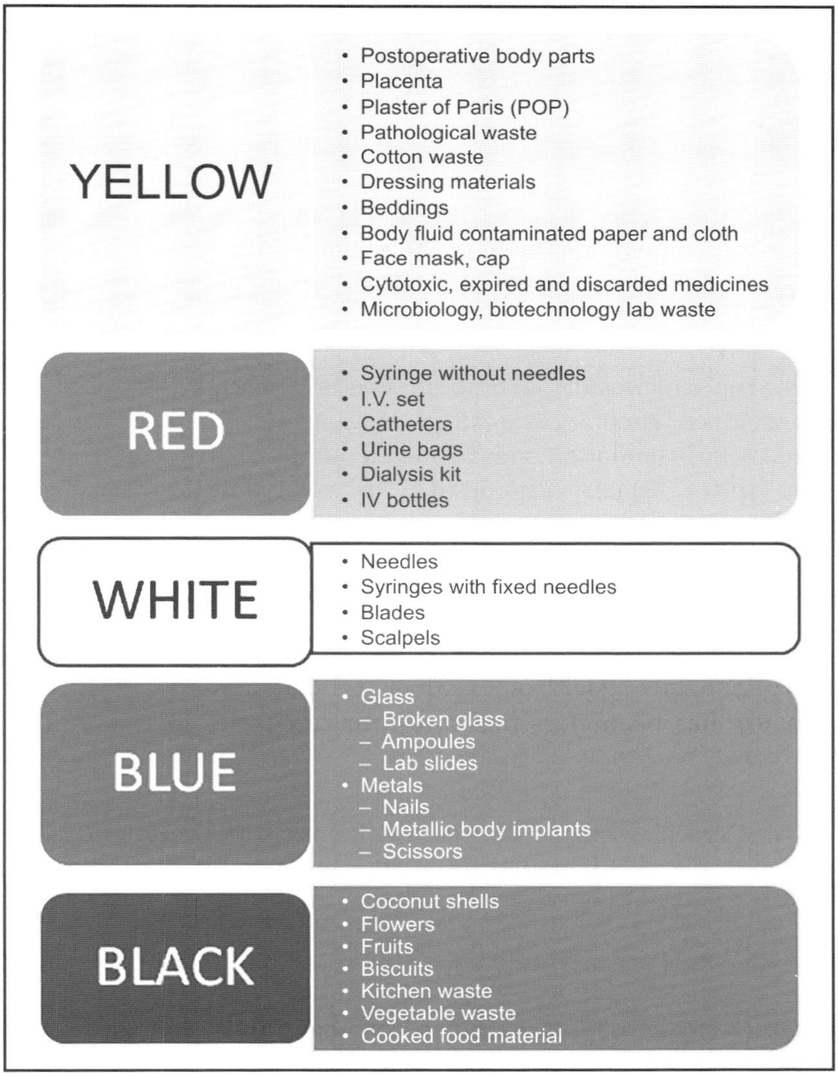

YELLOW
- Postoperative body parts
- Placenta
- Plaster of Paris (POP)
- Pathological waste
- Cotton waste
- Dressing materials
- Beddings
- Body fluid contaminated paper and cloth
- Face mask, cap
- Cytotoxic, expired and discarded medicines
- Microbiology, biotechnology lab waste

RED
- Syringe without needles
- I.V. set
- Catheters
- Urine bags
- Dialysis kit
- IV bottles

WHITE
- Needles
- Syringes with fixed needles
- Blades
- Scalpels

BLUE
- Glass
  - Broken glass
  - Ampoules
  - Lab slides
- Metals
  - Nails
  - Metallic body implants
  - Scissors

BLACK
- Coconut shells
- Flowers
- Fruits
- Biscuits
- Kitchen waste
- Vegetable waste
- Cooked food material

Steps for Effective BMW Management

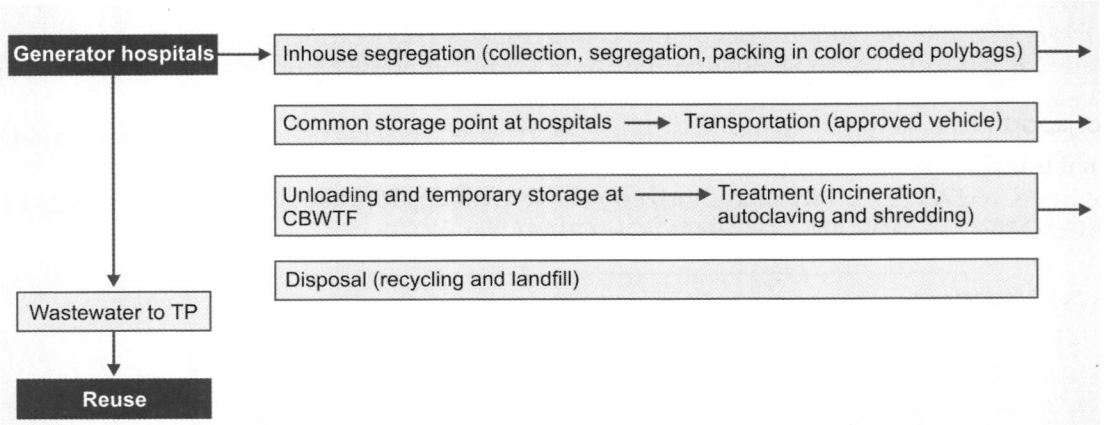

WASTE SURVEY

Waste survey is an important component of the waste management scheme. A survey helps in evaluating both the type and quantity of waste generated in hospitals.

Aims

- Differentiate the types of waste. Quantify the waste generated.
- Determine the points of generation and type of waste generated at each point.
- Determine the level of generation and disinfection within the hospital.
- To find out the type of disposal carried out.

Segregation

Segregation refers to the basic separation of different categories of waste generated at source and thereby reducing the risks as well as cost of handling and disposal. Segregation is the most crucial step in biomedical waste management. Effective segregation alone can ensure effective biomedical waste management. The BMWs must be segregated in accordance to guidelines laid down under Schedule 1 of BMW Rules, 2016.

Collection

The collection of biomedical waste involves use of different types of container. The containers/bins should be placed in such a way that 100% collection is achieved. Sharps must always be kept in puncture-proof containers to avoid injuries and infection to the workers handling them.

Storage

Once collection occurs then biomedical waste is stored in a proper place. Segregated wastes of different categories need to be collected in identifiable containers. The duration of storage should not exceed for 8–10 hours in big hospitals (more than 250 bedded) and 24 hours in nursing homes. Each container may be clearly labelled to show the ward or room where it is kept. The reason for this labelling is that it may be necessary to trace the waste back to its source. Besides this, storage area should be marked with a caution sign.

Transport

Final transport of BMW must be to common biomedical waste treatment storage and disposal facility (CBMWTSDF) only in authorized vehicle with appropriate documentation for further record.

Record Keeping

- MPCB consent and authorization. Formation of committee to establish a system to review and monitor the formation of committee to establish a system to review and monitor the activities related to biomedical waste management and maintain the record.
- Documents of tie-up with CBMWTSDF to safe dispose of BMW.
- Record of pretreatment of BMW and trade effluent.
- Records of training, health check up.
- Record of BMW generation and disposal through CBMWTSDF.
- Annual report.

BMW Treatment

Duties of HCFs/compliance

It shall be the duty of every occupier.

- To obtain Maharashtra pollution control board (MPCB) consent and authorization for its activity.
- To take all necessary steps to ensure the appropriate handling of BMW as per the guidelines of BMW (M) Rules, 2016.
- To make all the provisions of safe segregation, pre-treatment, storage and transport to CBMWTSDF.
- Pre-treatment of BMW.
- Phase out the chlorinated bags, gloves and blood bags.
- Not to give any BMW to municipal authority.
- Provide the training to all healthcare workers, staff at the time of induction and thereafter once in year and maintain the record of the same.
- Immunize all its healthcare workers and others time to time and maintain the record.
- Establish a bar-code system for bags or containers containing biomedical waste
- Ensure segregation of liquid chemical waste at source and ensure pre-treatment or neutralization.
- Ensure treatment and disposal of liquid waste before mixing with sewage water.
- Ensure complete treatment of sewage waste water and chlorination before discharge to drain.

- Ensure occupational safety of all its staff and monitor the same time to time.
- Conduct health check up at the time of induction and at least once in a year for all its healthcare workers and maintain the records.
- Maintain and update on day-to-day basis the biomedical waste management register and display the monthly record on its website.
- Report major accidents.
- Prepare the annual report for the period of January to December and submit the same till 30th June.
- Make available the annual report on its website.
- Form a committee to establish a system to review and monitor the activities related to biomedical waste management and maintain the record.

CONCLUSION

It is just not the law abide compliance but the social responsibility of every healthcare establishment to say...
- No to hazard of biomedical waste
- It will only take proper planning
- Spread awareness
- Involvement of everyone
- Segregation, pre-treatment at first stage
- Appropriate storage
- Timely disposal
- Maintain all records—and all clean.

Procedure for Registering Clinics/Hospitals/Industries Handling Biomedical Waste under Maharashtra Pollution Control Board

The authorization for collection/reception/treatment/transport/storage/disposal of bio-medical waste as defined under the "Authorisation under bio-medical waste (management and handling) rules, 1998" needs to be obtained from board, as the board has been declared as prescribed authority under the rules.

Website: http://www.mpcb.gov.in/consentmgt/authorize-bmw

Schedule for waste treatment facilities like incinerator/autoclave/microwave system after the rules were introduced in 1998.

A. Hospitals and nursing homes in towns with population of 30 lakhs and above or earlier	By 31st December 1999
B. Hospitals and nursing homes in towns with population of below 30 lakhs	
a. With 500 beds and above	By 31st December 1999 or earlier
b. With 200 beds and above but less than 500 beds	By 31st December 2000 or earlier
c. With 50 beds and above but less than 200 beds	By 31st December 2001 or earlier
d. With less than 50 beds	By 31st December 2002 or earlier
C. All other institutions generating biomedical waste not included in A	By 31st December 2002 or earlier

Fees for authorisation under Biomedical Waste (Management and Handling) Rules, 1998.

As per environment department, Government of Maharashtra, Resolution No. ENV/1098/559/P.K. 259 /T.C.1,dt. 10.04.2003

	Fees to be paid (p.a.)
a. Bed capacity	
1. Between 1–5	No fees
2. Between 6–25	Rs 1250
3. Between 26–50	Rs 2500
4. Between 50–200	Rs 5000
5. Between 201–500	Rs 10000
6. Above 501	Rs 15000
b. Treatment facility provider for biomedical waste	Rs 10000 per year
c. Transporter of biomedical waste	Rs 7500 per year
d. All other biomedical waste generating and handling agencies (except a, b, c above)	Rs 2500 per year

These fees are payable in the form of demand draft on any nationalised bank at the respective sub-regional or regional office or at headquarter along with completely filled prescribed forms.

For registration for biomedical waste management services the website to be accessed is: http://www.ecmpcb.in/registration/services

1. Go to the website www.empcb.in
2. Select the new industry option to login and fill the one time registration form with name, address, email address, phone number and details.
3. A notification email with credentials will be received after login.
4. Login with your credentials. Dashboard will appear.
5. Go to the applications section to get a list of application options
   - Select BMW authorization (combined consent)
   - For new applicants, the maitri portal opens to fill in details for registration including name, phone number, address, PAN and AADHAR details

   The options include:
   i. Less than 50 beds
   ii. More than 50 beds
   iii. Industry generation biomedical waste
   iv. CBMW facilitators

6. Go to the dashboard section to find your submitted application with a unique application number.
   - Download the application and proceed to payment.
   - In case of combined consent after filling the form, 2 unique identification numbers will be generated.
   - Both applications are linked to each other.

SOURCE REFERENCE AND SUGGESTED READING
- World Health Organization Blue Book 2014
- STP Amendment 2019
- Biomedical Waste Rules 2016
- Bar code notification

Chapter 41

Clinical Establishment Act in Day-to-Day Practice

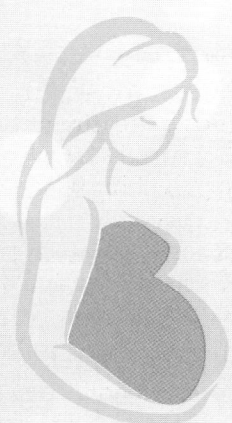

○ Girish Kumthekar

At present our medical fraternity is very much worried about the law which has been passed by Parliament and is being implemented by states one after another with modifications. Like many other acts this law, whether you like it or not, has come to stay and will be implemented one or the other day all over India. There is fear amongst health sector that this is detrimental to the small hospitals and clinics and is favouring corporate hospitals more. This is likely to bring end to affordable service the people of India get through small hospitals as more and more of them will pull down the shutters for inability to the compliance of the provisions. Though the fear is not unfounded, it is, to certain extent misplaced and exaggerated. Let us in brief try to get to the crux of the Act and think about the days to come. Bypassing the legal terms and enumerations of the bear act section wise, I will try to simplify things.

The Clinical Establishments Act (CEA) was passed by Parliament of India on 17th August 2010, to provide for registration and regulation of all clinical establishments in the country with a view to prescribing minimum standards of facilities and services which may be provided by them so that mandate of Article 47 of the constitution for improvement in public health may be achieved. The Act was notified vide Gazette notification dated 28th February, 2012 and initially came into force on 1st March, 2012 in the four states. At present, the Act is applicable in 10 states and 6 Union Territories.

The Ministry of Health and Family Welfare has notified the National Council for Clinical Establishments and the Clinical Establishments (Central Government) Rules, 2012 under this Act vide Gazette notifications dated 19th March, 2012 and 23rd May, 2012 respectively.

The Act is applicable to all kinds of clinical establishments from public and private sectors, of all recognized systems of medicine including single doctor clinics. The only exception is establishments run by the Armed forces which will not be regulated under this Act.

CEA aims to register and regulate clinical establishments based on minimum standards in order to improve quality of public healthcare in the country.

Definition: Clinical Establishment

i. A hospital, maternity home, nursing home, dispensary, clinic, sanatorium or an institution by whatever name called that offers services, facilities requiring diagnosis, treatment or care for illness, injury, deformity, abnormality or pregnancy in any recognized system of medicine established and administered or maintained by any person or body of persons, whether incorporated or not; or

ii. A place established as an independent entity or part of an establishment referred to in sub-clause (i), in connection with the diagnosis or treatment of diseases where pathological, bacteriological, genetic, radiological, chemical, biological investigations or other diagnostic or investigative services with the aid of laboratory or other medical equipment, are usually carried on, established and administered or maintained by any person or body of persons, whether incorporated or not, and shall include a clinical establishment owned, controlled or managed by a Government or
   a. Department of the Government;
   b. A trust, whether public or private;
   c. A corporation (including a society) registered under a Central, Provincial or State Act, whether or not owned by the Government;
   d. A local authority; and
   e. A single doctor

All clinical establishments—including diagnostic centres and single doctor clinics, across all recognized systems of medicine in both public and private sectors (exception: Establishments of the Armed Forces).

The Act recognizes all systems of medicine, i.e. Allopathic: Medical and Dental, AYUSH (Ayurvedic, Unani, Siddha, Homoeopathy, Yoga,) Naturopathy and Sowa

Registration

One must remember that no one can run a clinical establishment without registration. One has to register within one year from commencement of Act, every existing Clinical Establishment has to apply for registration within one year from commencement of Act and every new Clinical Establishment, i.e. which has come into existence after commencement of Act has to apply for registration within six months from the date of its establishment.

There are two types of registration as per the Act. You have to apply on the prescribed registration form

- **Provisional registration** is to be given by the appropriate authority within 30 days after application. If not given in 30 days, the establishment is deemed to be registered. The registration is valid for 1 year and renewable thereafter for 1 more year. For provisional registration the authority is not supposed to conduct inquiry prior to grant.
- **Permanent registration** is to be considered after notification of Minimum Standards. Clinical establishments will be required to meet minimum standards before grant of permanent

registration. The provisional registration shall not be renewed after a period of two years from the date of notification of minimum standards, in case of existing clinical establishments and the same shall not be renewed after a period of six months incase of new clinical establishments (i.e. which come into existence after date of notification of minimum Standards). Certificate of permanent registration is granted for five years at a time.

Conditions to be Fulfilled by every Clinical Establishment for Grant of Registration (Permanent) and Continuation

1. Minimum standards of facilities and services;
2. Minimum requirement of personnel;
3. Provision and maintenance of records and reports.
4. Every clinical establishment is required to provide treatment "within the staff and facilities available" to stabilize the emergency medical condition of an individual who comes or is brought to the clinical establishment.
5. Other conditions (as prescribed under Central Government Rules)
   - **Details of rates charged and facilities available** to be prominently displayed at a conspicuous place in local and in English language
   - **Maintain and provide electronic medical records or electronic health records of every patient as** may be determined and issued by Central/State Govt.
   - Clinical establishments shall **charge the rates for procedures and services within the range of rates** determined by the Central Government from time to time in consultation with the State Governments.
   - Clinical establishments shall ensure compliance to **standard treatment guidelines** as may be issued by Central/State Govt.
   - Every clinical establishments shall maintain **information and statistics** in accordance with all applicable laws and rules.

Fee for Registration, Renewal and Appeal

- Shall be specified by respective State Government/UT administration under Section 54.
- State/UT may charge fee category wise.
- Enhanced fee may be charged if renewal not applied within the prescribed time.
- State Government/UT administration may charge fee for appeal made to state/UT Council.

Time Period to Apply for Renewal of Registration

- 30 days before expiry of the validity of certificate in case of provisional registration
- 6 months before expiry of the validity of certificate in case of permanent registration

Cancellation of Registration of Clinical Establishment after Registration is Granted

1. If conditions of registration are not being complied
2. Person who is responsible for management of the clinical establishment has been convicted of offence under this Act.

3. If there is imminent danger to the health and safety of patients, then after cancellation, the authority may immediately restrain the clinical establishment.

Provision for Appeal against Cancellation of Registration

In case there is cancellation of registration by AA the **Section 34:** Allows any person, aggrieved by an order of the registering authority refusing to grant or renew a certificate of registration or revoking a certificate of registration to appeal within 30 days to the AA. However, sometime this limit is condoned for appropriate cause which convinces the AA.

Penalty for Contravention of the Law

The Act provides for punishment for contravention of the act in any form and for non registration. The penalty may vary from state to state as per amendments made but minimum penalty is Rs. five thousand for first offence to fifty thousand for further offences and cancellation of registration.

Important point here to remember is that a person who works in an establishment which is not registered is liable to a penalty up to twenty-five thousand.

Also if any clinical establishment refuses to co-operate with various directives under this law or shows disobedience or refuses or obstructs information sought by AA shall be punishable.

I have tried to cover only those aspects of the Act which are relevant to our day-to-day practice and clinical establishments working at present. Many technical section I have not touched upon as they are more of an executive nature and not required by us in full. Let us try to see some pros and cons of the Act in short.

Benefits of Act

- Comprehensive digital registry of clinical establishments and systematic collection of information
  - Policy formulation
  - Better surveillance, response and management of outbreak and public health emergencies
  - Engagement with private providers
- Clinical establishments categorized into categories which makes it feasible to prescribe uniform standards for a category
- Transparency:
  - Process of registration, data in public domain.
  - Details of **charges, facilities available would be prominently displayed** at a conspicuous place at each establishment
- Multi-stakeholder participation in institutional mechanisms (National and State Councils, District Registration Authority)—consensus-based decisions.
- **Effective regulation of** providers would occur
- **Improved quality** of healthcare as care is based on standard treatment protocols and minimum standards

- Increased patient confidence due to government registration
- Improved brand value of clinical establishments
- **Deterrent against quackery:** Under the Act, the registration is mandatory and allowed only for clinical establishments belonging to recognized systems of medicine
- **Better management of emergency** medical conditions
- **Better maintenance of records and reports**

Disadvantages or Hurdles Our Fraternity may Face
- Fear of Inspector and license raj which is not unfounded
- High maintenance costs for small hospitals
- Inability to meet the standards and hence small nursing homes may pull down shutters.
- Shortage of skilled staff which is a requirement of the Act, hence unable to get registration.
- Effectively increases the cost of medical treatment to public in general.
- Many more seen and unseen hurdles that affect a peaceful practice.

This all appears frightening for our fraternity and one will think twice before opening a hospital, clinic or nursing home but we have to accept the fact that the law is there and going to be there and as a responsible citizen we have to abide by it. However, the states are modifying the law suitable to their people in consultation with local organizations and citizens so that the health services to common people are not affected.

IMA and almost all specialty organizations are working hard to give inputs to state governments regarding making the law simplified and less punitive and have been successful to certain extent, but believe me the law is going to stay and we have to abide by it one or the other day.

SOURCE REFERENCE AND SUGGESTED READING
http://clinicalestablishments.gov.in

Index

Abortion Act 20
Accredited social health activists (ASHAs) 188, 282, 297
Action planning 82
Acute fatty liver of pregnancy (AFLP) 105
Adherent placenta 107
Admission register 6, 15
Admission test 74
Adolescence education program (AEP) 282, 320
Adolescent reproductive and sexual health (ARSH) 127, 281, 292
Adolescent reproductive and sexual health programm 318
Advisory committees (ACs) 25
AFE (amniotic fluid embolism) 74
AIDS 127
Albendazole 321
All India Council for Technical Education (AICTE) 359
Alprazolam 148
Altruistic surrogacy 226
American Society for Reproductive Medicine (ASRM) 219
Amniocentesis 24
Amniotic fluid embolism (AFE) 104
Ampicillin, metronidazole, gentamicin 126
Anaemia 327
Anaesthetic deaths 108
Analysis of maternal deaths 82
Anganwadi workers (AWWs) 127, 188
Antenatal care (ANC) 83, 125
Antithrombin 181
Appropriate authorities (AAs) 25
Approval of place 12
Areas of concern 38
ART (assisted reproductive technologies) 207
ART bank 240
ART bill 233
ART clinics 208
Artificial insemination with donor (AID) semen 239
Artificial insemination with husband's (AIH) semen 239
Arunkumar Manglik vs Chirayu Health and Medicare 66
ASHA package 309
ASHA workers 127
Assisted reproductive technology (ART) 217
Asthenozoospermia 241
Autopsies 116
Auxiliary nurse midwives (ANMs) 188

Bacterial vaginosis 140
Balika Samridhi Yojana (BSY) 282, 319
Balram Prasad versus Kunal Saha 64
Barriers to access 192

Barriers to quality 192
Basal body temperature (BBT) 208
Basic emergency obstetric care for medical officer 294
BCG 126
Benign ovarian tumours 181
Betadine 148
Biomedical waste 364
Biomedical waste (management) 246, 366
Block development officer (BDO) 127
Body mass index (BMI) 182
Bolam test 66
Bolitho test 66
Border district cluster strategy (BDCS) 277

Call to action (CAT) 291
Carbon dioxide (CO_2) 163
Cardiac arrest 167
Cardiovascular system 105
Carrier embryos 220
Case selection 196
Central Adoption Resource Authority (CARA) 313
Central nervous system 105
Central Supervisory Board (CSB) 25
Centre for Enquiry into Health and Allied Themes 188
Certificate of sterilization 199
Cervical intraepithelial neoplasia (CIN) 140
Cesarean section (CS) 74
Cetavalon 148
Chief District Medical Officer (CDMO) 202
Chief Medical Officer (CMO) 5, 202
Child Development Programme Officer (CDPO) 127
Child Health Programme-1 (RCH-1) 274
Child Health Programme-2 (RCH-2) 274
Child labor 252
Child Marriage Restraint Act 252
Child survival and safe motherhood (CSSM) 125, 274, 275
Cholecystectomy 140
Chorion villus biopsy 24
Civil Law 350
Civil Registration System (CRS) 80
Clinical assessment 137
Clinical Establishments Act (CEA) 372
Clinical process 146
Clinical risk management 72
Clomiphene citrate (CC) 214
Code of criminal procedure 46, 256
Column admission register 285
Commercial surrogacy 226
Common biomedical waste treatment storage and disp 369
Community-based MDSR 80
Community health centre (CHC) 186, 284

Comprehensive abortion care (CAC) services 189
Comprehensive emergency obstetric care (CEmOC) 83
Comprehensive lactation management centre (CLMC) 120
Confidential review (CR) 78
Confidentiality 211
Congenital absence of tubes 169
Congenital bilateral absence of the vas deferens 210
Consent form 6, 197, 211
Continuing medical education (CME) 332
Convention on elimination of all forms of discrimi 251
Counselling 136, 146, 211
Crimes against women 255
Criminal Law (amendment) Act 252, 255, 350
Criteria of female sterilization 149
Critical control points 124
Custody of forms 14

Data maintenance 74
Deemed renewal 52
Deep freezer 121
Deep vein thrombosis (DVT) 183
Delay in reaching first level health facility 89, 90
Delay in seeking care 89
Demographic information 138, 147
Dense adhesions 169
Dental Council of India (DCI) 359
Designer babies 220
Destruction of admission register 15
Diazepam 148, 160
Dilation and Curettage (D and C) 187
Direct obstetric deaths 88
District health officer (DHO) 5, 202
District level committee (DLC) 5, 13, 284
District level household survey III (DLHS III) 318
District Magistrate (DM) 87
District Medical Officer (DMO) 202
District Nodal Officer (DNO) 87
Domestic Violence Act 252, 265
Donor insemination 221
Donor population 121
District Quality Assurance Committee (DQAC) 202
Dr HL Shivpuri 19
Dr Laxman Balkrishna Joshi v/s Dr Trimbak Bapu God 59
Dr Payal Tadvi 357
Dr Sr Louie and Another versus Smt Kannolil Pathum 60
Drug abuse 252
Drug and Cosmetics Act 21
Dysmenorrhoea 181

E-waste (management) 366
Economic factors 188
Ectopic pregnancy 153, 170, 215
Education 328
Electrical vacuum aspiration (EVA) 187
Embryo donation 210
Embryo status 220
Embryo transfer 209
Embryos 212
Emergency obstetric and neonatal care 294
Emergency response centre (ERC) 267
Empowered action group (EAG) 306
Endometriosis 183
Entries in other registers 15
Essential obstetric care 294
Ethical considerations in gestational surrogacy 223
European society of human reproduction and embryol 219
Evisceration and organ dissection 104
Exercise 328
External examination 104
Extremely low birth weight babies (ELBW) 120

Facility-based MDSR 80
Facility nodal officer (FNO) 87
Facility-based maternal deaths reviews (FDMDR) 87
Falope ring loading 163
Family Planning Association of India (FPAI) 188
Family Planning Indemnity Scheme 200
FEBRASGO (Federacao Brasileira das Associacoes de Ginecologia e Obstetricia 113
Federacion Latinamerica na de Sociedades d (FLASOG) 113
Federation of Obstetrics and Gynaecological Societies of India(FOGSI) 189
Female sterilization 135, 139
Female vasectomy case 142
Fertilization and Embryology Act, UK 219
Fetus 107
First information report (FIR) 360
First referral units (FRUs) 83, 130, 188, 277
Follicle stimulating hormone (FSH) 214
Form C49 40
Family planning (FP) 202
Family Planning Indemnity Scheme (FPIS) 170
Fulminant hepatic failure (FHF) 109

Gametes 212
Gas embolism 168
Gastrointestinal system 105
GC (gestational carrier) 226
Gender equality 329
Gender selection 221
Genetic clinic (GC) 31
Genetic counseling centers (GCC), genetic laborato 25

Genetic counseling centre (GCC) 31
Genetic laboratory (GL) 31
Genital tract 106
Gestational surrogate (GS) 226
Global scenario 185
Gonadal dysgenesis 210
Good laboratory practice (GLP) 243
Grey areas 37
Guardians and Wards Act 316

Hazard analysis 124
HBV 241
HCV 241
Health care facilities (HCFs) 366
Health hazards 365
Health systems strengthening (HSS) 282
Healthy bones 328
Hematoma 168
Hepatitis B 126
Hepatitis E 105
High performing states (HPS) 281, 297
Highly vascular tubes 169
Hindu Adoptions and Maintenance Act 316
Histological examination 105
Histopathologic examination (HP) 108
HIV 241
Hospital management information systems (HMIS) 75
Human chorionic gonadotropin (hCG) 214
Human Fertilization and Embryology Act, UK 219
Human Fertilization and Embryology Authority (HFEA) 222
Human Genetics Commission (HGC) 220
Human leukocyte antigen (HLA) 221
Human menopausal gonadotropin (hMG) 214
Hyperlipidaemias 140
Hypo-osmotic swelling test (HOST) 242
Hypospermatogenesis 210
Hypothyroidism 182

Iatrogenic ovarian failure 210
ICMR Guidelines 229
Intracytoplasmic sperm injection (ICSI) 207
IMC Code 1.2.3 333
Improved access to safe abortion care 190
In vitro fertilization (IVF) 207, 209
In vitro fertilisation-embryo transfer (IVF-ET) 240
Incisional hernia 168
Indian Council of Medical Research (ICMR) 27, 207, 218
Indian Evidence Act 256
Indian Medical Association versus VP Shantha 59
Indirect Obstetric Deaths 89
Induced abortion 17
Infant mortality rate (IMR) 125
Information 211
Information, Education and Communication (IEC) 321

Informed consent 143, 196
Integrated child development services (ICDS) 127, 305, 275
Integrated Management of Neonatal and Childhood II 126, 274
Intended parents (IP) 226
Intended surrogate mother 238
Intending couple 238
Internal systemic examination 105
International Maternal and Child Health (IMCH) 189
Interval sterilization 179
Interval tubal ligation 152
Intimation of change 54
Intra-natal care 126
Intra-uterine insemination using donor (IUI-D) semen 240
Intra-uterine insemination using husband (IUI-H) 240
Intraoperative complications 153, 167
Intrauterine insemination (IUI) 242
Invasive techniques 27
Investigation tracking system for sexual offences 267
Iron deficiency anaemia 141
IT Act 257
IVF surrogacy 225

Jacob Matthew v/s State of Punjab 73
Janani Shishu Suraksha Karyakram (JSSK) 281, 295
Janani Suraksha Yojana (JSY) 128, 281, 295, 304
Judicial remedies 57
Justice Verma Committee 256
Juvenile Justice Act (care and protection of children) 44, 252, 316

Kishori Shakti Yojana (KSY) 282, 319
Kusum Sharma and Others versus Batra Hospital and Medical Research (2010) 64

Laboratory examinations 138, 147
Lactation management units (LMUs) 120
Lactation support units (LSUs) 120
Lady health visitors (LHVs) 128
Laminar air flow 121
Laparoscopic tubal ligation 156, 165, 179
LaQshya 295
Leave for illness 259
Leave for tubectomy 259
Legal agreement 228
Liver function tests 109
Liver tumours 182
Local anesthetic (LA) 159
Low birth weight (LBW) 126
Low performing states (LPS) 281, 297

Maharashtra Medical Council Act 333
Maharashtra pollution control board (MPCB) 369
Maintenance of records 14
Male sterilization 135, 139

Index

Male vasectomy case 142
Malignancy 169
Malignant hepatomas 182
Mandatory reporting 45
Manual vacuum aspiration (MVA) 187, 189
Martius scarlet blue (MSB) 106
Maternal child health (MCH) 125
Maternal death review 72, 88
Maternal death surveillance and response (MDSR) 78, 296
Maternal health 293
Maternal mortality ratio (MMR) 78, 129
MCI code 6.1.1 334
MCI code 6.1.2 334
MCI code 6.3 335
MCI code 6.4.1 334
MCI code 6.8 335
MCI code 7.17 335
MCI code 7.2 335
MCI code 7.20 335
MCI code 7.4 334
MCI code 7.7 335
Medically Aware and Responsible Citizens of Hyderabad (MARCH) 218
Medical Accreditation Board for Laboratories (NABL) 218
Medical Council of India (MCI) 332, 359
Medical ethics 331
Medical history 138, 147
Medical methods of abortion (MMA) 5, 187
Medical record office (MRO) 75
Medical Termination of Pregnancy (MTP) Act 185
Medicolegal issues 198
Menstrual hygiene 326
Microsurgical epididymal sperm aspiration (MESA) 210
Midazolam 160
Mild effects 160
Millennium development goal (MDG) 78, 86
Ministry of health and family welfare (MOHFW) 6, 195
Ministry of women and child development (MOWCD) 296
Modules 89
Monthly reporting format 285
Mother and child protection (MCP) 127
Mother's own milk (MOM) 119
MTP Act regulation 04 16
MTP Act regulation 06 16
MRKH syndrome 226
Multiple gestation 214
Municipal solid waste 366

Nabhan Farhan Sah versus Dr Latha Sharma 63
National Accreditation Board for Laboratories (NABL) 218
National AIDS Control Programme (NACP) 320
National Board for Assisted Reproductive Technology 233
National Commission for Women 22, 271

National Family Health Survey-2 (NFHS-2) 274
National Family Health Survey-4 268
National Family Planning Indemnity Scheme (NFPIS) 199
National Health Mission (NHM) 195, 290, 320
National Human Rights Commission 271
National Maternity Benefit Scheme (NMBS) 281, 304
National Population Education Project (NPEP) 282
National Population Policy (NPP) 188, 277
National Program for Youth and Adolescent Developmment 282
National Registry of Assisted Reproductive Technology 233
National Rural Health Mission (NRHM) 125, 290, 304, 318
National Scenario 186
National Social Assistance Programme (NSAP) 274
National Surrogacy Board 223
National Urban Health Mission (NUHM) 290
National Welfare Program 145
Nehru Yuva Kendra Sangathan (NYKS) 282
Nizam Institute of Medical Sciences versus Prasant 64
No-scalpel vasectomy (NSV) 195
Non-bailable 34
Non-compoundable 34
Non-hazardous waste 364
Non-obstetric causes 89
Non-use of machine 55
Nutritional rural livelihoods mission (NRLM) 327

Obstetric transition 82
Overseas Citizenship of India (OCI) 229
Oligozoospermia 241
Oocyte cryopreservation 218
Oocyte donation 210, 236
Opinion form 5
Ovarian drilling 242
Ovarian hyperstimulation syndrome (OHSS) 214
Ovarian tissue and oocyte cryopreservation 219
Overweight 328

Pan American Health Organisation (PAHO) 113
Panchayati Raj Institution (PRIs) 323
Partial zona dissection (PZD) 210
Pasteurization 123
Pasteurized donor human milk (PDHM) 119
Pathfinder International 190
Pelvic inflammatory disease (PID) 181
Pelvic tuberculosis 183
Penetrative sexual assault 45
Pentazocin 148
Permanent registration 373

Pethidine 148
Physical access 188
Physical examination 138, 147
Pitfalls in the Indian MTP Act 18
Pneumoperitoneum 162
POCSO Act 21, 252
Person of Indian Origin (POI) 229
Policy factors 187
Pooling of milk 122
Poonam Verma versus Ashwin Patel 60
Pornography 45
Postnatal care 294
Postoperative complications 153, 168
Postoperative monitoring 142
Postpartum haemorrhage (PPH) 115
Postpartum tubal ligation 151
Potentially infectious waste 364
Potentially toxic waste 364
Poverty line (BPL) 304
Practice Committee 219
Pradhanmantri Surakshit Matritva Abhiyan (PMSMA) 295, 298
Pre-conception and prenatal diagnostic techniques 23
Pre-conception techniques 24
pre-eclampsia 112
Pre-implantation genetic diagnosis (PGD) 220, 221
Pre-implantation genetic screening (PGS) 221, 237
Preoperative assessment 146
Preoperative instructions 146
Premature ovarian failure 210
Prenatal diagnoses (PND) 220
Preoperative instructions 138
Preoperative medication 139
Preservation of records 53
Preterm birth 215
Preterm labour 215
Primary (levels 1A and 1B) infertility clinic 233
Primary health centre (PHC) 186, 284, 319
Principle rules 31
Professional misconduct 333
Programme Implementation Plans (PIPs) 199
Prohibited scenarios 213
Prohibition of Child Marriage Act 252
Prolonged rupture of membranes (PROM) 141
Promethazine 148
Prospective adoptive parents (PAPs) 315
Protection for Women against Domestic Violence (PWDV) 270, 338
Protein C 181
Protein S 181
Prothrombin mutation 181
Provision of appeal 39
Provisional registration 373
Psychogenic impotence 245
Psychosocial concerns 228

Pt Parmanand Katara versus Union of India 60
Public information 55
Public interest litigation (PIL) 26
Pulmonary embolism (PE) 183
Pulmonary thromboembolism (PTE) 104

QAC: Quality Assurance Committee 202
Qualitative indicators 82
Quality antenatal care 293

Ragging 357
Rajiv Gandhi Scheme for Empowerment of Adolescent 282
Ramakant Rai v/s Union of India 196
Rashtriya Bal Swasthya Karyakram (RBSK) 320
Rashtriya Kishor Swasthya Karyakram (RKSK) 282, 292, 318
Record keeping 75, 124, 237
Record room 243
Recurrent pregnancy losses (RPL) 226
Referral chits 54
Registered medical practitioner (RMP) 50
Registrar General of India—Sample Registration System 293
Renewal of registration 39
Repeated implantation failure (RIF) 226
Reporting format 6
Reproductive and Child Health (RCH) 127, 319
Reproductive and Child Health phase II (RCH II) 318
Reproductive and Child Health Programme (RCH-II) 129
Reproductive, maternal, neonatal, child, and adolescent 290
Reproductive tract infections (RTI) 127
Res ipsa loquitur 64, 73
Research 212
Respiratory depression 167
Respiratory system 105
Restitutio in integrum 63
Risk analysis 114
Risk control 115
Risk identification 114
Risk treatment 115
RMNCH+A 282

Salient features 229
Samira Kohli versus Dr Manchanda 62
Sample Registration Survey (SRS) 318
Sarda Act 273
Sarva Shiksha Abhiyan 282
Sarwat Ali Khan versus Prof R Gogi 60
Savior siblings 221
Savitribai Phule Yojana 128
Screening of clients 137
Secondary (level 2) infertility clinic 233
Self help groups (SHG) 282, 327
Semen banks 222
Semen collection room 243
Semen processing laboratory 243
Sethuraman Subramaniam Iyer versus Triveni Nursing Home 61
Severe anemia 126
Severe effects 160
Sexual and reproductive health (SRH) 319
Sexual assault 45
Sexual harassment 45
Sexual harassment of women 252
Sexually transmitted diseases (STIs) 127
Shaker water bath 121
Shantilal Shah Committee 19
Shop and Establishment Act 246
Shyam Sunder versus State of Rajasthan 64
Sickle-cell disease 141
Skilled birth attendant (SBA) 130, 294
Skin sensitivity test 160
Social factors 187
Society of midwives, India (SOMI) 189
Sonohysterosalpingography 245
Special Juvenile Police Unit (SJPU) 46
Special Marriage Act 258
Specialized Adoption Agencies (SSA) 314
Sperm donation 235
Spontaneous abortion 215
Spring Medows Hospital and Another versus Harjol A 61
Staff Nurses (SNs) 129
State Level Monitoring and Review Committee for MD 83
State Level Taskforce (SLT) 83
State of Punjab versus Shiv Ram 61
State Quality Assurance Committee (SQAC) 202
Store room 243
Sub-zonal insemination (SUZI) 210
Subcutaneous emphysema 168
Submission of records 54
Subrogare 225
Superficial venous thrombosis 140
Surrogacy regulation bill 223
Surveillance systems 74

Sustainable development goal (SDG) 86, 129
Syphilis 241
Systemic lupus erythematosus (SLE) 183

Task force 219
Tertiary (Level 3) infertility clinic 233
Testicular sperm aspiration (TESA) 210
Tetanus 168
The Dowry Prohibition Act 251
The Employees State Insurance Act 259
The Equal Remuneration Act 258
The Factories Act 258
The golden hour 73
The Immoral Traffic (Prevention) Act 252
The Maternity Benefit Act 259
The National Commission for Women Act 260, 267
The National Health Service Litigation Authority 72
The negative autopsy 108
Third party reproduction (TPR) 223
Thyroid disorders 140
Traditional surrogacy 225
Training for health (ARTH) 188
Transport of milk 122
Transvaginal sonography (TVS) 242
Trichomonas vaginalis 140
Tubal ligation 145
Tubal pathology 169
Tubo-ovarian masses 169

Underweight 327
UNICEF 111
University Grants Commission (UGC) 358
Urinary system 105
Uterine perforation 168

Vaso-vagal attack 167
Very low birth weight (VLBW) 119
Village health and nutrition day (VHND) 296
Village health communities (VHC) 323
Violence free homes 271
Viral hepatitis 140
Vitamin A 126
Vitamin D 328
Voluntary counselling and testing centre (VCTC) 320

Weekly iron and folic acid supplement (WIFS) 282, 320
Women centered comprehensive abortion care (WCAC) 191
World health organisation (WHO) 44, 326
Wound sepsis 168